T0216206

Nutritional Psychiatry

Nutritional Psychiatry

A Primer for Clinicians

Edited by
Ted Dinan
University College Cork

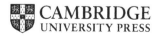

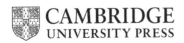

Shaftesbury Road, Cambridge CB2 8EA, United Kingdom

One Liberty Plaza, 20th Floor, New York, NY 10006, USA

477 Williamstown Road, Port Melbourne, VIC 3207, Australia

314–321, 3rd Floor, Plot 3, Splendor Forum, Jasola District Centre,
New Delhi – 110025, India

103 Penang Road, #05–06/07, Visioncrest Commercial, Singapore 238467

Cambridge University Press is part of Cambridge University Press & Assessment,
a department of the University of Cambridge.

We share the University's mission to contribute to society through the pursuit of
education, learning and research at the highest international levels of excellence.

www.cambridge.org
Information on this title: www.cambridge.org/9781009299848

DOI: 10.1017/9781009299862

First published 2023

A catalogue record for this publication is available from the British Library.

Library of Congress Cataloging-in-Publication Data
Names: Dinan, Timothy G., editor.
Title: Nutritional psychiatry : a primer for clinicians / edited by Ted Dinan, University College Cork.
Description: Cambridge, United Kingdom ; New York, NY : Cambridge University Press, 2023. | Includes
bibliographical references and index.
Identifiers: LCCN 2023022438 | ISBN 9781009299848 (paperback) | ISBN 9781009299862 (ebook)
Subjects: LCSH: Mental illness – Nutritional aspects. | Mental health – Nutritional aspects. | Nutrition –
Psychological aspects.
Classification: LCC RC455.4.N8 N88 2023 | DDC 616.89/0654–dc23/eng/20230607
LC record available at https://lccn.loc.gov/2023022438

ISBN 978-1-009-29984-8 Paperback

....

Contents

Contributors

Ivan Aprahamian
Geriatrics Division, Department of Internal Medicine, Jundiai Medical School, Jundiai, Sao Paulo, Brazil

Mary I. Butler
Department of Psychiatry and Neurobehavioural Science, University College Cork, Cork, Ireland

Ger Clarke
APC Microbiome Ireland and Department of Psychiatry, University College Cork, Cork, Ireland

Kathrin Cohen Kadosh
School of Psychology, Faculty of Health and Medical Sciences, University of Surrey, Guildford, UK

Caitlin Cowan
School of Psychology and Brain and Mind Centre, University of Sydney, Sydney, New South Wales, Australia

John F. Cryan
APC Microbiome Ireland and Department of Anatomy and Neuroscience, University College Cork, Cork, Ireland

Ted Dinan
Department of Psychiatry and APC Microbiome Ireland, University College Cork, Cork, Ireland

Eileen Gibney
School of Agriculture and Food Science, University College Dublin, Dublin, Ireland

Felice N. Jacka
Food and Mood Centre, The Institute for Mental and Physical Health and Clinical Translation (IMPACT), School of

Medicine, Deakin University, Geelong, Victoria, Australia; Centre for Adolescent Health, Murdoch Children's Research Institute, Parkville, Victoria, Australia; Black Dog Institute, Sydney, Australia

Jeanette M. Johnstone
Department of Psychiatry, Oregon Health and Science University, Portland, Oregon, USA

Nicola Johnstone
School of Psychology, Faculty of Health and Medical Sciences, University of Surrey, Guildford, UK

Bonnie J. Kaplan
Cumming School of Medicine, University of Calgary, Calgary, Alberta, Canada

John R. Kelly
Department of Psychiatry, Trinity College Dublin, Ireland and Tallaght University Hospital, Dublin, Ireland

Sabrina Mörkl
Department of Psychiatry and Psychotherapeutic Medicine, Medical University of Graz, Graz, Austria

Andréia de Oliveira Pain
Geriatrics Division, Department of Internal Medicine, Jundiai Medical School, Jundiai, Sao Paulo, Brazil

Rachelle Opie
Food for Thought Nutrition and Dietetics, Glen Iris, Victoria, Australia

Kenneth J. O'Riordan
APC Microbiome Ireland and Department of Anatomy and Neuroscience, University College Cork, Cork, Ireland

Noshene Ranjbar
University of Arizona College of Medicine,
Tucson, Arizona, USA

Sandra Maria Lima Ribeiro
Public Health School and The School of
Arts, Sciences and Humanities, University
of Sao Paulo, Sao Paulo, Brazil

Tetyana Rocks
Food and Mood Centre, The Institute for
Mental and Physical Health and Clinical
Translation (IMPACT), School of Medicine,
Deakin University, Geelong, Victoria,
Australia

Julia J. Rucklidge
School of Psychology, Speech and Hearing,
University of Canterbury, Christchurch,
New Zealand

Elizabeth Schneider
APC Microbiome Ireland, University
College Cork, Cork, Ireland

Lynda Sedley
Institute of Environment and Nutritional
Epigenetics, Coolum, Queensland,
Australia

Heidi M. Staudacher
Food and Mood Centre, The Institute
for Mental and Physical Health
and Clinical Translation (IMPACT),
School of Medicine, Deakin
University, Geelong, Victoria,
Australia

Scott Teasdale
Discipline of Psychiatry and Mental Health,
School of Psychiatry, University of New
South Wales, Sydney, New South Wales,
Australia

Amelia Villagomez
Department of Psychiatry, University of
Arizona College of Medicine, Tucson,
Arizona, USA

Preface

The management of mental illness over the past 100 years has seen many paradigm shifts. Around 1950, Charpentier synthesised chlorpromazine, which was demonstrated to possess antipsychotic activity within a year. A few years later, Paul Jansen and colleagues synthesised haloperidol. These developments revolutionised the management of psychotic illnesses. Iproniazid, which was used to treat tuberculosis, was noted to elevate mood. It was the first monoamine oxidase inhibitor used to treat depression. It was quickly followed by the synthesis of imipramine, the tricyclic antidepressant. It is reasonable to conclude that the 1950s was the decade of pharmacological advancement. However, there has been very little in the way of pharmacological developments within the past 20 years.

The closure of long-stay psychiatric institutions represented another significant paradigm shift with the recognition that such institutions had profound negative effects on patients. These closures represented the dawn of appropriate social interventions in the management of patients with severe mental illnesses.

There have also been advances in psychotherapy – probably none more so than the development of cognitive behaviour therapy. In the 1960s, the American psychiatrist Professor Aaron T. Beck noticed psychological patterns in his depressed clients. In general, they held negative views of themselves, others and their future. Based on this observation, he developed strategies for the effective treatment of depression and anxiety disorder. Cognitive behaviour therapy is now the most widely used psychological therapy for these disorders.

The brain–gut–microbiota axis has been described as a new paradigm in psychiatry. It is a bidirectional communication system linking the brain and the gut microbiota, the collection of microorganisms in the intestine. Research over the past 20 years on this axis has hastened developments in nutritional psychiatry. In clinical practice, very few psychiatrists or psychologists provide nutritional advice for their patients, despite evidence that such advice complements drug and psychological therapies. Nutritional advice for many psychiatric patients may be as relevant as that provided by cardiologists for patients with heart disease. However, at both undergraduate and postgraduate levels, nutritional training is rarely offered, leaving many psychiatrists and psychologists ill-equipped to deal with the recent advances in this field. Few textbooks of psychiatry cover the topic of nutrition.

The gut microbiome as a potential therapeutic target for mental illness is a hot topic in psychiatric research. Trillions of bacteria reside in the human gut and have been shown to play a crucial role in gut–brain communication. Patients with various psychiatric disorders, including depression and schizophrenia, have been shown to have significant alterations in the composition of their gut microbiome. Enhancing beneficial bacteria in the gut, for example through the use of psychobiotics, prebiotics or dietary change, has the potential to improve mood and reduce anxiety in both healthy people and patient groups.

Appropriate nutrition impacts the brain directly and impacts it indirectly through the gut microbiota. This book provides an overview of the relevant aspects of nutrition from a psychiatric perspective. Topics such as the basic principles of nutrition are covered, as well as the relevance of the brain–gut–microbiota axis in mental health. The importance of nutrition in the common mental illnesses seen in adults, such as depression, anxiety disorder and schizophrenia, is covered together with disorders seen in children and older adults. The Mediterranean diet is the most extensively studied from a mental health perspective, and this diet is covered in detail. So, too, are the benefits of psychobiotics and general fermented foods. Chapter 10 explores how nutrition can influence genetic activity by epigenetic modulation. This is an evolving area of biology with major relevance to branches of medicine from psychiatry to oncology.

The book will be of interest to psychiatrists and psychologists, as well as behavioural scientists, neuroscientists and nutritionists. A wealth of titles have been published recently on diet and mental health aimed at a general reader, but this is the first guide for clinicians.

Chapter 1

Basic Principles of Nutrition

Eileen Gibney

Summary
The basic principle of nutrition is the provision of adequate nutrients for populations or groups within populations. Adequate nutrition requires that all nutrients are consumed in adequate amounts and in the correct proportions. Energy is one of the most important things we obtain from food. In the body, energy consumed is used to support metabolic processes. Energy expenditure is made up of three components: basal metabolic rate, thermic effect of food and physical activity. Within the diet, the role of carbohydrates is to be a source of fuel, but overall carbohydrates are also part of energy stores, structural components of cell walls, part of nucleic acids (RNA and DNA) and part of many proteins and lipids. Protein is the most abundant nitrogen-containing compound in the diet. It is a major functional and structural component of all body cells. Fats, also known as lipids, are composed of a carbon skeleton with hydrogen and oxygen substitutions. Understanding the pathway for each nutrient allows for the development of dietary reference values, which aim for optimal levels of a nutrient for each population group. The types of foods eaten in different countries are influenced by factors such as ethnicity, culture, dietary habits, food preferences, intake patterns and food availability, and so the classification and types of foods contained in the major 'food groups' can vary somewhat from country to country.

Introduction

Centuries ago, scientists first noticed the link between foods that were lacking in the diet and conditions or illnesses such as scurvy, pellagra and anaemia (1, 2). Occurrences of illnesses were associated with the lack of specific and essential components in the overall diet (i.e. deficiency of nutrients) (1, 2). In this way, some of the basic concepts which lay the foundations of the science of human nutrition were discovered – the need for adequate nutrition for the maintenance of body function and consequently good health (3, 4, 5). In more recent decades, human nutrition has evolved beyond mere avoidance of nutrient deficiency and developed so that we can aim to consume a diet that will support optimum health (6, 7). Nutritional advice has broadened to include the prevention of lifestyle-related chronic diseases such as cardiovascular disease and type 2 diabetes and so has led to the concept of balanced nutrition for optimal health (8). However, these modern-day afflictions of excess often co-exist alongside the immensely serious problem of undernutrition, which is still widespread in developing countries and among vulnerable groups of people living in developed countries (9).

1

Adequate nutrition requires that all nutrients are consumed in adequate amounts and in the correct proportions. Adequate nutrition is required for functions such as growth and development in utero; physical growth in infancy, adolescence and other life stages; reproduction, pregnancy and lactation; repair of body tissues; and resistance to infection, among others (6, 7). At birth, breast milk provides the perfect balance of nutrients. However, when we start to rely on a variety of foods, we require a balanced diet to maintain good health. In the following sections, we will consider important nutrients and other attributes within an optimal diet.

Energy

Energy is one of the most important things we obtain from food. In the body, energy consumed is used to support metabolic processes (digestion, absorption, excretion, growth) (10, 11). Energy intake is the sum of the energy content of macronutrients in the foods consumed – the total of carbohydrate, protein, fat and alcohol – with fat being the most energy dense (Table 1.1). When considering energy intake, it is important to ensure we consume enough for our specific requirements (10, 11). If we consume too much, we store excess energy for use in periods of energy deficit, leading to increased adiposity. To maintain a stable body weight, we need to balance intake and expenditure – this is known as energy balance.

Energy expenditure is made up of three components – basal metabolic rate (BMR), thermic effect of food (TEF) and physical activity (PA) (12). BMR refers to the energy required to maintain essential functions (e.g. heart rate and respiration). It is by far the largest component of energy requirements, accounting for approximately 70% of required energy. It varies by age, sex and body size. Alongside BMR, there is a specific component of energy associated with the digestion of food known as the TEF. This is caused by an increase in metabolic processes involved in the digestion, absorption and metabolism of foods that are consumed. This accounts for approximately 10% of our energy requirements. PA is used to describe physical movement, which includes movement during normal daily activities, as well as exercise. This can be the most variable aspect of energy expenditure, accounting for anywhere between 20% and 50% of our total energy requirements (12, 13). The recommended intake of energy will be discussed later, but it is important to note that excess energy consumed that is not utilised can be stored as fat (adipose tissue) or glycogen (muscles and liver). The adipose tissue is the largest energy store and, unlike glycogen, it has no limit and can continue to accumulate while the body is in positive energy balance. Excessive adiposity is known to cause increased risk of diseases such as type 2 diabetes and cardiovascular disease (14).

Table 1.1 Macronutrient energy equivalents

Macronutrient	Energy equivalent/g
Carbohydrate	16 KJ, 3.8 kcal
Fat	37 KJ, 9.0 kcal
Protein	17 KJ, 4.0 kcal
Alcohol	29 KJ, 6.9 kcal

KJ = kilojoule, kcal = kilocalorie

Carbohydrate

Within the diet, the role of carbohydrates is to be a source of fuel, but overall carbohydrates are also part of energy stores, structural components of cell walls, part of nucleic acids (RNA and DNA) and part of many proteins and lipids (3). There are many different types of carbohydrates which differ by their basic structure. This difference in structure also affects how easily they are digested, with more complex structures taking longer to digest than simple carbohydrates, which are readily broken down during digestion (3, 15, 16). Fibre is part of the carbohydrate family – and a very important but quite complex nutrient. The exact definition of fibre is often open to question. Generally, it is an indigestible complex carbohydrate found in plants. Fibre can either be classified as 'soluble' or 'insoluble' and 'digestible' or 'indigestible'. Insoluble fibre is essentially a bulking agent which helps to prevent constipation and maintain gut health. A low fibre intake is known to be associated with constipation and gut disease (15, 16). The recommended intake for adults varies slightly according to different national guidelines but ranges between 18 g and 25 g per day (17). In the diet, the main sources of carbohydrate include starchy foods such as bread, cereal, potatoes, rice and pasta and foods and drinks containing sugars such as milk, fruits and confectionery. Carbohydrates are the most important form of energy in the diet, usually contributing between 40% and 60% of energy intake. Major sources of fibre are fruits, vegetables, pulses or legumes, wheat bran, seeds, brown rice and whole-grain products such as breads, cereals and pasta (18, 19, 20).

Protein

Protein is the most abundant nitrogen-containing compound in the diet. It is a major functional and structural component of all body cells. Proteins consist of one or more chains of amino acids, with each protein having a unique sequence of amino acids. Amino acids have the same central structure with a carboxylic acid (COOH) and amino nitrogen (NH_2) group. Proteins' roles in the body include acting as enzymes and messengers/signallers (hormones), as well as having essential parts to play in growth, gene expression and immune function (3, 21, 22). Protein requirements have been defined by the World Health Organization (WHO) as

> the lowest level of dietary protein intake that will balance the losses of nitrogen from the body, and thus maintain the body protein mass, in persons at energy balance with modest levels of physical activity, plus, in children or in pregnant or lactating women, the needs associated with the deposition of tissues or the secretion of milk at rates consistent with good health. (23)

However, it is also important that protein intakes are considered in terms of both the amount and quality, with an appropriate consumption of required amino acids. Amino acids may be categorised as essential (they need to be provided in the diet as the body cannot synthesise them), conditionally essential (there is a measurable limitation to the rate at which they can be synthesised) or non-essential (they can be synthesised in adequate amounts in the body) (Table 1.2) (22).

Protein can also provide energy and typically provides 10–15% of dietary energy. Food sources are generally split into proteins of animal origin and proteins of plant origin. Good dietary sources of animal protein are meat, cheese, eggs and fish. Good dietary sources of plant protein are beans, pulses, nuts and cereal products (24).

Table 1.2 Amino acid classification

Essential	Non-essential	Conditionally essential
Leucine, isoleucine, valine, phenylalanine, tryptophan, methionine, lysine, histidine, threonine	Tyrosine, cysteine, arginine, glutamine, glycine, proline	Selenocysteine, glutamate, aspartate, asparagine, alanine, serine

Fat

Fats, also known as lipids, are composed of a carbon skeleton with hydrogen and oxygen substitutions. They can be classified into four categories, namely simple (e.g. triacylglycerol or cholesterol esters vitamin A and D), complex (e.g. phospholipids or lipoproteins), derived (e.g. fatty acids) and miscellaneous (e.g. carotenoids and vitamins E and K) (3, 25, 26). With respect to diet, the main components of dietary fat are fatty acids (FAs). FAs are defined by the number of carbon atoms, the number of double bonds and the position of the first double-bond acids. How we name FAs is quite complex, with both common names and structured naming systems applied. The basic rule is that there are three parts: first, the number of carbons; second, the number of double bonds; and finally, the position of the first double bond (3, 26). For example, the common dietary saturated FA stearate is C18:0 because it has 18 carbons and no double bonds. FAs can be both saturated (all single bonds) and unsaturated (one or more double bonds). The presence of double bonds leads to a change in the structure of the FAs. FAs with a single double bond are known as monounsaturated FAs, and two or more double bonds are known as polyunsaturated FAs. Lipids have three major functions – structural, storage and metabolic. Structural fat can include lipids associated with cell membranes (3, 25, 26). These consist of a continuous double layer of lipid molecules into which proteins are embedded. There are three major classes of lipids in cell membranes – phospholipids, cholesterol and glycolipids, with phospholipids being the most common. Dietary fat is predominantly stored in the form of triacylglycerols (TAGs). TAGs are formed by linking FAs with an ester linkage to three alcohol groups in glycerol. These are the form in which fat is stored in adipose tissue and can be used as a fuel source during lipolysis, where fat stores are broken down. An example of a lipid with metabolic functions would be as a precursor to hormones such as steroids and eicosanoids (3). Fats in the diet are found in meat, in processed cooking fats such as oils, butter and spreads and in dairy products such as milk, cheese and cream. The average daily energy derived from fat in a typical diet ranges between 35% and 40% of total energy and consists mainly of triglycerides. The recommended intake of fat is between 20% and 35% of total energy intake (27, 28, 29). The intake of saturated fats is recommended to be less than 10% of total dietary energy (30, 31, 32). However, recent evidence has opened a debate on the intake of saturated fat in particular (33). In a large review and meta-analysis, de Souza examined associations between intake of total fat and saturated fat with all-cause mortality and morbidities. From their analysis, they suggested that saturated fat intake was not associated with all-cause mortality or other metabolic diseases (33). Others have also examined this relationship by specific food groups, with similar findings (34, 35). Despite these more recent findings, the most recent review of published literature by the UK Scientific Advisory Committee on Nutrition (SACN), the body who provides independent scientific evidence for the development of public health guidelines in the UK, concluded that there is a significant body of evidence demonstrating a relationship between intake of saturated fats and cardiovascular disease and coronary heart disease events (36). They noted that, irrespective of the lack of evidence for an effect on mortality, non-fatal cardiovascular disease and coronary heart disease events have a serious adverse impact on health and quality of life, and that existing public health recommendations for saturated fat, at <10% total energy, are to be maintained (36).

Vitamins and Minerals

Vitamins and minerals are essential components of the diet. There are a number of known vitamins, which can be broadly split into water-soluble vitamins and fat-soluble vitamins. B vitamins, vitamin C, biotin, folic acid, niacin and pantothenic acid are water soluble (3, 37). Vitamins A, D, E and K are fat soluble (3, 37, 38). This solubility has a significant influence on the metabolism, storage and functioning of the vitamin. If we do not consume enough of each of these vitamins, we can become deficient in that vitamin, which means that whatever function it is supposed to do in the body is neglected (3, 37, 38). For example, vitamin C is an essential cofactor in numerous enzymatic reactions such as the biosynthesis of collagen and the regulation of gene expression. Severe vitamin C deficiency has been known for many centuries as scurvy (39). By the late 1700s, it was commonly known that scurvy could be cured by eating oranges or lemons, even though vitamin C was not isolated until much later, in the 1930s (39).

Non-nutrients

Regular consumption of fruits, vegetables, whole grains and other plant foods has been shown to have an inverse relationship with the risk of developing chronic diseases, and these foods provide not only a range of vitamins, minerals and fibre but also a range of different bioactive compounds, including phytochemicals (40, 41). There are over 5,000 different phytochemicals identified to date and they each have specific roles in plant reproduction, growth, metabolism and defence, as well as contributing to plant colour (40, 41). Taking polyphenols as an example, polyphenol intake is hard to estimate because of large variations in plants influenced by season, harvesting conditions, processing and many more factors. While there is limited data on the consumption of phytochemicals overall, there has been a huge amount of research on the relationship of polyphenols to health outcomes, and emerging research suggests that consuming a diverse range of phytochemicals from fruits, vegetables, pulses and whole grains is beneficial for health (42, 43). Therefore, consumers should obtain their nutrients, antioxidants, bioactive compounds and phytochemicals from a balanced diet with a wide variety of fruits, vegetables, whole grains and other plant foods for optimal nutrition, health and well-being.

Nutrient Requirements

Establishing nutrient requirements was and still is considered one of the major steps in the derivation of food-based dietary guidelines (FBDGs). Nutrient requirements are quantitative nutrient intake goals or targets, known as recommended daily allowances (RDAs) or dietary reference values (DRVs), set to meet the needs of the majority of the population (44). During the 1950s, research in nutrition led to the emergence of the concept of the role of diet in health promotion, as opposed to mere prevention of nutrient deficiency. This in turn led to the recognition that guidance was needed on consumption of energy and some macronutrients (total and saturated fat), as well as components in the diet such as sugar, salt and fibre. This led to the idea of dietary guidelines advising populations to reduce fat, salt or sugar. In more recent decades, research focussing on the role of other nutrients (including vitamins and minerals) in health promotion and prevention of chronic conditions such as obesity, cardiovascular disease, type 2 diabetes, osteoporosis and some cancers has led to increasing recognition that even micronutrients may be required in optimal amounts (44, 45, 46, 47). Therefore, although RDAs were originally designed to help protect against deficiency of nutrients, the association of nutrition with the development of chronic disease led to them also defining optimal levels of intake (44, 45, 46, 47).

To more fully understand what is meant by optimal levels of intake, it is important to consider the levels of nutrient adequacy (48). For most nutrients, a stepwise understanding of nutrient adequacy can be established, ranging from optimisation of body stores or status to prevention of clinical deficiency (Figure 1.1). When considering body stores, we can store some nutrients within cells and organs within our body. When we have fluctuating intakes, we use these stores. If we have no intake, the stores go down – like a petrol tank. If you do not put the petrol in, the light comes on saying petrol is low, and eventually there is none left. Our body has biochemical measures that act similarly to the petrol light to tell us we are low but still have some petrol/nutrient in the tank. If not repleted, body stores will continue reducing and the function associated with that nutrient cannot be completed. Keeping with the car analogies, if we run out of petrol, we cannot drive; if we run out of water to clean our windscreen, we cannot clean it. Both are separate; each has a specific function which cannot be completed without the petrol/water. In the case of the water, the car/body can still function (because it has petrol) but it is not working at its best. With each nutrient, before we see signs of deficiency there are mild/undetectable symptoms, and these are the symptoms that begin to appear when stores are low and the body is not working as well as it should (44, 45, 46, 47, 48) (Figure 1.1). For example, when our body is low in iron, say, we could feel tired and sluggish before we show overt signs of anaemia. Understanding this pathway for each nutrient allows for the development of dietary reference values, which aim for optimal levels of a nutrient for each population group (48).

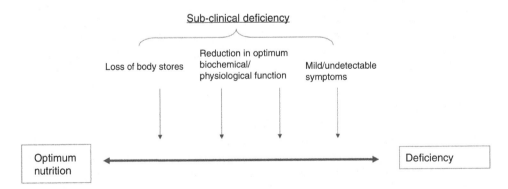

Figure 1.1 Stages in nutrient deficiency.

DRVs are the complete set of quantitative nutrient reference values for nutrients, indicating the specific amount of a nutrient that healthy people need depending on their age and sex (44, 45). DRVs include recommendations for average, upper and lower levels of intake (Table 1.3). Recommendations are given by nutrients, not foods. Instead of recommending portions of meat, fish or eggs, DRVs recommend a certain amount of protein intake in grams or recommended intake of folate in µg. It is also important to note that DRVs should not be viewed as recommendations for individuals. Rather, they are reference intakes for a population average (44, 45).

Recommendations about nutrient intakes are based on data and the distribution of the specific variable in a population (45, 47, 49). A combination of random genetic and environmental factors causes individuals to cluster near the average for many traits we measure, with fewer at extremes away from the average. Plotting this information for any given trait in a population results in a curve known as a normal distribution curve (Gaussian distribution). We use this concept of normal distribution curves in determining nutrient requirements, where the peak of the curve is equal to the average requirement for that population, with half of the population having requirements above and half of them having requirements below this point. This is normal for many measurements in a population – each individual will vary so that some require more, some less. Statistical calculations calculate the mean (or average) and the statistical variation around that average, called the standard deviation (SD). The mean of a normal distribution plus two standard

Table 1.3 Dietary reference value definitions and nomenclature

Name (abbreviation)	Description
Population reference intake (PRI)	The level of (nutrient) intake that is enough for nearly all healthy people in a population/group. Several terms are used interchangeably with the PRI such as recommended dietary allowance (RDA), reference nutrient intake (RNI), recommended intake (RI) and adequate intake (AI).
Average requirement (AR)	The level of (nutrient) intake that is enough for half of the people in a healthy group, given a normal distribution of requirement.
Lower-threshold intake (LTI)	The level of intake below which almost all individuals will be unlikely to maintain optimum metabolic function according to a criterion chosen for each nutrient.
Adequate intake (AI)	An AI is the average observed daily level of intake by a population (group) of apparently healthy people that is assumed to be 'adequate'. It is the value estimated when a PRI cannot be established because an AR cannot be determined.
Reference intake range (RI)	The reference intake range for macronutrients, expressed as % of the daily energy intake, defined by a lower and upper bound. This applies to ranges of intakes that are adequate for maintaining health and associated with a low risk of selected chronic diseases.
Upper intake level (UL)	The maximum level of total chronic daily intake of a nutrient (from all sources) judged to be unlikely to pose a risk of adverse health effects to humans.

deviations means that 97.5% of the population's requirements or needs are met, so only the top 2.5% fall outside this. Using this approach, the statistical distribution of each individual nutrient can be calculated. As shown in Figure 1.2, the average requirement is set at the mean, with the PRI at the mean plus two standard deviations – so the requirements for 97.5% of the population will be met. The lowest threshold is set at the mean minus two standard deviations and the tolerable upper limit, which is above the PRI (45, 47, 49).

Consumption of most nutrients greater than requirements is generally not harmful (except for energy) (3, 10, 11). For energy, we do not recommend intakes at the mean plus two standard deviations as this would mean that 97.5% of population needs are being met, but many people are consuming more than they need. Therefore, if we set the energy needs for the population near to the highest requirement, we would be asking most of the population to be consuming above their requirements, resulting in weight gain. Over time, small imbalances in energy intake (EI) to energy expenditure (EE), where EI is greater than EE, can lead to overweight and obesity (3, 10, 11). Energy recommendations are therefore given at the average for the population and we use the estimated average requirement (EAR) (3, 10, 11) (Figure 1.2).

RDAs are set for healthy populations and are not applicable to those who have different illnesses or conditions as their nutrient requirements are completely different (45, 47, 49). Nutrient requirements vary with age, sex and physiological condition because of differences in growth for younger age groups and age-related changes in nutrient absorption and body functions and/or functional capacity. For this reason, DRVs are developed for different life stages and sex groups (45, 47, 49). Separate reference values are also established for pregnant and lactating women, taking into account the additional nutrient requirement for the formation of new tissues or to compensate for the nutrients lost to the body in the form of human milk, respectively, and considering the physiological adaptations that occur during these conditions. The European Food Safety Authority (EFSA) provides ongoing scientific opinions on DRVs to ensure they are underpinned by the latest available knowledge. In 2020, EFSA launched an interactive tool called the DRV Finder that searches by population group or nutrient based on their published opinions (50).

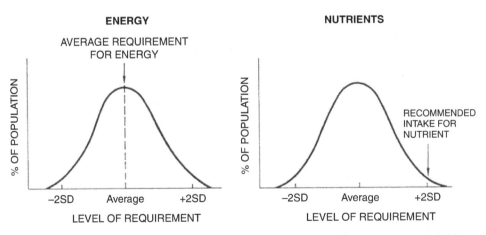

Figure 1.2 Nutrient and energy distribution curve. Source: National Academy of Sciences, *Recommended Dietary Allowances*, 10th ed.

Food-Based Dietary Guidelines

While we accurately derive and set specific population nutrient requirements, people eat food, not nutrients – yet it is the combination of nutrients in food that determines the health of the individual. Nutritionists think of the foods that we eat in terms of the nutrients they provide. A balanced diet must provide the following basic nutrients: proteins, fats, carbohydrates (including fibre), vitamins, minerals and water, but the difficulty is that all of these nutrients are necessary in different quantities. So, how do nutritionists communicate the concept of good nutrition to the public? It is ironic that this most fundamental cornerstone in human nutrition simultaneously remains one of the most challenging areas for nutrition scientists. The translation of nutrient requirements for good health into the foods that people should eat is a complex and indeed sometimes contentious process. FBDGs are the translation of nutrients to food and are often referred to as 'healthy eating guidelines' or 'healthy eating advice'. The nutrients needed for health are translated into the *amounts* and *types* of foods that are required to achieve a balanced diet. Government organisations and nutrition scientists are usually responsible for formulating and conveying these recommendations for healthy eating to the population (51, 52, 53, 54).

FBDGs are to be used by governments as part of their national health strategies for health promotion. In 1992, the United Nations Food and Agricultural Organization (FAO) and the WHO identified that one major strategy to improve the nutritional status of populations was to call upon governments to provide quantitative and qualitative dietary advice to the public for different age groups and lifestyles. Later in 1995, the WHO/FAO jointly organised an expert consultation titled 'Preparation and use of food-based dietary guidelines', where it was concluded that FBDGs needed to take account of factors such as current dietary practices and habits and prevailing public health problems rather than nutrient requirements alone (55). The resulting WHO/FAO expert consultation report highlighted the rationale for FBDGs. There was established evidence for nutrition in health and disease prevention and complex science needed to be translated into practical guidance for people. The original concept of FBDGs took into account both the scientific evidence and epidemiological data linking specific food consumption patterns with low incidence of certain diseases, while not requiring a complete understanding of the underlying biological mechanisms. This report noted some important points that form the basis of the development of FBDGs (55). Foods make up diets but foods are more than just a collection of nutrients. There is already good evidence from studies (animal, clinical and epidemiological) that specific dietary patterns are associated with a reduced risk of specific diseases. For certain micronutrients, evidence suggests that intake higher than present nutritional recommendations may help to lower the risk of non-communicable diseases. However, scientific evidence has not yet identified the potential health outcomes of some non-nutrient food components (55).

More recently, in 2010, an expert panel of EFSA issued specific recommendations to be followed for a stepwise approach for the derivation of FBDGs (56). In the European Union, there are 27 member nations with very diverse populations. Therefore, each government needs to identify their priorities in terms of public health issues. The diet–disease relationships that exist in a particular country or region need to be established and FBDGs need to be developed that are in line with other existing policies relevant to health promotion. For example, there may be physical activity or alcohol policies already in existence and FBDGs need to be integrated where possible with these. The inclusion of stakeholders early on in the development of the guidelines is an important step in ensuring that the final outcome is acceptable (56). The final result should be a food guide that is consistent, easily understood and memorable. The key recommendations of this report were as follows:

1   Identify diet–health relationships relevant to a particular nation
2   Identify nutrients of public health importance
3   Identify foods relevant to FBDGs
4   Identify food consumption patterns
5   Test/optimise FBDGs
6   Consider graphic representation of FBDGs
7   Implement and monitor FBDGs' impact

While the science has evolved, the rationale for the development of FBDGs remains the same. Most importantly, FBDGs need to be underpinned by strong scientific evidence written or produced in a very simple, easy-to-understand format. In practice, when considering food-based recommendations, foods that are similar are grouped into food groups. This means we can give recommendations based on food groups rather than a mix of individual foods. Each food group provides specific nutrients or has a specific function in the body. The major food groups often depicted or considered in FBDGs include the specific food groups, or variations of these, depending on the source. The key attributes and nutrients associated with each food group are also listed (see Table 1.4) (56).

Food items providing energy but few nutrients are grouped into the food group 'Foods and drinks high in sugar, fat and salt' – these include foods such as confectionery, cakes, biscuits, chocolate, crisps, savoury snacks and so on. Recommended intakes of these food groups are given as portions per food group and often depicted in a visual way to help the consumer understand which food groups to eat more or less. On this basis, using a pyramid as a visual, the food group 'Vegetables, salads and fruit' would be depicted at the bottom, with the greatest recommended intake of portions, and the food group 'Foods and drinks high in sugar, fat and salt' depicted as the smallest food group at the top (56).

The types of foods eaten in different countries are influenced by factors such as ethnicity, culture, dietary habits, food preferences, intake patterns and food availability, and so the classifications and types of foods contained in the major food groups can vary somewhat

Table 1.4 Food groups used in food-based dietary guidelines

Food group	Primary contribution to diet
Vegetables, salads and fruit	Providing mainly vitamins, minerals, fibre and other beneficial substances (e.g. phytochemicals)
Wholemeal breads, cereals, pasta, rice and other starchy foods such as potatoes	Providing mainly carbohydrate, fibre and B vitamins
Milk, yoghurt and cheese	Providing mainly calcium and other micronutrients
Meat, poultry, fish, eggs, beans and nuts	Providing mainly protein and iron
Fat, spreads and oils	Providing mainly fat and saturated fat
Foods and drinks high in sugar, fat and salt	Providing sugar, fat and salt

from country to country (51). For example, in Ireland and the UK, potatoes are consumed as a major staple, contributing mainly to carbohydrate intake, and so are included in the group 'Wholemeal breads, cereals, pasta, rice and other starchy foods'. However, in other countries, where they are eaten less frequently, they may be considered only in the group 'Vegetables, salads and fruit' (56). Similarly, the number of food groups used may differ in different national food guides. For instance, the USA and Canada split their 'Vegetables, salads and fruit' group into one food group for 'Fruit' and a separate food group for 'Vegetables'. The pictorial display of the guidelines varies from country to country and can be in the form of a plate (UK), a pyramid (USA, Ireland), a rainbow (Canada), a pagoda (China, Korea) or a circle (Australia, Germany, Sweden) (51).

Conclusion

The basic principle of nutrition is the provision of adequate nutrients for populations or groups within populations. Recommendations for nutrient intakes are based on scientific evidence, using a variety of information to determine recommended intake, as well as higher and lower levels. Each nutrient's recommended intake is linked to its function and specific requirements in the body. While these are precise and specific, they lack relevance for the general public, and as such are translated into FBDGs. These aim to provide consumer-friendly food recommendations for people to achieve a nutritionally adequate balanced diet for optimal health and reduced risk of disease.

References

1. Murphy, S. P., Yates, A. A., Atkinson, S. A., Barr, S. I. and Dwyer, J., 2016. History of nutrition: the long road leading to the Dietary Reference Intakes for the United States and Canada. *Advances in Nutrition, 7* (1), pp. 157–68.

2. Keusch, G. T., 2003. The history of nutrition: malnutrition, infection and immunity. *The Journal of Nutrition, 133*(1), pp. 336S–340S.

3. Lanham-New, S. A., Hill, T. R., Gallagher, A. M. and Vorster, H. H. eds., 2019. *Introduction to human nutrition.* John Wiley & Sons.

4. Afshin, A., Sur, P. J., Fay, K. A., et al., 2019. Health effects of dietary risks in 195 countries, 1990–2017: a systematic analysis for the Global Burden of Disease Study 2017. *The Lancet, 393*(10184), pp. 1958–72.

5. Kocarnik, J. M., Compton, K., Dean, F. E., et al., 2022. Cancer incidence, mortality, years of life lost, years lived with disability, and disability-adjusted life years for 29 cancer groups from 2010 to 2019: a systematic analysis for the Global Burden of Disease Study 2019. *JAMA Oncology, 8* (3), pp. 420–44.

6. Forouhi, N. G. and Unwin, N., 2019. Global diet and health: old questions, fresh evidence, and new horizons. *The Lancet, 393*(10184), pp. 1916–18.

7. Kirkpatrick, S. I., Vanderlee, L., Dias, G. M. and Hanning, R. M., 2019. Can dietary guidelines support the transformation of food systems to foster human and planetary health? UNSCN News 44, 122–8.

8. Pomerleau, J., McKee, M., Lobstein, T. and Knai, C., 2003. The burden of disease attributable to nutrition in Europe. *Public Health Nutrition, 6*(5), pp. 453–61.

9. Perez-Escamilla, R., Bermudez, O., Buccini, G. S., et al., 2018. Nutrition disparities and the global burden of malnutrition. *British Medical Journal, 361,* k2252.

10. Shetty, P., 2005. Energy requirements of adults. *Public Health Nutrition, 8*(7a), pp. 994–1009.

11. Roberts, S. B., Heyman, M. B., Evans, W. J., et al., 1991. Dietary energy requirements of young adult men, determined by using the doubly labeled water method. *The*

American Journal of Clinical Nutrition, *54* (3), pp. 499–505.

12. Levine, J. A., 2005. Measurement of energy expenditure. *Public Health Nutrition*, *8*(7a), pp. 1123–32.

13. Donahoo, W. T., Levine, J. A. and Melanson, E. L., 2004. Variability in energy expenditure and its components. *Current Opinion in Clinical Nutrition & Metabolic Care*, *7*(6), pp. 599–605.

14. Franco, M., Ordunez, P., Caballero, B., et al., 2007. Impact of energy intake, physical activity, and population-wide weight loss on cardiovascular disease and diabetes mortality in Cuba, 1980-2005. *American Journal of Epidemiology*, *166*(12), pp. 1374–80.

15. Buttriss, J. L. and Stokes, C. S., 2008. Dietary fibre and health: an overview. *Nutrition Bulletin*, *33*(3), pp. 186–200.

16. Seal, C. J., 2006. Whole grains and CVD risk. *Proceedings of the Nutrition Society*, *65* (1), pp. 24–34.

17. Agostoni, C. V., Bresson, J. L., Fairweather Tait, S., et al., 2010. Scientific opinion on dietary reference values for carbohydrates and dietary fibre. *European Food Safety Authority Journal*, *8*(3), p. 1462.

18. McGowan, C., O'Sullivan, E., Kehoe, L., et al., 2022. Intakes and sources of dietary fibre in a nationally representative sample of teenagers (13–18 years) in Ireland. *Proceedings of the Nutrition Society*, *81* (OCE4), p. E125.

19. McCarthy, R., Kehoe, L., Flynn, A. and Walton, J., 2020. The role of fruit and vegetables in the diets of children in Europe: current state of knowledge on dietary recommendations, intakes and contribution to energy and nutrient intakes. *Proceedings of the Nutrition Society*, *79*(4), pp. 479–86.

20. Kehoe, L., Walton, J., McNulty, B. A., Nugent, A. P. and Flynn, A., 2021. Energy, macronutrients, dietary fibre and salt intakes in older adults in Ireland: key sources and compliance with recommendations. *Nutrients*, *13*(3), p. 876.

21. Young, V. R., Gersovitz, M. and Munro, H. N., 2018. Human aging: protein and amino acid metabolism and implications for protein and amino acid requirements. In Moment, G. R., Adelman, R. C. and Roth, G. S. (eds.), *Nutritional approaches to aging research* (pp. 47–81). CRC Press.

22. Wu, G., 2010. Functional amino acids in growth, reproduction, and health. *Advances in Nutrition*, *1*(1), pp. 31–7.

23. Food and Agriculture Organization and World Health Organization Ad Hoc Expert Committee, 1973. *Energy and protein requirements*. In FAO Nutrition Meetings Report Series (no. 52). Food and Agriculture Organization.

24. Hone, M., Nugent, A. P., Walton, J., McNulty, B. A. and Egan, B., 2020. Habitual protein intake, protein distribution patterns and dietary sources in Irish adults with stratification by sex and age. *Journal of Human Nutrition and Dietetics*, *33*(4), pp. 465–76.

25. Hayes, K. and the Expert Panel, 2010. Fatty acid expert roundtable: key statements about fatty acids. *Journal of the American College of Nutrition*, *29*(suppl. 3), pp. S285–S288.

26. Foster, R., Williamson, C. and Lunn, J., 2009. *Culinary oils and their health effects*. British Nutrition Foundation. Briefing papers.

27. Feeney, E. L., Nugent, A. P., McNulty, B., et al., 2016. An overview of the contribution of dairy and cheese intakes to nutrient intakes In the Irish diet: results from the National Adult Nutrition Survey. *British Journal of Nutrition*, *115*(4), pp. 709–17.

28. Li, K., McNulty, B. A., Tiernery, A. M., et al., 2016. Dietary fat intakes in Irish adults in 2011: how much has changed in 10 years? *British Journal of Nutrition*, *115* (10), pp. 1798–1809.

29. Linseisen, J., Welch, A. A., Ocke, M., et al., 2009. Dietary fat intake in the European Prospective Investigation into Cancer and Nutrition: results from the 24-h dietary recalls. *European Journal of Clinical Nutrition*, *63*(4), pp. S61–S80.

30. Jacobson, T. A., Maki, K. C., Orringer, C. E., et al., 2015. National Lipid Association recommendations for

patient-centered management of dyslipidemia: part 2. *Journal of Clinical Lipidology*, 9, pp. S1–S122.

31. Eckel, R. H., Jakicic, J. M., Ard, J. D., et al., 2014. 2013 AHA/ACC guideline on lifestyle management to reduce cardiovascular risk: a report of the American College of Cardiology/American Heart Association Task Force on Practice Guidelines. *Journal of the American College of Cardiology*, 63, pp. 2960–84.

32. United States Department of Agriculture, 2015. Scientific report of the 2015 Dietary Guidelines Advisory Committee: advisory report to the Secretary of Health and Human Services and the Secretary of Agriculture. Available online: https://health.gov/sites/def ault/files/2019-09/Scientific-Report-of-the-2 015-Dietary-Guidelines-Advisory-Committee.pdf.

33. De Souza, R. J., Mente, A., Maroleanu, A., et al., 2015. Intake of saturated and trans unsaturated fatty acids and risk of all cause mortality, cardiovascular disease, and type 2 diabetes: systematic review and meta-analysis of observational studies. *British Medical Journal*, 351, h3978.

34. Drouin-Chartier, J.-P., Brassard, D., Tessier-Grenier, M., et al., 2016. Systematic review of the association between dairy product consumption and risk of cardiovascular-related clinical outcomes. *Advances in Nutrition*, 7, 1026–40.

35. Alexander, D. D., Bylsma, L. C., Vargas, A. J., et al., 2016. Dairy consumption and CVD: a systematic review and meta-analysis. *British Journal of Nutrition*, 115, 737–50.

36. Scientific Advisory Committee on Nutrition. 2019. Saturated fats and health. Available online: https://assets.publishing.service.gov .uk/government/uploads/system/uploads/att achment_data/file/814995/SACN_report_o n_saturated_fat_and_health.pdf.

37. Dattola, A., Silvestri, M., Bennardo, L., et al., 2020. Role of vitamins in skin health: a systematic review. *Current Nutrition Reports*, 9(3), pp. 226–35.

38. Maqbool, M. A., Aslam, M., Akbar, W. and Iqbal, Z., 2018. Biological importance of vitamins for human health: a review. *Journal of Agriculture and Basic Sciences*, 2 (3), pp. 50–8.

39. Carr, A. C. and Rowe, S., 2020. Factors affecting vitamin C status and prevalence of deficiency: a global health perspective. *Nutrients*, 12(7), p. 1963.

40. Mitra, S., Tareq, A. M., Das, R., et al., 2022. Polyphenols: a first evidence in the synergism and bioactivities. *Food Reviews International*, pp. 1–23.

41. XTruzzi, F., Tibaldi, C., Zhang, Y., Dinelli, G. and D' Amen, E., 2021. An overview on dietary polyphenols and their biopharmaceutical classification system (BCS). *International Journal of Molecular Sciences*, 22(11), p. 5514.

42. Tomas-Barberan, F. A. and Andres-Lacueva, C., 2012. Polyphenols and health: current state and progress. *Journal of Agricultural and Food Chemistry*, 60(36), pp. 8773–5.

43. Rajha, H. N., Paule, A., Aragonès, G., et al., 2022. Recent advances in research on polyphenols: effects on microbiota, metabolism, and health. *Molecular Nutrition & Food Research*, 66(1), p. 2100670. www.efsa.europa.eu/en/topi cs/topic/dietary-reference-values.

44. Barr, S. I., 2006. Introduction to dietary reference intakes. *Applied Physiology, Nutrition, and Metabolism*, 31(1), pp. 61–5.

45. Murphy, S. P., Yates, A. A., Atkinson, S. A., Barr, S. I. and Dwyer, J., 2016. History of nutrition: the long road leading to the Dietary Reference Intakes for the United States and Canada. *Advances in Nutrition*, 7 (1), pp. 157–68.

46. National Academies of Sciences, Engineering, and Medicine, 2017. Guiding principles for developing Dietary Reference Intakes based on chronic disease. National Academies of Sciences, Engineering, and Medicine.

47. Jensen, G. L. and Binkley, J., 2002. Clinical manifestations of nutrient deficiency.

Journal of Parenteral and Enteral Nutrition, 26, pp. S29–S33.

48. Meyers, L. D., Hellwig, J. P. and Otten, J. J. eds., 2006. *Dietary reference intakes: the essential guide to nutrient requirements.* National Academies Press.

49. EFSA Dietary Reference Finder, n.d. https://multimedia.efsa.europa.eu/drvs/index.htm.

50. Herforth, A., Arimond, M., Álvarez-Sánchez, C., et al., 2019. A global review of food-based dietary guidelines. *Advances in Nutrition,* 10(4), pp. 590–605.

51. Smitasiri, S. and Uauy, R., 2007. Beyond recommendations: implementing food-based dietary guidelines for healthier populations. *Food and Nutrition Bulletin,* 28(1_suppl1), pp. S141–S151.

52. Erve, I., Tulen, C. B. M., Jansen, J., et al., 2017. Overview of elements within national food-based dietary guidelines. *European Journal of Nutrition and Food Safety, 7,* pp. 1–56.

53. Turrini, A., Leclercq, C. and D'Amicis, A., 1999. Patterns of food and nutrient intakes in Italy and their application to the development of food-based dietary guidelines. *British Journal of Nutrition, 81* (S1), pp. S83–S89.

54. Food and Agriculture Organization and World Health Organization, 1998. *Preparation and use of food-based dietary guidelines.* World Health Organization.

55. EFSA Panel on Dietetic Products, Nutrition, and Allergies (NDA), 2010. Scientific opinion on establishing food-based dietary guidelines. *EFSA Journal,* 8(3), p. 1460.

56. Flynn, M. A., O'Brien, C. M., Ross, V., Flynn, C. A. and Burke, S. J., 2012. Revision of food-based dietary guidelines for Ireland, Phase 2: recommendations for healthy eating and affordability. *Public Health Nutrition,* 15(3), pp. 527–37.

Diet and the Microbiome–Gut–Brain Axis
Feeding Your Microbes for Mental Health Benefit

Kenneth J. O'Riordan, Elizabeth Schneider, Ger Clarke and John F. Cryan

Summary

The assortment of trillions of microorganisms resident along the human gastrointestinal tract, our gut microbiota, has co-evolved with us over thousands of years. It can influence a plethora of aspects of human physiology, including host metabolism, immunity and even brain function, cognition and behaviour across the lifespan. The gut microbiota and the brain can communicate with one another, directly and indirectly, through immune system modulation, tryptophan metabolism, vagus nerve activity, the enteric nervous system and bioactive microbial by-products, or metabolites produced by the gut microbiome. Indeed, the gut microbiota are responsible for a rich reservoir of novel metabolites and bioactive substances that can have pleiotropic functionalities for the host. Moreover, diet, an easily accessible and thus powerful interventional tool, can act as a modulator of gut-microbial composition and activity, impacting on host physiology. As such, nutrition is seen as one of the major modulators of the gut microbiota. Intriguingly, although psychiatric conditions often include a dietary aspect, much research investigating this link in clinical populations ignores this relationship, missing a key therapeutic avenue. This has led to the concept of nutritional psychiatry, where we can use food and supplements to support mental health and brain function. As a result, it is critical to consider emerging microbiome-targeted dietary approaches with the greatest potential to improve health outcomes in a psychiatric population.

Introduction

Our gut microbiota, the collection of trillions of microorganisms residing within the human gut, influences various aspects of human physiology, including host metabolism and immune function, and is now well recognised for its ability to influence brain function, cognition and behaviour (1). Diet is a key modulator of gut-microbial composition and marks a potentially easily accessible but powerful interventional tool to manipulate the gut microbiota and affect the host's physiological responses (2–4). Although nutrition is one of the major modulators of the gut microbiota, and psychiatric conditions often include a dietary aspect, studies investigating the gut-microbiota composition in clinical populations often ignore this relationship (5). This has led to the concept of nutritional psychiatry (6), using food and supplements to support mental health and brain function, which is gaining considerable traction (7, 8). In this chapter, we will survey the clinical research landscape to ascertain the current level of knowledge, identify the main knowledge gaps and list potential future research that would be beneficial to the field, focussing on emerging microbiome-targeted dietary approaches with the greatest potential to improve health outcomes in a psychiatric population.

The Gut Microbiome

The human gut microbiome, the collective term for the hundreds of trillions of bacteria, viruses, phage and archaea (gut microbiota) residing in the gastrointestinal tract, including the full compilation of associated genetic material, has been a part of human biology from the very beginning. In fact, microbial organisms existed long before humans came along, and thus there has never been a time when humans have not been influenced by microbes or the brain has been without signals from the gut. This at times symbiotic relationship has co-evolved over thousands of years and plays a critical role in health, well-being and host physiology; therefore, understanding the core mechanisms involved is vital for appreciating how our microbiome contributes to our health, and in particular our neurological function. Moreover, diet remains the most direct and easily modifiable form of interaction with the gut microbiota, presenting nutrition as a viable option to modulate host gut–microbiome interactions to promote health and treat disease (9, 10).

Research into the gut microbiome has advanced exponentially in recent years. Although much of it has explored hypotheses in pre-clinical models, more studies are beginning to examine human gut–microbiome changes in healthy and clinical populations. One of the main reasons for the boom in microbiome research is the development of microbiome bioinformatic pipelines for analysis, reduced costs and advances in sequencing; that is, 'omics technologies' (specifically *genomics*, full genetic characterisation of an organism; *transcriptomics*, analysis of the mRNA transcripts indicating active cellular processes; *proteomics*, a measure of currently active proteins; and *metabolomics*, a measurement of the complete set of metabolites in a sample). Such technological advances have enabled scientists to fully explore how microbes affect human biology. In fact, we have since determined that over 99% of our genes are microbial. For every human gene counted, there are over 100 non-human (microbial) genes measured. Given that microbes are far more genetically dense than a human cell, current estimates have determined that there are ~1.3 microbial cells to every human cell in a human body from 500 to 1,000 different bacterial species. As such, our composition is more non-human than human. Furthermore, while the inherited genome is mostly stable throughout the lifetime of the host, the microbiome is large, diverse, adaptable and infinitely modifiable, presenting itself as a potential target for therapeutic intervention.

The most abundant type of microbe in the gastrointestinal tract is bacteria, and as such this is the most studied to date. However, archaea, yeasts, single-celled eukaryotes, helminth parasites and viruses, including bacteriophage, also share our gastrointestinal tract with bacteria. In fact, the gut virome (predominantly composed of bacterial viruses such as bacteriophage) remains a relatively unexplored area, with much of our current understanding based mostly on sequencing information from faecal samples, which represents only a static snapshot of the colonic virome. However, there does appear to be a strong association in measures of diversity between the gut virome and gut bacteriome.

Gastrointestinal bacterial classification follows the normal Linnaean taxonomic rank: species, genus, family, order, class and phylum; they are largely defined by two bacterial phylotypes, *Bacteroidetes* and *Firmicutes*. However, *Actinobacteria*, *Proteobacteria*, *Fusobacteria* and *Verrucomicrobia* phyla are present in relatively low abundance. Human gut-microbial colonies have been classified into three distinct enterotypes, which are distinguished by high levels of a single microbial genus: *Bacteroides*, *Prevotella* or *Ruminococcus*.

It is important to note, however, that our understanding of the gut microbiome and its involvement in host physiology is still in its infancy, and currently we are only able to characterise the functional output of relative shifts in the microbiome under study. Current work can only report on broad correlations between large, obvious gut-microbial compositional changes; it is not yet feasible to define a causal role for these correlational observations. This is further complicated by the fact that we cannot yet define the cocktail of a healthy gut microbiome, as this appears to be unique to each individual and experiences many shifts during the host lifespan. Although temporal intra-individual differences are seen to be smaller than inter-individual differences, the maintenance or disruption of the host gut homeostasis is seen as a fundamental determinant in health and disease. Where possible, we will try to indicate if observed changes in a study are causative or correlative. Nonetheless, current collective understanding highlights the importance of homeostasis for each balanced compositional signature within a host, where disruption of this results in increased susceptibility to disease.

In Silico Methods Used to Study the Gut Microbiome

While we are capable of collecting vast amounts of data such as the microbes that are present, where they are present and what they are doing, understanding what questions to ask is central to understanding the functional relevance of our microbial friends. With the advent of high-throughput sequencing and the technological explosion over the last 10–15 years allowing for the use of artificial intelligence and deep machine learning, it is now possible to broaden the multi-disciplinary efforts and involve bioinformatic and sequencing approaches. Analysing and interpreting microbiome data outputs can be challenging, in part because of the sheer number of specialist software tools needed to pre-process and analyse the data (11). It is important to note that microbiome data is compositional and thus undergoes compositional data analysis (CoDA) (12). Further, because microbiome count data typically has many zeros, and the logarithm of a zero is undefined, we cannot ignore zero counts in our data; indeed, this remains under heated discussion in the open forum and several reasonable solutions have been proposed (e.g. the ALDEx2 framework).

Bioinformatics

Bioinformatic investigations, which include biostatistics, data analysis and computational biology of data garnered from pre-clinical and human studies, involve complex computational algorithms. The earliest attempts at understanding databases of information accrued from large studies include the Human Microbiome Project and MetaHIT, which have been instrumental in training researchers on how to handle big data. Statistical modelling methods such as multi-dimensional scaling and consortia abundance and diversity are now commonplace in gut-microbiome sequencing and analysis. While it is common to model genetic sequences (genomics), studies also often look at the transcriptome, proteome and metabolome. As such, large complex modelling algorithms and dataset handling pipelines become critical tools in the research.

Genomic Sequencing

There are two main methods regularly used in microbiome sequencing, 16S (or amplicon) sequencing and whole-genome shotgun (WGS) sequencing (13), both of which have distinct and complementary advantages. Both techniques are biased towards detecting specific genetic sequences and thus, by extension, specific microbial taxa. Much recent effort has been driven towards consolidating analysis pipelines across the field by standardising sequencing and analysis protocols with the aim of improving output quality and comparability across different studies.

16S sequencing has been very popular, mostly as it is much cheaper to perform than WGS and is therefore available to more laboratories across the world. It includes methods where an evolutionarily preserved genomic sequence is targeted and sequenced. 16S uses next-generation sequencing (NGS) technology to measure the relative abundance of microbes present in a sample. The protocol involves the ubiquitous polymerase chain reaction (PCR) technique to amplify a specific and highly conserved genetic sequence (amplicon) that is present in all bacterial members of the sample. These sequences cluster based on their genetic relatedness and sum to give a metric of relative abundance. Technically, any sequence can be amplified, but usually known and highly conserved 16S ribosomal RNA subunit sequences are used. This information allows us to classify and differentiate microbes within a sample. From this information, we can predict the functional potential of the microbiota within the sample from the 16S output using well-verified and highly implemented bioinformatic tools such as PICRUSt (Phylogenetic Investigation of Communities by Reconstruction of Unobserved States), Tax4Fun (14) and Piphillin (15).

However, it is important not to ignore the obvious limitations of the 16S method. It cannot identify novel microbial species, nor can it account for intraspecies variation and mutations. This is because the technique can only compare against a reference genome defined in a database. Secondly, some amplicons will amplify more efficiently than others using the PCR method, something that cannot be avoided or controlled for, which imparts bias on the sample output. When aligning operational taxonomic units (OTUs) or amplicon sequence variants (ASVs) to a database, the Silva and Greengenes databases are widely recognised as the most extensive and accurate (16). Further, the QIIME2 platform is an excellent and well-maintained Python-based resource for microbiome analysis (17).

WGS, on the other hand, is far more expensive and thus usually limited to well-funded research projects or government/industry-based programmes of research. Here, all genetic material in a sample is targeted and sequenced. The output is of a far higher resolution and specificity as the technique constructs *de novo* genomes or aligns the sequences garnered from NGS to a reference database. Thus, taxonomic and functional classification of shotgun metagenomics data is more computationally intensive and provides strain-level resolution of both microbial abundance and the functional capacity of a sample. Common tools used in WGS to process raw data include bioBakery, Kraken2 and Bracken.

The main advantages of WGS over 16S include the omission of the PCR step in sequencing a sample, thus removing the inherent potential for bias. Also, as the whole genome is sequenced and not just an amplicon, the output read is far more reliable an identifier of what is in the sample and its functional relevance. It also allows us to identify novel strains or mutations and save sequence reads for future analysis when more information on unknown sequences will inevitably be available. So why would one choose 16S over WGS, apart from the cost advantage? 16S is the preferable option in samples that are heavily contaminated by off-target DNA (host cells/tissues). Further, the 16S subunit ribosomal RNA is a unique prokaryotic sequence, so host DNA contamination is not a problem. Because of the nature of the exponential amplification of the sequence in the PCR technique, 16S may be preferable when working with lower amounts of genetic material.

Methods of Describing the Microbiome

Because the gut microbiome is essentially a highly complex ecosystem, working with the output data provides many challenges when converting vast quantities of high-dimensional data into understandable metrics. As a result, bioinformaticians draw upon techniques and methods described previously by ecologists and statisticians who have dealt with these challenges for decades. Such methods include multi-dimensional scaling and describing the abundance and diversity of an ecosystem, albeit modified to suit data from microbiome samples. These methods are readily adapted to our needs as long as we maintain the understanding that both 16S and WGS techniques produce compositional data, which only contains information about ratios between parts (microbial species) of a whole (the complete sample), but does not contain information about absolute counting numbers (18). Further, the properties of compositional data are different from classical datasets, and thus statistical tools such as Pearson's correlation coefficient cannot be employed here. For example, the initial comparison examined in most studies is comparative relative abundance. However, we are never dealing with absolute counts of organisms, but rather the relative abundance of one genus/species to another. Therefore, we cannot ignore the fact that relative abundance may change substantially where absolute numbers may not.

The next metric usually examined is microbiome diversity, where the degree of heterogeneity within a sample or between two samples is measured. Using a variety of different statistical formulae, diversity metrics are reported as α-, β- and γ-diversity (19, 20). α-diversity is used to describe the differences found within a sample, whereas β-diversity describes the dissimilarity between samples measured. γ-diversity is then used to explain the total species diversity across all samples in an experiment but is not as useful as α and β descriptors for microbiome research. The different formulae employed use different weighting of factors such as species distribution. However, it should not be taken as a principle that a higher α-diversity necessarily means it is better, as many examples in the literature have indicated that an elevated α-diversity is associated with abnormal or unhealthy states relative to healthy controls. α-diversity is also at the mercy of PCR bias, and measures are sensitive to the number of rare taxa that are present in a given sample and thus sequencing depth. For example, after an antibiotic treatment, α-diversity may appear higher, which could be due to the emergence of more rare taxa appearing that otherwise would have been filtered out of the original data management pipeline.

It is important to appreciate the assumptions and limitations inherent in trying to describe the differences between two different complex ecosystems and attempting to distil that into a single number. The most commonly used methods of measuring these differences in modern microbiome bioinformatic pipelines include Jaccard's index (describing the proportion of unique taxa shared between two samples without taking abundance into account); Euclidean distance (measuring the geometric distance by applying the Pythagorean theorem, where every microbe is a separate dimension); Bray–Curtis dissimilarity (a combination of Jaccard's index and Euclidean distance); UniFrac (unweighted/weighted, making use of phylogenetic information to measure differences between samples); and PhILR (using a log-ratio transformation called the isometric log-ratio (ILR) transformation; uses a phylogenetic tree to recast the microbiome variables as a series of log-contrasts/balances). It must be noted, however, that β-diversity should not be calculated on centred log-ratio (CLR) or similar transformed data because features are inherently negatively correlated. One possible method suggests that after the CLR transformation, the values of features can take on any value (unlike count data); therefore, classical statistical approaches should be applied only after transformation.

Another important metric that needs to be considered is volatility: the degree of change in the microbiome over time that is inversely related to stability. It essentially encompasses a change in a sample's α- or β-diversity over time. As a rule, it is considered that a higher level of volatility is associated with negative health outcomes, and vice versa (16). A common measurement is comparing β-diversity between two or more points in time from the same sample donor, and it has been recently demonstrated that microbiome composition partially explains microbiome volatility.

Once we have the statistical data to hand, it is necessary next to visualise metrics such as relative abundance. This is performed by applying a multi-dimensional scaling (MDS) algorithm or a principal component analysis (PCA). The PCA plots distances between every combination of two points in a set as coordinates in a two- or three-dimensional plot. These are then used as input determinants to plot each sample in an experiment to visualise the dissimilarity of individual samples: the closer two samples are, the more similar they are. To understand why we need this level of resolution and detail in our studies of the gut microbiome, we now turn our attention to the potential impact this collection of microbes has on human physiology.

The Microbiome–Gut–Brain Axis

The microbiome–gut–brain axis is a relatively recent concept that describes the mechanisms involved in the bidirectional communication pathways between the gut microbiome and the brain. Much research is currently focussed on illuminating these communication pathways, which include direct and indirect signalling mechanisms through immune system modulation, tryptophan metabolism, vagus nerve activity, the enteric nervous system and bioactive microbial by-products, or metabolites, produced by the gut microbiome. Indeed, the gut microbiota offer the potential of a rich reservoir of novel metabolites and bioactive substances that can have pleiotropic functionalities for the host (21).

Earlier gut-to-brain (bottom-up) communication work focussed on digestive function and satiety; more recently, attention has turned towards higher-order cognitive and psychological effects in both bottom-up and brain-to-gut (top-down) mechanisms. This research has highlighted the pathophysiological consequences of a dysfunctional reciprocal gut–brain network, exacerbated by gut inflammation disorders, altered responses to both chronic and acute stressors and altered behavioural states. Pre-clinical studies involving lower animals such as worms, fish and rodents have been instrumental in such research, where germ-free (completely devoid of any microbial colonisation) and antibiotic-treated mice (strongly ablated gut microbiota) have helped parse the role of microbiome–gut–brain signalling across the lifespan. Although translationally limited, such pre-clinical models provide unique insight into how the gut microbiota can shape the behaviour, physiology and neurobiology of its host (22).

Germ-Free

The first report of germ-free animals dates back to an aseptic C-section performed in 1897 where the animals were kept germ-free for up to two weeks (23). This technique did not become a regular model used in research until the mid-1940s, when successive generations of germ-free rodents were routinely produced. Similar methods are used today to produce a variety of genetically distinct germ-free rodents. While the initial colony is delivered via C-section, subsequent generations can be delivered *per vaginum* germ-free. More recently, a new method to produce germ-free animals involves embryonic transfer at the two-cell stage into a germ-free host mother (24).

These germ-free animals have extraordinarily different physiology and neurodevelopment than conventionally colonised animals. Lacking a gut microbiome across early life development results in reduced body weight, impaired intestinal function, lower concentrations of most gastrointestinal luminal amino acids and, intriguingly, longer lifespans than their conventional counterparts. Germ-free mice tend to have an impaired immune system, altered metabolism, dysregulated hormone signalling and differences in neurotransmission, although the germ-free phenotype varies across species (mouse vs. rat), sex, research group and strain, thus demonstrating that host genetics and the gut microbiome are important influencers of the phenotype. While these animals have limited translatability to human situations, they have nonetheless been an integral starting point in examining whether the gut microbiome is involved in a given process or not. A strong advantage of the germ-free model is the ability to mono-colonise the germ-free mouse with individual strains of bacteria (generation of gnotobiotic mice) or cocktails of known consortia, including performance of a faecal microbial transplantation (FMT) from another mouse or human donor.

Antibiotics

Researchers have also used antibiotics as a means to temporally and specifically ablate a conventional animal's gut microbiota to study the impact of microbiota perturbations on brain and behaviour. Antibiotics can be given acutely (days) or chronically (weeks) at any stage across an animal's lifespan across varying dosages, providing greater control over the extent of microbial depletion. Singular antibiotics with known specific effects can be used or cocktails designed to substantially ablate the entire microbiota. More recently, non-absorbable antibiotics (e.g. vancomycin, neomycin and bacitracin) have been the method of choice to ensure targeted effects on gut microbiota with minimal direct effect on the host. They avoid potential central and systemic effects while allowing direct assessment of the effect of a perturbation of the gut microbiota on the brain. The field is moving away from using the likes of metronidazole and minocycline as they can enter systemic circulation and potentially have a direct effect on the brain and behaviour. Moreover, antibiotics allow us to more closely model the clinical scenario in humans. Such translational relevance and experimental flexibility allow antibiotics to be a hugely valuable tool in the study of the microbiome–gut–brain axis and form a key component of studies in the field.

Faecal Microbial Transplantation

Another technique commonly used is FMT. Here, intestinal microbiota from one individual (human or rodent) is transferred into a donor mouse (germ-free or antibiotic-treated) or from human to human. Successful engraftment of the donor consortia is achieved via administration of specially prepared faecal material via oral gavage in rodents or colonoscopy in humans. This establishes a donor-like microbiome in the gastrointestinal tract of the recipient. Such a technique allows for stronger inferences to be made regarding the causal relationships between gut microbiome and host outcomes.

While FMT is a frequently used pre-clinical technique, it is not a new procedure. Currently, FMT is being trialled as a viable treatment option in inflammatory bowel disorder (IBD), irritable bowel syndrome (IBS) and chronic constipation. However, clinical trials are limited because of potential safety concerns (25). Pre-clinically, FMT is an effective method for 'humanisation' of the rodent microbiota in a laboratory setting, thus enhancing translatability.

FMT has revealed the transferral of behavioural phenotypes from rodent or human to rodent, including anxiety-like and depressive symptomatology, which highlights the role the gut microbiome plays in regulating anxiety and depression. Germ-free mice are known to have a reduced body weight; when humanised with an inoculum from obese individuals, these mice gained a significant amount of body weight compared to control animals given an FMT from lean individuals, indicating the importance of the donor characteristics and nutrition. FMT is usually performed in germ-free mice or conventional animals that have been pre-treated with antibiotics, increasing the likelihood of a successful engraftment but with the proviso of markedly altered physiology.

Pathways of Communication

There are many pathways that connect the gut microbiome to the brain, and vice versa, both directly and indirectly. While we have learned a lot about these mechanisms to date, we still do not fully understand the underlying mechanisms involved in bidirectional signalling between the gut microbiome and the brain. However, it is clear that there is perpetual communication between both in the regulation of host homeostasis and health. The main systems involved include endocrine, nervous, immune and small-molecule signalling.

Neural Pathways of Communication

The central nervous system (CNS) and peripheral nervous system (PNS) are both involved in relaying direct and indirect information between the gut and the brain (Figure 2.1). Specifically, the autonomic nervous system (ANS) acts as a neural relay network managing corporeal functions that require no conscious effort, such as breathing, heartbeat and digestion. The ANS itself comprises sympathetic and parasympathetic branches that, when combined with the enteric nervous system (ENS) under central control, are responsible for regulating host homeostasis and together comprise a vast, complex neural network throughout the body connecting the brain with the gastrointestinal tract. In particular, the ANS oversees important gut functions including gut motility and permeability, epithelial fluid maintenance, secretion of bile, luminal osmolarity, carbohydrate-level maintenance, mechanical manipulation of the mucosa, and bicarbonate and mucus production, as well as the intestinal-fluid handling and mucosal immune response (26).

From a bottom-up perspective, incoming visceral information from the gut to the brain travels along the ANS to the central networks, where positive and negative feedback loops are activated, providing the gut with immediate and direct top-down responses to manage homeostasis, as well as reactions to visceral pain and stress (27). Both sympathetic and

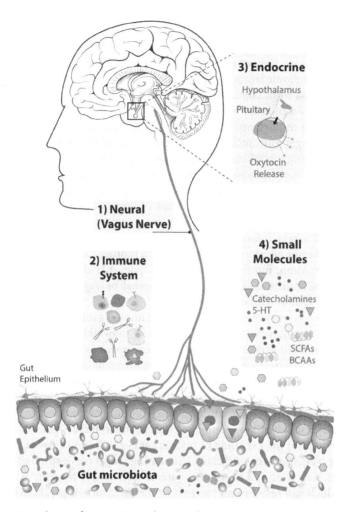

Figure 2.1 The main pathways of communication between the gut microbiome and the brain.

parasympathetic innervation can influence ENS activity controlling motility and the rate of delivery of nutrition from the diet along the gastrointestinal tract. Such activity can also be triggered by interoceptive afferent feedback from the gut, instigating bottom-up responses.

The gastrointestinal tract is innervated by sympathetic neurons including postganglionic vasoconstrictor cells and secretion and motility suppression neurons. These neurons are amenable to modulation which results in altered transit, motility and secretion, mostly through cholinergic activation mechanisms and smooth muscle sphincter contraction. The sympathetic nervous system in the gut is also believed to control the intestinal mucous layer, which is a critical structure involved in the local immune response and microbial composition maintenance.

There are two main neuroanatomical pathways of neural signalling from the gut to the brain. One is pain sensation carried by the splanchnic nerve, and the non-painful signalling mechanisms, conveyed by the vagus nerve. The vagus nerve is the 10th cranial nerve and extensively innervates visceral tissues, rapidly relaying signals from brain and gut, and vice versa. It is composed of 80% afferent and 20% efferent fibres which transmit vital information from the gut, respiratory and cardiovascular systems and provide central feedback to the viscera. In particular, the gut is home to the hepatic and celiac branches of the vagus nerve, where intraganglionic laminar endings and intramuscular arrays and terminal axonal endings in the mucosa form connections with the muscle wall, enteroendocrine cells and neuropods. Vagus afferents are polymodal in that they perform many different tasks including responding to hormonal, chemical and mechanical signals. This system is also home to the vago-vagal anti-inflammatory reflex loop, which can modulate circulating levels of proinflammatory cytokines and macrophage activation.

Pain, discomfort, inflammation and injury sensory information is carried by spinal mechanisms, specifically spinoreticular, spinomesencephalic, spinohypothalamic and spinothalamic tracts to the brain. Under conditions of homeostasis, nociceptive signalling is under gated control, where associated neurons are quiescent until a stimulation threshold has been surpassed, where information is then conveyed. Vagal and spinal signal conduction mechanisms do not necessarily operate under a mutually exclusive tone; physiological events such as distension, motility, inflammation, pain, pH change, cellular damage and temperature can be transmitted through either spinal or vagal neurons via the nucleus tractus solitarius (NTS) of the brainstem.

Sensory vagal neurons synapse on nuclei in the nodose ganglia and brainstem, whereas fibres from the gut mostly synapse on the NTS where information signals to the hypothalamus, nucleus accumbens and ventral tegmental area, as well as other brainstem nuclei. The NTS also has the capacity to influence noradrenaline and serotonin neurotransmitter signalling mechanisms. This is highly relevant for identification of neural pathways involved in gut modulation of behavioural responses, as the NTS has been shown to orchestrate the integration of interoceptive feedback information transmitted via the vagus nerve from gut to brain and vice versa, essentially acting as a hub for microbiome–gut–brain signalling.

A useful mechanism for the study of microbiome–gut–brain signalling mechanisms is either removing (vagotomy) or artificially stimulating (vagal nerve stimulation (VNS)) the vagus nerve (28). Vagotomy is a technique that has been used in humans as a treatment for peptic ulcers, which can result in an increase in the incidence of psychiatric disorders. In rodents, vagotomy has been shown to alter motility and anxiety-like and fear-related behaviour, as well as stress responsiveness. At a cellular level, vagotomy has been reported to reduce hippocampal neurogenesis, a brain structure critical for learning and memory. Conversely, VNS has been used as a viable treatment method for refractory depression and chronic pain in humans, indicating its involvement in mood regulation. In rodents, VNS increases hippocampal neurogenesis and regulates neurotransmitter (norepinephrine, 5-HT and dopamine) release in brain regions associated with depression and anxiety, thus indicating the potential for gut microbes to use the vagus signalling mechanisms to alter host emotional and behavioural responses.

At this critical interface between host and gut luminal contents, the gastrointestinal neuronal network of the ENS is intricately integrated into microbiome–gut–brain axis signalling pathways. There are two main ENS structures largely responsible for coordinating motility and the movement of fluid along the tract: the submucosal and myenteric plexus. Intestinofugal neurons signal sensory information to sympathetic ganglia that continue along spinal and vagal afferent routes, providing an opportunity for gut luminal contents to influence gut function and signal to the CNS. However, it is still unclear if microbial factors can directly signal to the ENS in a healthy host. Interestingly, germ-free mice have significant ENS ultrastructure and neurochemistry abnormalities and deficits in intrinsic sensory signalling, which was reversed upon recolonisation. Here, recolonisation increased enteric neural serotonin and serotonin receptor expression, ultimately restoring normal gut physiology, implying a role for the gut microbiota in serotonin signalling to the ENS, as well as neurogenesis, neural cell differentiation and cell turnover.

The use of antibiotic treatment in rodents to study the involvement of the gut microbiota in ENS signalling resulted in wide-ranging effects, including changes in neuronal and glial architecture, neurochemistry and fundamental ENS function. In an autism mouse model, similar ultrastructural and neurochemical changes in the ENS, combined with changes in the faecal bile acid profile to those in antibiotic-treated animals, were noted. Further, recolonisation of germ-free mice with individual bacterial strains or supplementation of conventional animals with microbial metabolites has been demonstrated to influence ENS function (29). Indeed, different microbial strains appear to have differential effects on neuronally driven secretomotor responses.

Immune System Signalling

The densest concentration of immune cells in the human body exists along the gastrointestinal tract, at the interface of microbes and host, which can communicate via direct physical contact or through the release of secreted compounds. This single-cell layer of gut tissue is tasked with limiting contact of the visceral tissue with the gut luminal microbiome and contents; it achieves this by secreting a protective viscous mucus layer from epithelial goblet cells. The vast majority of host–microbe interaction takes place at this mucosal-luminal interface where recognition of self and non-self-antigens help to prime the immune system to identify potential pathogens. Here enterocytes, secretory cells, chemosensory cells and gut-associated lymphoid tissue (GALT) interact with lymphocytes and release mucous from goblet cells, antimicrobials from Paneth cells, and cytokines and neuroendocrine compounds (e.g. ghrelin, somatostatin, cholecystokinin, peptide YY and serotonin) from enteroendocrine cells.

Host immune cells have evolved to identify bacteria by polysaccharides, peptidoglycans and other antigens expressed both intracellularly and on their outer membrane. Pattern recognition receptors expressed on gut epithelial cells recognise the unique bacterial molecular patterns expressed that help identify commensal from pathogen. Moreover, bacterial metabolites (bacteriocins, bile acids, neuromodulators and short-chain fatty acids (SCFAs)) can act as immunomodulatory compounds, having anti-inflammatory effects via astrocytes, and are involved in the modulation of microglial function. Activation in the gut can lead to a release of chemokines, cytokines, neuropeptides, neurotransmitters and endocrine messengers, which can infiltrate the blood and lymphatic systems. It has been shown that the gut microbiome can influence the local release of innate immune cells (e.g. basophils, monocytes, macrophages, eosinophils, neutrophils, mast cells, platelets and natural killer cells); however, the interaction between gut microbes and resident innate immune cells in the brain has not been investigated until recently (30).

Much current work is focussed on examining microglia–microbiota interactions as potentially key mechanisms underlying microbiota–immune–brain interactions. Brain-bound microglia make up about 5–12% of all cells in the brain and are immune sentinels solely responsible for mounting an immune response in the brain against potentially pathogenic intruders. Even though they reside at a distance from the gut, microglia maturation, activation and differentiation are amenable to signals from microbes in the gut, as established from research using germ-free and antibiotic-treated rodents. Surprisingly, these alterations were reversed after cessation of antibiotic treatment or recolonisation of the germ-free gut. Therefore, a healthy and diverse gut microbiome is required for proper brain immune function. Microglia have also been shown to recruit monocytes from the periphery to the brain to help with the neuroimmune response and clear debris, a process that was modulated by supplementation with probiotics. Thus, gut microbes have the capacity to indirectly modulate centrally mediated events through regulation of monocyte trafficking to the brain, including subsequent microglia activation.

Not only is the innate immune response influenced by gut-microbial signalling but adaptive immune programming can also be shaped by host exposure to microbes. In a pre-clinical model, B and T lymphocytes were modulated after supplementation with a synbiotic containing *L. reuteri* and a tryptophan-rich diet. Indeed, gut-derived immunoglobulins (e.g. IgA) were discovered in the CNS after exposure to experimental autoimmune encephalomyelitis, a pre-clinical model for multiple sclerosis; these cells were found to suppress inflammation through interleukin-10 (IL-10). IL-10+T-regulatory and T-helper cells also appeared to be regulated by levels of abundance of *Clostridium*, emphasising that gut microbes may be working synergistically with the adaptive immune system and the CNS. Further, specific bacterial antigens were demonstrated to respond to dietary components, suggesting that diet and nutrition could be a viable therapeutic avenue in need of exploration.

Enteroendocrine Signalling Mechanisms

Enteroendocrine cells (EECs) are important sensory cells resident in the gut epithelium involved in the maintenance of gut homeostasis, where they coordinate alterations in the gut-nutrient luminal content with metabolic and behavioural responses (e.g. regulation of insulin secretion; food intake). Enteroendocrine L cells and enterochromaffin cells are the two most-studied EECs and are most abundant in the distal small and large intestines, alongside the greatest concentration of bacteria in the gut. They span the gut epithelium from the apical to the luminal side where they interact with luminal contents including microbial metabolites. EECs have a long lifespan, allowing them to integrate with the local ENS and immune system responses.

Enteroendocrine L cells secrete two very important and potent anorexigenic hormones, glucagon-like peptide-1 (GLP-1) and peptide YY (PYY), in the postprandial state, controlling host eating habits. Receptors for these hormones exist both locally on gut enteric neurons and in the CNS. In particular, the neuropod, a basolateral cytoplasmic process of EEC L cells, has been shown to synapse to local ENS glia cells and vagus nerve afferents, indicating that they could signal directly from gut to brain. L cells can respond to gut-derived carbohydrates via sodium-coupled glucose transporter (SLC5A1), long-chain fatty acids via free fatty acid receptors (FFAR1 and FFAR4) and monoacylglycerols via G-protein-coupled receptors (GPR119). Colonic EEC L cells tend to be exclusively activated by bacterial-derived metabolites such as SCFAs, which in turn can stimulate the secretion of GLP-1 and PYY through the FFARs (31).

Bacterial fermentation of non-digestible food ingested by the host continues at a slow pace between meals, supporting colonic L-cell activity and the secretion of anorexigenic hormones for hours afterwards. This results in a basal secretion of GLP-1 and PYY, which plays an important role in the control of food intake by the host, indicating important implications for metabolic disorders and obesity. Thus, this suggests an avenue for controlling appetite through careful formulation and delivery of fermentable foodstuffs through the diet (e.g. prebiotics, probiotics) to decrease food intake and body weight and improve overall glucose tolerance. Already, prebiotics such as the polysaccharide inulin, as well as fructooligosaccharides (FOS) and galactooligosaccharides (GOS), have been shown to increase GLP-1 and PYY production. Similarly, specific *Lactobacillus* strains can stimulate GLP-1 production. Altogether, these findings demonstrate the importance of bacterial metabolites and adequate diet in the maintenance of metabolic health, and that gut microbes can regulate the secretion of GLP-1 and PYY.

The majority (>95%) of serotonin in a human is produced by enterochromaffin cells (ECs) in the gut through metabolism of dietary tryptophan. However, gut-derived serotonin cannot cross the blood–brain barrier (BBB) and therefore is unlikely to have a direct effect on the brain. Nonetheless, gut-derived serotonin likely impacts gut–brain signalling by modulating local vagal and immune pathway activity. In the gut, serotonin activates intrinsic and extrinsic afferent nerve fibres to mediate gastrointestinal functions such as electrolyte secretion, intestinal peristalsis, pain perception and inflammatory responses. However, we know very little about the interaction between ECs and the gut microbiome. Using the germ-free model, recent work has indicated that certain strains of bacteria can upregulate expression of the rate-limiting enzyme in the production of serotonin (tryptophan hydroxylase 1 (TPH1)), modulating gut-based serotonin biosynthesis and increasing intestinal transit.

The hypothalamic–pituitary–adrenal (HPA) axis is one of the main neuroendocrine systems and a key non-neuronal signalling mechanism of gut–brain communication. It is principally known for its role in the stress response in priming the fight-or-flight response. Germ-free animals exhibit a hyper-responsive HPA axis, characterised by increased plasma levels of corticosterone, indicating a role for the gut microbiome in HPA axis modulation. Interestingly, IBS patients have exaggerated adrenocorticotrophic hormone (ACTH) and cortisol responses to corticotrophin-releasing factor (CRF) infusion, resulting in altered HPA axis activation. Interestingly, VNS can increase the levels of ACTH and corticosterone, as well as the expression of CRF mRNA in animals, highlighting an interplay between the vagus nerve and HPA axis activity. Therefore, more research is needed to understand this relationship.

Small-Molecule Signalling Mechanisms

It has long been understood that microbes in the gut use neuromodulatory metabolites to communicate with each other, similar to those used by the host nervous system. These molecules include neurotransmitters such as tryptophan precursors and metabolites, serotonin (5-hydroxytryptamine (5-HT)), γ-aminobutyric acid (GABA) and catecholamines (noradrenaline, norepinephrine and dopamine), all of which can influence host mood, behaviour and cognition (32, 33). Therefore, it is of utmost interest to the field to ascertain at what level these microbially derived bioactive neurotransmitters interact with the host nervous system. For example, the microbially derived metabolite 4-ethylphenylsulfate is sufficient to induce anxiety-like behaviour in mice and can also modulate motor activity in fruit fly (*drosophila*). It is important to note, however, that many of the host–microbe metabolite interactions that occur at the luminal interface could also affect indirect action in the brain.

Many other microbial metabolites are beginning to come under the microscope for their dual role in the microbe and host. For example, catecholamines, which are involved in the stress-induced fight-or-flight response in the host, promote pathogenesis and growth in bacteria. It has been shown that host production of norepinephrine can induce bacterial virulence gene expression, driving infection and mortality in the host. While the ENS can synthesise dopamine and norepinephrine, it cannot make the enzyme that converts norepinephrine into epinephrine (phenylethanolamine N-methyltransferase); however, the bacterial enzyme β-glucuronidase has been shown to play a critical role in converting host norepinephrine and dopamine, further emphasising the synergistic nature of humans and their microbial passengers. Indeed, many gut-based bacterial strains can produce catecholamines (e.g. *Escherichia* = norepinephrine; *Bacillus* = norepinephrine and dopamine), which are identical in structure to those produced by the host. Moreover, both host- and gut-derived bacterial strains have the capacity to convert glutamate into GABA, the major inhibitory neurotransmitter of the host nervous system. For example, *Lactobacillus spp.* and *Escherichia spp.* have been shown to synthesise GABA, as well as glutamic acid, although its importance is unclear. Further, five different bacterial strains isolated from the human gut were discovered to be capable of converting monosodium glutamate into GABA. Recent work has even proposed that the faecal microbiome has the ability to encode the enzyme that converts glutamic acid into GABA (glutamate decarboxylase).

Other gut-bound neurotransmitters important for host–microbe communication include histamine, tryptophan and kynurenine. Histamine is an important neurotransmitter that plays a role in host physiology, including modulating wakefulness; thus, bacterial production of histamine has been scrutinised as microbial-derived histamine may interact with the host nervous system. For example, the commensals *Escherichia coli* and *Morganella morganii* have been shown to produce histamine, and many colonic bacteria express the histidine decarboxylase gene, conferring the capacity to synthesise histamine within the host gut.

Clostridium perfringens has been demonstrated to modulate gut production of serotonin via host-derived TPH1. Microbial metabolite SCFAs can also modulate host TPH1, indicating that there may be a microbial feedback loop regulating host gastrointestinal motility through modulation of the host gut serotonergic system. Conversely, host serotonin has been shown to modulate bacterial motility and can induce the expression of bacterial virulence genes via a quorum-sensing mechanism. Not all tryptophan ends up being converted into serotonin; 90% of available tryptophan is actually funnelled into the kynurenine pathway. Kynurenine, and the metabolites kynurenic acid and quinolinic acid, have been implicated in mental health. Bacterial indole production from the metabolism of L-tryptophan can also affect host physiology by altering host barrier integrity and modulating intestinal inflammation. As such, further studies are required to reveal the functional dynamics and importance of such neuroactive molecules as mediators of host–microbe crosstalk. Considering many of these molecules are involved in several human behavioural and physical illnesses, it is important to understand how the microbiota influence neurotransmitter production and metabolism along the microbiome–gut–brain axis.

Other than neurotransmitters, branched-chain amino acids (BCAAs: valine, leucine and isoleucine), along with SCFAs, are involved directly and indirectly in many biochemical functions in the PNS and CNS and are in high concentrations in the gut. BCAAs are essential amino acids in that the host needs to ingest them in their diet because of the inability to synthesise them *de novo*. BCAAs and SCFAs are coming under increased scrutiny as potential bioactive molecules for nutritional supplementation to promote host health. Gut-derived BCAAs have been shown to be involved in protein synthesis, energy production, insulin secretion, amino acid uptake and luminal immunity, in both humans and animals. BCAAs are also a key nitrogen donor for the host. BCAAs are readily transported across the BBB and could therefore be a method of indirect signalling from the gut to the brain and warrant further examination. SCFAs are involved in many host physiological processes, including gastrointestinal function, blood-pressure regulation, circadian rhythm control and neuroimmune function, although less is known about their role in brain physiology and behaviour. All SCFAs act as histone deacetylase (HDAC) inhibitors, with butyrate being the most potent inhibitor of class I and IIa HDACs, therefore indicating microbial potential for host epigenetic modulation. SCFAs can also potently activate FFARs, indicating a potential route for microbial modulation of vagus nerve activation and enteroendocrine activity. It is possible that SCFAs cross and interact with the BBB, having been reported in the cerebrospinal fluid at active concentrations and modulating tight-junction proteins.

While all these pathways and mechanisms have been studied mostly in adults, it is becoming increasingly clear that more attention needs to be directed towards other stages of life, specifically early life and ageing. Next, we will examine the current knowledge of the differences between the functions of the adult microbiome–gut–brain axis to the extremes of life.

Microbiome–Gut–Brain Axis: Across the Lifespan

Although still somewhat contested, it is generally accepted that initial colonisation begins at birth, where the delivery process exposes the infant to a unique microbial signature obtained from the mother, either by C-section or *per vaginum*. The consortia of gut microbiota are not a static ecosystem throughout the lifespan of the host; in fact, the gastrointestinal microbial composition is in a constant state of flux, with small day-to-day changes growing into larger cycles when viewing the population as a whole. For the most part, the adult gut microbiome is more stable than at both extremes of the lifespan, where both abundance and diversity are characteristically different. As a result, both early life and ageing are seen as sensitive periods for the consortia of microbes resident in the gut, where they are much more amenable to external influences and therefore influential for important host functions such as language and cognition. The fact that sensitive periods in colony development or decline coincide with sensitive developmental periods for the host suggests gut microbes are very important in healthy ageing.

Early Life

While the topic of *in utero* colonisation is still debated (34), even if it does occur, it appears that it has limited impact on early postnatal microbial composition development when compared to the contribution of the natural birthing process. Here, germ-free mice have made an invaluable contribution towards deciphering the role of the microbiome–gut–brain axis during initial development. Germ-free mouse embryos exhibit increased BBB permeability, which was restored after recolonisation, indicating an influential role for the gut microbiome in ensuring normal development of the BBB. While there is no definitive make-up of a healthy microbiome in early life, soon after birth important early colonising species lay the groundwork for a stable long-term composition. Bacteria that play an important part here include high levels of *Enterobacteriaceae*, *Bifidobacteriaceae* and

Clostridiaceae and low levels of *Lachnospiraceae* and *Ruminococcaceae* at the family level. Throughout maturity, strict anaerobes begin to dominate, alongside an increase in overall diversity (likely due to an increase in nutritional diversity). An adult-like consortia begins to embed between the ages of 1 and 3, which coincides with a change in diet and a shift to solid foods. This changeover is observed in mice too, as this age in humans coincides with weaning in rodents, alongside a shift from mothers' milk to solid foods (35). Nonetheless, microbial composition and function remains different from a true adult-like consortia as measured in 7–12-year-olds. However, the growing gut microbiome is highly susceptible to a large variety of external influences, including birth method (natural vs. C-section), birth location (hospital vs. home) and infant nutrition (breastfeeding vs. infant formula).

Maternal health parameters can also play an influential part, including gestational diet and weight gain, presence of a pet in the home, general state of health, medication and/or antibiotic usage, and levels of maternal stress. Some of these early life factors can have enduring effects on the physical and mental health of the host, altering trajectories of mental and physical health and/or cognitive performance (36). Promisingly, early data from clinical trials of probiotic interventions for children at risk of developing gastrointestinal problems later in life has resulted in outcomes highlighting a reduction in risk. Studies are also examining the efficacy of probiotic interventions in ameliorating the risk of developing autism spectrum disorder (ASD) and attention-deficit/hyperactivity disorder (ADHD). Several groups have shown that early probiotic intervention can mitigate the deleterious effects of antibiotic-treated and C-section-delivered infants, maternal high-fat diet and immune activation, and early life stress (37, 38).

Adolescence into Adulthood

Leading on from early life and childhood, adolescence is a period when the brain experiences widespread reshaping that includes synaptic pruning, alterations in myelination levels, changes in area volumes and functional connectivity (39). Concomitantly, the body undergoes rapid physical development as the host traverses a diverse range of social networking challenges, circadian rhythm disruptions and potential initial exposure to alcohol and drugs, all of which have been linked to alterations in the microbiome–gut–brain axis in adults (40, 41). Few studies have compared the adolescent gut microbiome to that of the adult, but some work has indicated that the profile of older adolescents resembles that of an adult population; noted differences include higher relative abundances of *Bifidobacterium* and *Clostridium* in adolescents but lower relative levels of *Prevotella* and *Sutterella*. This follows on from similar studies in childhood indicating that these genera may play a formative role in gut-microbiome maturation from childhood through to adulthood, although more work is needed. However, this highlights the paucity of research surrounding age specificity.

In rodents, work performed at a comparable age illustrated that any sex differences in gut-microbiome amelioration only emerge after puberty onset, indicating a role for the endocrine system. Stress-induced changes in the timing of puberty onset can also be modulated by probiotic treatment. Further, antibiotic ablation of the gut microbiota in adolescent mice impacted anxiety, cognition and social behaviour in adult mice. In this study, researchers reported that multiple metrics were affected, including brain-derived neurotrophic factor (BDNF) expression, oxytocin and vasopressin levels, and tryptophan metabolism.

Ageing

While throughout adulthood the human gut microbiome is relatively stable when unperturbed, the beginning of the ageing process is marked by a loss in stability (42). Two major determinants of gut-microbiota stability, diet and exercise, usually also mark the beginning of the steady decline at the end of life. As this is heavily dependent on the individual, the timing of this transition into an elder type is not as acutely demarcated as that from childhood into adulthood. The relationship between ageing and the gut micro-biome is thought to be bilateral, where the gut microbiome can also contribute to healthy ageing. Ageing-associated gut-microbiota changes result in increased gut permeability, modifications in the production of gut-microbiota-derived metabolites and alterations in the host immune system. The process of ageing has been classified as a sensitive period for the gut microbiome where it is susceptible to environmental triggers and intrinsic factors in the host. While much of the current work has reported on large differences between individuals within-study, the consortia differences between studies have proven to be far greater, likely due to the cultural, geographical or inherent methodological variances (37). Nonetheless, a common theme across studies indicates that reduced microbial diver-sity correlates with adverse outcomes in adults through to old age and frailty. Some specific microbial alterations noted include a reduction in the prime beneficial commensals *Lactobacillus* and *Bifidobacterium* and a reduced *Firmicutes* to *Bacteroidetes* ratio (a metric that is a correlational and observational output of microbiome analysis given that *Firmicutes* and *Bacteroidetes* represent over 99% of the known bacterial species in the gut) in some ageing populations. Conversely, a higher abundance of *Akkermansia* has been associated with long life, a metric of healthy ageing. Indeed, a mantra developing from the results of such studies states that the more diverse the diet, the more diverse the microbiota, as microbiota diversity has been linked to improved health and reduced frailty in ageing. Other taxa linked with healthy ageing include *Bacteroidetes*, *Clostridium* cluster XIVa and the butyrate-producing bacterium *Faecalibacterium prausnitzii* that also has anti-inflammatory properties. Similarly, *Porphyromonadaceae* was linked to cognitive decline and the emergence of affective disorders.

Pre-clinical studies using various models targeting the gut microbiome have demonstrated a role for the gut microbiome in regulating neuroimmunity from middle to old age in mice. This work has helped characterise the process of 'inflammageing', which describes an increased proinflammatory state coupled with reductive adaptive immunity throughout the ageing process. This is an almost self-perpetuating phenomenon where general ageing and stress weaken the integrity of the barriers (BBB and gut barrier) increasing permeability, further feeding the inflammageing cycle. A key player in the brain's neuroinflammatory response, microglia (the brain's resident immune cells), play an active role in shaping neural circuitry, synaptic plasticity and cellular processes such as phagocyt-osis, supporting the growth of neuronal progenitor cells and longevity of neurons. As the ageing process begins, microglia become highly reactive and unbalanced, a state that promotes cellular dysfunction, resulting in cognitive and behavioural deficits. Intriguingly, these processes were reversed and promoted healthy ageing when aged mice were fed the probiotic *Bifidobacterium* for 14 weeks. Indeed, *Bifidobacterium* species correlate negatively with pro- and anti-inflammatory cytokine levels in humans, highlight-ing the potential of *Bifidobacteria* to reduce the inflammatory response associated with unhealthy ageing. Further, transplantation from young donors to aged recipients via FMT reversed any observed ageing-associated differences in peripheral and brain immunity and altered the hippocampal metabolome and transcriptome in the ageing mice. This transfer of a healthy ageing phenotype from the young to aged mice also attenuated age-associated impairments in cognitive behaviour.

From a nutritional standpoint, dietary restriction has proven to be the most effective strategy supporting healthy ageing and increased lifespan; this phenomenon has been recorded across many species. Any type of caloric restriction in rodent models has resulted in a longer overall lifespan, coinciding with structural changes in the gut microbiome, including *Lactobacillus* strongly correlating with longer life, accompanied by changes in SCFA levels in the gut. Next, we will delve deeper into potential microbiome–gut–brain axis modulating dietary interventions for promoting health.

Gut-Microbiome-Targeted Dietary Interventions

There are many avenues through which the gut microbiome can communicate with the brain that are amenable to nutritional/dietary modulation. Although much of this information has been collected via pre-clinical methods, there is a strong impetus to use these interactions for clinical outcomes/therapies. These include administration of a candidate species (or cocktail) of live bacteria (probiotics), substrates that are selectively used by host microorganisms (prebiotics), a carefully calculated combination of both (synbiotics) or waste left over after digestion of prebiotics and probiotics (postbiotics), all of which individually confer beneficial health effects upon the host and specifically have beneficial effects on the brain and behaviour (psychobiotics). Commonly used psychobiotic therapies include administration of probiotic organisms such as *Bifidobacterium* and *Lactobacillus* strains, alone or combined.

Prebiotics

The official International Scientific Association for Probiotics and Prebiotics (ISAPP) definition of a prebiotic is 'a substrate that is selectively utilised by host microorganisms conferring a health benefit'. They mainly include dietary fibres such as inulin, FOS, GOS, resistant starches and other soluble dietary fibres, although it is important to point out that not all dietary fibres are prebiotic. Foods commonly found to be high in prebiotics include fruits and vegetables (e.g. asparagus, leek, banana), chicory, and grains (e.g. oats, wheat). The reduced prebiotic intake of the typical Westernised diet correlates with an increase in the incidence of inflammatory diseases, metabolic syndrome, obesity, anxiety and stress. While prebiotics do not necessarily alter the composition or activity of the resident gut microbiota in a selective or predictable manner, they have been shown to reduce anxiety- and depressive-like behaviours and stress responsiveness, facilitate changes in hippocampal synaptic efficacy, and increase hippocampal BDNF expression, general hypothalamic neuronal activity and overall cognition and learning.

Resistant starches are a common source of prebiotic for the gut microbiota. This form of undigested carbohydrate has been shown to induce differential alterations in gut-microbial composition in animals, such as increasing in the *Firmicutes* to *Bacteroidetes* ratio. Inulin is another very common prebiotic that is predominantly found in a variety of vegetables, fruit and wheat. Inulin has been shown to boost the growth of powerful commensals *Bifidobacterium spp.* and *Faecalibacterium prausnitzii* and increase the numbers of butyrate-producing bacteria (e.g. *Coprococcus* and *Faecalibacterium*). Inulin has been shown to reduce the symptoms of colitis in a sodium-induced colitis mouse model, probably through increasing *Lactobacillus* composition. In humans, exposure to a mixed prebiotic supplementation during pregnancy has been correlated with an increase in protection against food allergies linked to a reduction in histamine levels and intestinal permeability in the offspring, where increased gut permeability has been associated with poorer indices of health.

FOS and GOS are now well-established prebiotics that have been found to be present in high quantities in breast milk. A form of GOS (Bimuno-galactooligosaccharide (B-GOS®) (Bimuno™, Clasado Biosciences Ltd, Buckinghamshire, UK)) increased the abundance of the commensals *Bifidobacteria* and *Lactobacilli* when compared to unsupplemented infants. The same supplement increased *Bacteroides* and *Bifidobacterium spp.* in elderly individuals. Not only has GOS been shown to impact microbial populations directly but many immune metrics have also been reported altered in individuals on a GOS-supplemented diet, including a reduction in pre-clinical anxiety, but not major depressive disorder (MDD). The anti-inflammatory cytokines IL-10 and IL-8 were increased and proinflammatory cytokines reduced in the same elderly population on B-GOS supplementation, which also acted as an early anxiolytic-like phenotype in healthy individuals. In mice, B-GOS prevented proinflammatory cytokine release undergoing a stress procedure where lipopolysaccharide (LPS) treatment increased cortical interleukin-1β and serotonin 2A receptor levels.

FOS, on the other hand, are found in high levels in fruit, and numerous reports have shown them to strongly affect gut-microbial commensal strains. *Bifidobacterium* and *Faecalibacterium prausnitzii* were enhanced in a double-blind intervention study in obese women supplemented with FOS, with both strains correlating strongly with improved health outcomes. Commonly, FOS and GOS are used together to boost commensal levels as a prebiotic treatment. In a randomised, double-blind, crossover study, 2 weeks of supplementation of both FOS and GOS significantly increased *Bifidobacterium* levels, coupled with a reduction in butyrate-producing bacteria. Further, this prebiotic combination reduced anxiety-like behaviours and stress-induced corticosterone release in mice, while also altering caecal SCFAs, microbial metabolites believed to have beneficial health outcomes in certain contexts. Polyphenol consumption has also been described as having a strong prebiotic effect in healthy and clinical populations and reducing depressive symptoms, although more investigation into their potential is needed.

Probiotics and Psychobiotics

A variety of probiotic strains has already been shown to alter metrics of metabolism, immunity and endocrine function in both humans and rodents. It has even demonstrated the ability to alter neurogenesis, neuropeptide expression levels, neurotransmission, neuroinflammation and ultimately behaviour. Probiotic supplements are believed to interact with host gut microbiota and the intestinal epithelium directly, even slowing ageing in pre-clinical studies. In healthy populations, probiotic supplementation has resulted in reductions in stress, depression and anxiety, improved symptoms of depression (using *Lactobacillus helveticus* R0052 and *Bifidobacterium longum* R0175 (CEREBIOME)) and reduced anxiety using a multi-strain probiotic (*B. longum, B. bifidum, B. lactis* and *L. acidophilus*) in clinical populations. However, even though there are promising results, many more randomised controlled trials (RCTs) are desperately needed.

Pre-clinically, a single bacterial strain, *Faecalibacterium prausnitzii* (ATCC 27766), demonstrated potential to act as an anxiolytic and psychobiotic in rats, ameliorating a depressant-like phenotype, probably through modulating caecal SCFA, anti-inflammatory cytokine and corticosterone levels. Such treatments of individual strains, or cocktails of commensal bacteria, have demonstrated efficacy in improving behavioural symptoms in models of depression, anxiety and autism, leading to the concept of psychobiotics, with the intended use as treatment for neurological and psychiatric disorders through targeting the gut microbiota. Although probiotics were considered the original psychobiotic, approaches now commonly include prebiotics, postbiotics, synbiotics, FMT and dietary components.

In humans, a landmark study investigating ingestion of a fermented milk drink that combined four different probiotic strains showed altered functional brain activity in adult healthy women. Specifically, midbrain connectivity centred on the periaqueductal gray (PAG), along with the prefrontal cortex (PFC), precuneus, basal ganglia and parahippocampal gyrus, was altered relative to controls not consuming the drink. A more recent study linked members of the *Actinobacteria* phylum to cognitive test scores when comparing subjects with and without obesity; specifically, alterations in neural activity in the thalamus, hypothalamus and amygdala were seen, implicating the gut microbiota in cognitive performance in humans.

While there are sparse reports of studies using both pre- and probiotics in human trials, recent work has demonstrated improvements in depression, stress and anxiety in patients undergoing haemodialysis, in those with coronary artery disease and in professional athletes. Regardless of the need for more RCTs, candidate pre- and/or probiotics may have an impact on the host commensal microbiome overall, potentially altering consortia complexity and diversity.

Postbiotics and Microbial Metabolites

The gut microbiome represents a vast reservoir of metabolites (e.g. SCFAs) and postbiotics (inanimate microorganisms and/or their components) that could have beneficial health effects for the host (7, 43). The presence and activity of these bacterial metabolites can act on host tissue locally or distally from their site of production, impacting host behaviour and health. SCFAs are the most-studied gut-microbiota-derived metabolite and are a product of bacterial fermentation of complex polysaccharides ingested through diet that would otherwise be indigestible by the host. Ninety-five per cent of gut-derived SCFAs are in the form of acetate, propionate and butyrate, in increasing order of chemical complexity. Foods containing high levels of SCFAs include dairy products such as cheese and butter, while other foods with appreciable levels include inulin, cellulose, resistant starches, beans, lentils, peas and whole grains. Fermented foods such as sauerkraut, pickles and tempeh also contain a small amount of SCFAs. Intriguingly, germ-free animals and antibiotic-treated mice have been shown to have markedly lower SCFA levels.

There are now a plethora of studies purporting SCFA regulation of a variety of host physiological processes. As a result, there is considerable interest in probing the therapeutic potential of SCFA-producing microbial genera that are commonly found in the gut and could form part of a nutritional plan, which include: *Ruminoclustridium, Akkermansia, Bifidobacterium, Fusicatenibacter, Lactobacillus, Lactocaseibacillus, Ruminococcus, Ligilactobacillus, Blautia, Bacteroides, Enterococcus, Roseburia, Eubacterium, Prevotella, Faecalibacterium, Clostridium* and *Coprococcus* (44).

A diet high in fibre has been shown to increase the diversity and abundance of SCFA-producing microbe *Bifidobacterium pseudocatenulatum*, which is also capable of modulating clinically relevant host outcomes in type 2 diabetes. The same strain was subsequently shown to significantly reduce weight gain, body fat accumulation, fasting glucose levels and insulin resistance and improve postprandial glycaemic response in a mouse model. These promising neuroprotective and anti-inflammatory properties make SCFAs a potentially good candidate as a nutritional therapeutic agent promoting health.

Conclusions

It is becoming increasingly clear that the gut microbiome plays a key factor in host physiology communicating along the bidirectional gut–brain axis. While communication pathways continue to be examined for direct or indirect involvement, much more work is still needed. A growing number of studies are examining the effects of the gut microbiome on host physiology and homeostasis, yet no consensus has been reached regarding whether a specific healthy gut-microbiome signature exists. Even though there has been much interest in the field, caution needs to be exercised as much of the available clinical data is largely derived from small cohorts lacking a longitudinal perspective. More mechanistic studies are urgently needed to understand how changes in the gut microbiome can moderate health and disease and to implement and ascertain safety efficacy for potential therapeutics. Even with a growing body of pre-clinical research supporting the hypotheses, definitive evidence supporting the translatability of these findings to a human population is sorely lacking, although early evidence is encouraging. There are still too few adequately powered longitudinal clinical observational and interventional studies, and more are needed. Appropriate selection of participants and adequate management of confounding variables must be a part of future study designs. It is now evident that we need to gather more information to understand whether tailoring host nutrition to increase/decrease modulating factors of the gut microbiota can improve health and cognitive outcomes. It could very well be that microbial accessibility (i.e. fermentability) is the key for designing specific dietary needs for a positive influence of nutrition on brain health. Therefore, future research needs to take into consideration the investigation of mechanisms involved, including host metrics such as genetics, the gut-microbiome profile and other pertinent lifestyle factors. Better dietary habits supporting mental health need to be advocated. More high-quality longitudinal data is also needed, specifically surrounding brain function, behaviour and physiology. These factors should be championed to aid in establishing evidence-based health claims to develop efficacious therapeutic interventions.

Acknowledgements

Professor Cryan is funded by Science Foundation Ireland SFI/12/RC/ 2273_P2, the Saks Kavanaugh Foundation, EU H2020 project DLV-848228 DIS-COvERIE and Swiss National Science Foundation project CRSII5_186346/NMS2068. Professor Cryan has received research funding from 4D Pharma, Cremo, Dupont, Mead Johnson, Nutricia and Pharmavite; has been an invited speaker at meetings organised by Alimentary Health, Alkermes, Ordesa and Yakult; and has served as a consultant for Alkermes and Nestle. Professor Clarke has received honoraria from Janssen, Probi and Apsen as an invited speaker; is in receipt of research funding from Pharmavite and Fonterra; and is a paid consultant for Yakult and Zentiva. Dr O'Riordan has been an invited speaker for Sanofi Genzyme and Danone. This support neither influenced nor constrained the contents of this chapter. Dr Schneider declares no competing interests.

References

1. Cryan, J. F., O'Riordan, K. J., Cowan, C. S. M., et al., 2019. The microbiota-gut-brain axis. *Physiological Reviews*, 99(4), 1877–2013.

2. Butler, M. I., Bastiaanssen, T. F. S., Long-Smith C., et al., 2020. Recipe for a healthy gut: intake of unpasteurised milk is associated with increased lactobacillus abundance in the human gut microbiome. *Nutrients*, 12(5).

3. Schverer, M., O'Mahony, S. M., O'Riordan, K. J., et al., 2020. Dietary phospholipids: role in cognitive processes across the lifespan. *Neuroscience & Biobehavioral Reviews*, 111, 183–93.

4. Dinan, T. G., Stanton, C., Long-Smith, C., et al., 2019. Feeding melancholic microbes: MyNewGut recommendations on diet and mood. *Clinical Nutrition*, 38(5), 1995–2001.

5. Cryan, J. F., O'Riordan, K. J., Sandhu, K., Peterson, V. and Dinan, T. G., 2020. The gut microbiome in neurological disorders. *Lancet Neurology*, 19(2), 179–94.

6. Berding, K., Carbia, C. and Cryan, J. F., 2021. Going with the grain: fiber, cognition, and the microbiota-gut-brain-axis. *Experimental Biology and Medicine*, 246(7), 796–811.

7. Berding, K. and Cryan, J. F., 2022. Microbiota-targeted interventions for mental health. *Current Opinion in Psychiatry*, 35(1), 3–9.

8. Berding, K., Vlckova, K., Marx, W., et al., 2021. Diet and the microbiota-gut-brain axis: sowing the seeds of good mental health. *Advances in Nutrition*, 12(4), 1239–85.

9. Casertano, M., Fogliano, V. and Ercolini, D., 2022. Psychobiotics, gut microbiota and fermented foods can help preserving mental health. *Food Research International*, 152, 110892.

10. Dinan, T. G., Butler, M. I. and Cryan, J. F., 2021. Psychobiotics: evolution of novel antidepressants. *Modern Trends in Psychiatry*, 32, 134–43.

11. Bastiaanssen, T. F. S., Quinn, T. P. and Loughman, A., 2022. Treating bugs as features: a compositional guide to the statistical analysis of the microbiome-gut-brain axis. https://arxiv.org/pdf/2207.12475.pdf.

12. Knight, R., Vrbanac, A., Taylor, B. C., et al., 2018. Best practices for analysing microbiomes. *Nature Reviews Microbiology*, 16(7), 410–22.

13. Claesson, M. J., Clooney, A. G. and O'Toole, P. W., 2017. A clinician's guide to microbiome analysis. *Nature Reviews Gastroenterology & Hepatology*, 14(10), 585–95.

14. Asshauer, K. P., Wemheuer, B., Daniel, R. and Meinicke, P., 2015. Tax4Fun: predicting functional profiles from metagenomic 16S rRNA data. *Bioinformatics*, 31(17), 2882–4.

15. Iwai, S., Weinmaier, T., Schmidt, B. L., et al., 2016. Piphillin: improved prediction of metagenomic content by direct inference from human microbiomes. *PLoS One*, 11(11), e0166104.

16. Bastiaanssen, T. F. S., Gururajan, A., van de Wouw, M., et al., 2021. Volatility as a concept to understand the impact of stress on the microbiome. *Psychoneuroendocrinology*, 124, 105047.

17. Armstrong, G., Martino, C., Morris, J., et al., 2022. Swapping metagenomics preprocessing pipeline components offers speed and sensitivity increases. *mSystems*, 7 (2), e0137821.

18. Aitchison, J., 1986. *The statistical analysis of compositional data*. Chapman and Hall.

19. Tuomisto, H., 2010. A diversity of beta diversities: straightening up a concept gone awry. Part 1. Defining beta diversity as a function of alpha and gamma diversity. *Ecography*, 33(1), 2–22.

20. Tuomisto, H., 2010. A diversity of beta diversities: straightening up a concept gone awry. Part 2. Quantifying beta diversity and related phenomena. *Ecography*, 33(1), 23–45.

21. van der Hee, B. and Wells, J. M., 2021. Microbial regulation of host physiology by short-chain fatty acids. *Trends in Microbiology*, 29(8), 700–12.

22. Cryan, J. F. and Mazmanian, S. K., 2022. Microbiota-brain axis: context and causality. *Science*, 376(6596), 938–9.

23. Nuttall, G. H. F. and Thierfelder, H., 1987. Thierisches Leben ohne Bakterien im Verdauungskanal. (II. Mittheilung). *Hoppe Seylers Z. Physiol Chem.*, 2, 62–73.

24. Bibiloni, R., 2012. Rodent models to study the relationships between mammals and their bacterial inhabitants. *Gut Microbes*, 3 (6), 536–43.

25. Chinna Meyyappan, A., Forth, E., Wallace, C. J. K. and Milev, R., 2020. Effect of fecal microbiota transplant on symptoms of psychiatric disorders: a systematic review. *BMC Psychiatry*, 20(1), 299.

26. Margolis, K. G., Cryan, J. F. and Mayer, E. A., 2021. The microbiota-gut-brain axis: from motility to mood. *Gastroenterology*, 160(5), 1486–1501.

27. Wilmes, L., Collins, J. M., O'Riordan, K. J., et al., 2021. Of bowels, brain and behavior: a role for the gut microbiota in psychiatric comorbidities in irritable bowel syndrome. *Neurogastroenterology and Motility*, 33(3), e14095.

28. Fulling, C., Dinan, T. G. and Cryan, J. F., 2019. Gut microbe to brain signaling: what happens in vagus. *Neuron*, 101(6), 998–1002.

29. Clarke, G., Sandhu, K. V., Griffin, B. T., et al., 2019. Gut reactions: breaking down xenobiotic-microbiome interactions. *Pharmacological Reviews*, 71(2), 198–224.

30. Lynch, C. M. K., Clarke, G. and Cryan, J. F., 2021. Powering up microbiome-microglia interactions. *Cell Metabolism*, 33(11), 2097–9.

31. Leeuwendaal, N. K., Cryan, J. F. and Schellekens, H., 2021. Gut peptides and the microbiome: focus on ghrelin. *Current Opinion in Endocrinology, Diabetes and Obesity*, 28(2), 243–52.

32. Spichak, S., Bastiaanssen, T. F. S., Berding, K., et al., 2021. Mining microbes for mental health: determining the role of microbial metabolic pathways in human brain health and disease. *Neuroscience & Biobehavioral Reviews*, 125, 698–761.

33. Needham, B. D., Funabashi, M., Adame, M. D., et al., 2022. A gut-derived metabolite alters brain activity and anxiety behaviour in mice. *Nature*, 602(7898), 647–53.

34. Walter, J. and Hornef, M. W., 2021. A philosophical perspective on the prenatal in utero microbiome debate. *Microbiome*, 9(1), 5.

35. Ratsika, A., Codagnone, M. C., O'Mahony, S., Stanton, C. and Cryan, J. F., 2021. Priming for life: early life nutrition and the microbiota-gut-brain axis. *Nutrients*, 13(2).

36. Callaghan, B. L., Fields, A., Gee, D. G., et al., 2020. Mind and gut: associations between mood and gastrointestinal distress in children exposed to adversity. *Development and Psychopathology*, 32(1), 309–28.

37. Cowan, C. S. M. and Cryan, J. F., 2021. The microbiome-gut-brain axis in neurocognitive development and decline. *Modern Trends in Psychiatry*, 32, 12–25.

38. Cowan, C. S. M., Dinan, T. G. and Cryan, J. F., 2020. Annual research review: critical windows – the microbiota-gut-brain axis in neurocognitive development. *Journal of Child Psychology and Psychiatry*, 61(3), 353–71.

39. Lach, G., Fulling, C., Bastiaanssen, T. F. S., et al., 2020. Enduring neurobehavioral effects induced by microbiota depletion during the adolescent period. *Translational Psychiatry*, 10(1), 382.

40. Crouse, J. J., Carpenter, J. S., Song, Y. J. C., et al., 2021. Circadian rhythm sleep-wake disturbances and depression in young people: implications for prevention and early intervention. *Lancet Psychiatry*, 8(9), 813–23.

41. Carbia, C., Lannoy, S., Maurage, P., et al., 2021. A biological framework for emotional dysregulation in alcohol misuse: from gut to brain. *Molecular Psychiatry, 26* (4), 1098–1118.

42. Claesson, M. J., Cusack, S., O'Sullivan, O., et al., 2011. Composition, variability, and temporal stability of the intestinal microbiota of the elderly. *Proceedings of the National Academy of Sciences of the United States of America, 108*(suppl. 1), 4586–91.

43. O'Riordan, K. J., Collins, M. K., Moloney, G. M., et al., 2022. Short chain fatty acids: microbial metabolites for gut-brain axis signalling. *Molecular and Cellular Endocrinology, 546*, 111572.

44. Dalile, B., Van Oudenhove, L., Vervliet, B. and Verbeke, K., 2019. The role of short-chain fatty acids in microbiota-gut-brain communication. *Nature Reviews Gastroenterology & Hepatology, 16*(8), 461–78.

The Mediterranean Diet and Mental Health

Mary I. Butler and Sabrina Mörkl

Summary
The Mediterranean diet is widely acknowledged as one of the best nutritional approaches for improving health and longevity. In recent years, the evidence for such beneficial effects has extended beyond the realm of metabolic and cardiovascular health to include the brain and mental health. At a population level, adherence to a Mediterranean diet is associated with lower risk of depression and cognitive disorders. In people suffering with depression, switching to a Mediterranean-style diet is an effective treatment strategy. The Mediterranean diet is a safe and sustainable dietary pattern which should form part of the toolkit of any mental health professional wishing to incorporate nutritional approaches. In this chapter, we review the evidence for the use of the Mediterranean diet for mental health and explore the biological mechanisms involved. We provide practical advice for mental health professionals wishing to use this nutritional approach as part of a treatment plan.

Introduction

The Mediterranean diet is hailed as one of the best nutritional approaches to enhance health and longevity. It is recognised as being beneficial for cardiovascular and metabolic function, for autoimmune disease, for cancer prevention and, more recently, for brain and mental health. While nowadays we rely on cohort studies and randomised controlled clinical trials to assess the impact of the Mediterranean diet, humans have intuitively practised this way of eating for many centuries. Historical references to food consumption in ancient Greek and Roman literature reveal many similarities to our modern description of the Mediterranean dietary pattern. However, the concept of a particular 'Mediterranean diet' only came into being in the mid-twentieth century. Ancel Benjamin Keys was an American physiologist who became interested in nutrition during World War II. He was tasked with designing portable food rations for soldiers and later with determining the best approaches for re-feeding starving civilians in war-torn Europe. Keys noticed that rates of heart disease in European men were dramatically lower than in the United States, and he wondered about the potential link between food and cardiovascular disorders. He had observed that southern Italy had the highest concentration of centenarians in the world and he hypothesised that this might be related to their diet. Keys undertook a large longitudinal cohort study, known as the Seven Countries Study (1), which concluded that cholesterol levels were strongly related to coronary artery disease mortality. He subsequently promoted the idea that a Mediterranean-style diet, low in animal fat and rich in fruit and vegetables, protected against heart disease and that a diet high in animal fats led to heart disease. This work could be regarded as the beginning of 'lifestyle medicine' and an appreciation of the importance of lifestyle factors such as diet and nutrition in determining health.

In the decades since Ancel Keys' study, his work has received many criticisms, from claims that countries were selectively included based on the desired outcome to a failure to consider sugar as a confounding factor. Indeed, there is currently much controversy in relation to the link between animal fats, cholesterol and heart disease, and contradictory studies have resulted in widespread public confusion about how and what to eat. In contrast, the evidence concerning the wide-ranging health benefits of the Mediterranean diet has remained relatively stable and consistent, making it an attractive whole-dietary pattern that clinicians can confidently recommend to many people for improving health status. Such evidence, which began in the realm of cardiovascular and metabolic health, has now extended to the brain and mental health.

What Is the Mediterranean Diet?

What exactly does the term 'Mediterranean diet' denote? Over 20 diverse countries border the Mediterranean Sea, including Greece, Italy, Spain, France, Croatia, Lebanon, Turkey and several North African countries, all with unique and varied culinary cultures. However, reference to the Mediterranean diet classically describes the diet of people in the olive-producing regions of Crete, Greece and southern Italy around the 1950s to 1970s. There are several guidelines currently in use outlining Mediterranean dietary principles in the form of food pyramids. Although there are slight differences with regards to specific quantities, the key features are, for the most part, consistent. Firstly, high levels of fruits and vegetables along with wholegrain breads, cereals, beans, nuts and seeds represent the core components. Secondly, olive oil is the principal source of fat and consumed in large quantities every day. This should preferably be extra virgin olive oil (EVOO), meaning that it is cold-pressed and unprocessed. Thirdly, dairy products, fish, poultry and eggs are consumed in moderate amounts while the use of red meat and sweets is occasional. Red wine is another distinct feature, consumed regularly in small amounts with meals. The Greek dietary guidelines, published in 1999 by the Ministry of Health and Welfare in Greece, reflect a traditional Mediterranean diet (2), while a more recent food pyramid compiled by the Mediterranean Diet Foundation was designed to present greater flexibility and updated recommendations to reflect the lifestyle, dietary, sociocultural, environmental and health challenges faced by present-day Mediterranean populations (3). The primary features of both guidelines are outlined in further detail in Table 3.1.

From a nutritional perspective, the predominantly plant-based nature of the Mediterranean diet makes it abundant in antioxidants, polyphenols and fibre, as well as being low in saturated fats and animal proteins. Polyphenols are a large family of naturally occurring organic compounds which are abundant in plants. They are categorised into four classes: phenolic acids, flavonoids, stilbenes and lignans. Polyphenols are present in all the main key foods of the Mediterranean diet; EVOO, nuts, red wine, legumes, vegetables, fruits and wholegrain cereals. Polyphenols have antioxidant and anti-inflammatory effects and it is thought that long-term consumption may protect against a wide variety of chronic illnesses. The fat component of the Mediterranean diet is also important. While saturated and trans-fats are considered unhealthy fats, unsaturated fats (monounsaturated or

Table 3.1 Comparison of the Greek dietary guidelines (1999) and the Mediterranean Diet Foundation guidelines (2011) regarding the components of a Mediterranean diet

Greek Dietary guidelines (1999)		Mediterranean Diet Foundation guidelines (2011)
Main added lipid, use daily	**Olive oil**	Every meal
6 servings vegetables per day 3 servings fruit per day	**Fruit and vegetables**	≥2 servings vegetables per meal 1–2 servings fruit per meal
8 servings per day	**Breads and cereals (preferably wholegrain)**	1–2 servings per meal
5–6 servings per week	**Fish, seafood**	≥2 servings per week
3–4 servings per week	**Legumes and nuts**	1–2 servings per day
2 servings dairy per day 4 servings poultry per week 3 servings eggs per week	**Dairy, poultry, eggs**	2 servings dairy per day 2 servings poultry per week 2–4 servings eggs per week
3 servings sweets per week 4 servings red meat per month Wine in moderation	**Red meat, sweets, other**	<2 servings red meat per week ≤2 servings sweets per week Wine in moderation

polyunsaturated) are recognised as having many health benefits. Olive oil is a rich source of monounsaturated fatty acids (MUFAs), while nuts and fish provide a plentiful supply of the polyunsaturated fatty acids (PUFAs) omega-3 and omega-6. An important feature of the Mediterranean diet with regards to fat intake is the relative proportion of omega-3 to omega-6 PUFAs. The Western diet generally has high levels of omega-6 as it is abundant in vegetable oils such as corn oil, which is widely used in cooking and added to many processed foods. Although PUFAs are considered healthy fats, an unbalanced omega-3 to omega-6 ratio is thought to be unfavourable and possibly proinflammatory. The typical Western diet has an omega-3 to omega-6 ratio of up to 1:20, while the recommended ratio is much lower, closer to 1:4 or less. Thus, increasing omega-3 PUFAs is vital and an important nutritional feature of the Mediterranean diet.

The Mediterranean Diet and Mental Health

What is the evidence that the Mediterranean diet is beneficial for mental health? Importantly, does the value of this diet extend beyond the realm of general population-level preventative health promotion and actually have therapeutic potential for those suffering with specific mental health disorders? In the years since the seminal Seven Countries study, the Mediterranean diet has been the focus of much research across a variety of disease states. It has been associated with reduced risk of many chronic diseases including type 2 diabetes, cardiovascular disease, cancer and cognitive-related illnesses. Interest in the potential of the Mediterranean diet to improve mental health was spurred on by the seminal PREDIMED (Prevención con Dieta Mediterránea) study, a large Spanish multi-centre trial investigating the Mediterranean diet in primary cardiovascular prevention (4). Although the trial was not powered to investigate depression outcomes, secondary analyses suggested reduced risk of depression with the Mediterranean diet, in particular in patients with type 2 diabetes (5). Additional subgroup analyses demonstrated an association with improved cognitive function (6–8). Unfortunately, later revelations regarding serious protocol deviations cast a shadow on the PREDIMED trial but interest in the link between the Mediterranean diet, depression and cognitive function had been established.

Depression and Anxiety

Over the past decade, many cross-sectional and cohort studies have been undertaken exploring the association between diet and depression. There is now reasonably robust evidence, at a systematic review and meta-analysis level, that a healthy diet, including the Mediterranean and other traditional dietary patterns, is associated with a lower risk of depressive symptoms (9–12). Additionally, observational studies suggest that the Mediterranean diet is protective when it comes to anxiety symptoms (13). However, disentangling the diet–mental health link using cross-sectional and cohort studies is fraught with difficulties given the possibility of reverse causation and the many confounding factors to consider, including socioeconomic influences, comorbidity, obesity and metabolic health. In addition, most studies have involved non-clinical cohorts self-reporting depressive and anxiety symptoms, and the association between a healthy diet and depression is less clear when considering a strict clinical diagnosis of depression as the outcome (9, 14, 15). While the public health importance of improving diet to reduce overall population-level depression and anxiety risk is clear, randomised controlled trials are vital to further explore this area. Excitingly, several such trials using a Mediterranean diet intervention for depression have been undertaken in recent years, all based far from the Mediterranean in Australia.

The first of these trials, published in early 2017, was the SMILES (Supporting the Modification of lifestyle In Lowered Emotional States) trial led by a research team at Deakin University, Geelong (16). This 12-week, parallel-group, single-blind, randomised trial enrolled 67 participants with major depression, 33 of whom were allocated to a Mediterranean diet intervention; the remaining 34 underwent a social support control intervention. The dietary intervention involved seven one-to-one educational sessions with a dietician providing personalised dietary advice and nutritional counselling support. Additionally, participants received a food hamper, incorporating the main components of the diet, along with recipes and meal plans. Notably, this was an adjunctive intervention with the majority of participants also being treated with pharmacotherapy and/or psycho-therapy. The social support control condition comprised a 'befriending' protocol which involved trained personnel discussing neutral topics of interest or engaging in activities such as cards or board games. The befriending sessions involved the same visit schedule and length as the dietary support intervention. At the 12-week endpoint, the dietary group demon-strated significantly greater reductions in depression scores than the control group, as measured by the Montgomery-Asberg Depression Rating Scale (MADRS). Encouragingly, remission from depression was achieved in 32.3% of the diet group compared to only 8.0% of the control group.

The following year a similar study was published, this time from the University of South Australia, Adelaide (17). This was a larger study with 152 participants which extended to a 6-month follow-up. The study design was similar, although the dietary intervention involved group cooking workshops (fortnightly for 3 months) as opposed to individual sessions. Participants in the dietary arm also received fish oil supplements. Again, the dietary group had greater reduction in depression scores, as well as improved mental health quality of life scores at 3 months. These improvements were sustained at the 6-month follow-up. An important factor to consider in this trial was the fish oil supplementation. Such supplements in themselves are known to promote brain health, thus making it impossible to ascertain the overall effect of the Mediterranean diet intervention. Authors measured the impact of fish oil supplementation using erythrocyte omega-3 and omega-6 fatty acid content. Although no significant correlation between increased omega-3 and improved depressive symptoms was seen, improved depression scores were associated with a decreased ratio of omega-6 to omega-3. This is consistent with evidence that the balance between omega-3 and omega-6 is an important determinant of health.

More recently, researchers at the University of Technology Sydney, New South Wales reported that an adjunctive Mediterranean diet intervention specifically target-ing clinically depressed young men was effective in reducing depressive symptoms and improving quality of life compared to a befriending group (18). The intervention here was less intensive than the two aforementioned studies, with only two online nutri-tional education sessions at baseline and week 6, along with a food hamper. An even more basic intervention, incorporating Mediterranean diet components, was used by a team at Macquarie University, Sydney (19). This consisted of food hampers along with a 13-minute dietary video followed up with 5-minute phone calls on day 7 and day 14 of the 3-week intervention. Despite the limited intervention, participants showed significantly greater reductions in self-reported depressive symptoms compared to an inactive control group.

In addition to studies involving a whole-diet change, numerous randomised controlled trials have been undertaken investigating the use of polyphenols in the treatment of depression. The most commonly investigated compounds have been isoflavone, curcumin and hypericum extract. Meta-analyses confirm a beneficial effect of polyphenols on depressive symptoms, although they appear to be less effective in reducing anxiety (20). The anti-depressive effect of polyphenols appears to be particularly marked in peri- or post-menopausal women, attributable to the fact that isoflavone is a phytoestrogen and improves symptoms of menopause (21).

Thus, it appears that the Mediterranean diet not only plays a prophylactic role in protecting against the development of depressive symptoms but can also have a therapeutic effect in those suffering with established depression. It is interesting that quite limited interventions, based on Mediterranean diet principles, appear to yield significant beneficial results for improving mood. Clearly, from a health economics perspective, such interventions could be cost-effective, resource-friendly, low-risk strategies for reducing the burden of depression. At a time when almost one in five adults in the UK is taking a prescribed antidepressant (22), the need for alternative treatment approaches is vital. The SMILES trial undertook a prospective economic evaluation and demonstrated that the dietary intervention was cost-effective as an adjunctive treatment for depression from both health sector and societal perspectives (23). Additionally, at an individual level, a cost analysis showed that the weekly cost of the Mediterranean diet was cheaper than the cost of participants' baseline diet (24). Interventional studies exploring the Mediterranean diet in other psychiatric conditions such as anxiety disorders, bipolar disorder or psychosis are currently lacking.

Cognition

There is much interest in the potential of the Mediterranean diet to reduce age-related cognitive decline and prevent cognitive disorders such as Alzheimer's disease. As with depression, there is robust observational evidence that adherence to a Mediterranean diet is inversely associated with the development of cognitive disorders (25). Such observational evidence has been supported by a handful of clinical trials. One trial involving a subgroup of elderly participants from the PREDIMED study, all cognitively healthy but at high cardiovascular risk, demonstrated improved cognitive scores in the Mediterranean diet group (with either EVOO supplementation or nuts) after a median follow-up of 4 years (6). This trial extended the findings of two other PREDIMED sub-studies which reported better cognitive performance after the Mediterranean diet intervention, although baseline cognition had not been assessed in either study (7, 8). The Mediterranean – Dietary Approaches to Stop Hypertension (DASH) Intervention for Neurodegenerative Delay (MIND) study is a 3-year, multi-centre, randomised controlled trial to test the effects of the MIND diet on cognitive function in 604 individuals at risk for Alzheimer's disease (26). It used a dietary approach which combined principles from the Mediterranean diet and the DASH diet, emphasising those components which had the most compelling evidence in the diet–dementia field. The study has been completed but results are awaited and will be a valuable addition to the evidence.

There is promising evidence that polyphenols have the potential to improve cognition and increase resistance to age-related cognitive decline, although their impact on established dementia remains to be seen (27). It appears that the quality of the olive oil component of the Mediterranean diet may be particularly important for cognition. A small pilot study in Greece explored the effect of Greek High Phenolic Early Harvest EVOO versus Moderate Phenolic EVOO and Mediterranean Diet (without extra olive oil supplementation) in people with mild cognitive impairment. The quality of the olive oil was carefully chosen to reflect varying levels of phenols and polyphenols. Following 12 months of the intervention, they found that those participants with the highest-quality olive oil demonstrated better performance across almost all cognitive domains (28), suggesting that the phenolic constituents are vital for cognitive function. Given the enormous and growing burden of cognitive disorders, there is an urgent need to identify lifestyle measures such as the Mediterranean diet to reduce their incidence.

Mechanisms of Action

Many questions remain in relation to what mechanisms are involved in mediating an improvement in mental health with a Mediterranean diet. One could speculate that associated eating-related behaviours traditionally seen in Mediterranean populations might have been key factors in the early observations of health and longevity in these groups. People from Greece and Italy traditionally focussed on sourcing local, seasonal foods, prioritised home-cooking and engaged in slow, relaxed social meals with family and friends, often outdoors in the sunshine. While it is highly likely that such lifestyle factors contribute to well-being, it does appear that the diet itself has inherent health-promoting properties. A Mediterranean diet intervention has now been investigated in many different countries and settings and is consistently associated with health improvements. Numerous biological pathways appear to be involved. Modulation of inflammatory mechanisms and oxidative stress undoubtedly play a role, as do diet-induced changes to the gut microbiota. A Mediterranean diet can lead to changes in tryptophan metabolism, vagal activity and the cortisol-mediated stress response. Central changes may also be important, including influences on microglia and neuroinflammation, as well as on brain-derived neurotrophic factor (BDNF) activity. Much research is underway to explore these mechanisms further and uncover how exactly a Mediterranean diet impacts brain health. The pathways of relevance are summarised in Figure 3.1 and outlined in more detail in the following sections.

Inflammation

Inflammation appears to be a key player in the mechanistic link between diet and mental health. It is well recognised that depression and other neuropsychiatric conditions, including bipolar disorder, schizophrenia and post-traumatic stress disorder, are associated with chronic low-grade inflammation. The source of this inflammation is unclear but it is likely that it is mediated by a wide variety of influences, one of which may be diet and nutrition. A large population-based study demonstrated that people with severe mental illness have more inflammatory diets than the general population, with higher intake of proinflammatory foods and significantly lower consumption of anti-inflammatory nutrients (29). For people with metabolic syndrome or with elevated cardiovascular risk, switching to a Mediterranean diet resulted in a reduction in inflammatory markers (30), and this nutritional pattern could represent a safe and effective way to reduce the chronic inflammation seen in psychiatric conditions.

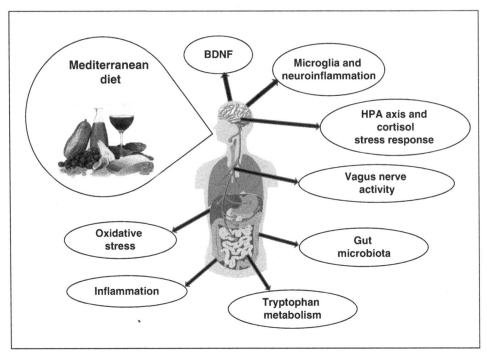

Figure 3.1 Biological pathways involved in mediating the impact of the Mediterranean diet on the brain and mental health.
(BDNF: brain-derived neurotrophic factor; HPA: hypothalamic pituitary adrenal)

Oxidative Stress

Oxidation is a ubiquitous process in all human cells. It results in the production of free radicals which are neutralised by antioxidants, maintaining a careful homeostatic balance. Oxidative stress arises when there is an imbalance between free radical production and antioxidant capacity. Although oxidative stress plays important physiological roles, when persistent it is thought to contribute to a variety of disease processes. There is clear evidence that antioxidant levels are lower and serum-free radical levels are higher in depressed patients (31). Similarly, antioxidant capacity appears to be reduced in patients with bipolar disorder (32) and schizophrenia (33). The diet is a rich and important source of antioxidant substances and thus a potential target for improving oxidative status. Plant-based foods are far higher in antioxidants than animal-based foods, with the highest antioxidant potential seen in nuts, seeds, coffee, dark chocolate, spices, herbs and berries. Unsurprisingly, given that it is a predominantly plant-based diet, the Mediterranean diet is associated with higher levels of plasma antioxidant capacity, which may represent one mechanism by which it mediates a mental health benefit.

The Gut Microbiota

The trillions of bacteria that inhabit the human gut, collectively termed the gut microbiota, have a far-reaching impact on human health and disease. The gut–brain axis is a bidirectional system which allows extensive bottom-up and top-down communication via a variety of neuroendocrine, immune and metabolic pathways. It is now recognised that the gut microbiome is a key node in the gut–brain communication system and plays a role in many physiological processes. The gut microbiome is altered in many psychiatric conditions including depression, anxiety, bipolar disorder, autism spectrum disorder and psychosis (34), and for many patients with such conditions achieving optimal gut health could be an important part of holistic treatment.

Diet is one of the major determinants of gut microbiota composition. However, the interplay between diet, the gut microbiota and human health is a complex and dynamic process and many questions remain as to how to achieve optimum gut microbiota through dietary means. Adherence to a Mediterranean diet appears promising in this regard. A large multi-centre European study investigated a 1-year Mediterranean diet intervention on gut microbiota and frailty status in 612 elderly people (35). Adherence to the Mediterranean diet led to increased abundance of specific taxa that were associated with lower frailty and improved cognitive function, while being negatively associated with inflammatory markers. Such taxa included *Faecalibacterium prausnitzii* and *Roseburia* (*R. hominis*). Reduced levels of *Faecalibacterium* are a repeated finding across various psychiatric disorders, including depression, bipolar disorder and schizophrenia (36), while high levels of this taxa are positively associated with quality of life measures (37). Additionally, *Roseburia* levels are consistently depleted in patients with schizophrenia and bipolar disorder (38). Both *Faecalibacterium* and *Roseburia* are butyrate-producers and exhibit anti-inflammatory effects, which are likely key mechanisms driving their health-promoting influence.

An interesting finding from the aforementioned study is that the taxa changes were shared across the five European countries, demonstrating that the Mediterranean diet alters the gut microbiota in a consistent manner despite different baseline dietary patterns. Even more encouraging is the fact that another study, which also used a Mediterranean diet intervention in healthy obese or overweight subjects, reported similar findings, namely an increase in *Faecalibacterium prausnitzii* and *Roseburia* (39). Thus, it appears that an important mechanism by which the Mediterranean diet can promote good mental health is through the promotion of healthy gut microbiota and an increase in levels of specific bacterial groups known to be depleted in psychiatric conditions.

Brain-Derived Neurotrophic Factor

Another mechanism by which the Mediterranean diet may improve mental health is the modulation of BDNF expression. BDNF is a protein found predominantly in the brain. It plays an important role in neuronal development during early life and continues to impact neuronal transmission and synaptic plasticity throughout the lifespan. Stress, a key risk factor for many psychiatric disorders, results in reduced levels of BDNF and hippocampal atrophy. Serum BDNF levels are reduced in depression and various antidepressant medications increase BDNF expression. While there are many inconsistencies across animal and human studies of BDNF, it does appear to represent a biomarker of depression and treatment response (40). Interestingly, nutritional factors, particularly polyphenols, can increase plasma BDNF, which may in part account for the antidepressant effects of a Mediterranean diet. Analysis of a randomly selected subgroup from the PREDIMED trial revealed that, among participants with prevalent depression at baseline, significantly higher BDNF levels were found for those assigned to a Mediterranean diet supplemented with nuts (41). A more recent study used the MIND diet, as described earlier, in healthy obese women. Researchers reported that, although no differences in mean plasma levels of BDNF were found after 3 months of intervention in volunteers allocated to the MIND diet group, higher overall plasma BDNF levels were seen in the MIND diet group as compared with the control group (42).

Cortisol and the Stress Response

The stress response is mediated by the hypothalamic–pituitary–adrenal axis which culminates in the production of cortisol. Dysregulation of this system can be a long-term consequence of early life trauma and is a prominent feature of many psychiatric conditions. An observational study of 240 European adolescents demonstrated that increased adherence to a Mediterranean diet was inversely associated with cortisol levels and moderated the relationship between cortisol and inflammatory biomarkers, suggesting that it may counteract stress-induced inflammation (43). Another cross-sectional study, involving over 10,000 participants, suggested that the Mediterranean diet was positively associated with higher psychological resilience (44). To date, there have been no published human clinical trials investigating the impact of a Mediterranean diet intervention on the cortisol stress response. However, an interesting study using female macaques has recently explored this area. Thirty-eight animals were randomised to consumption of a Western- versus Mediterranean-type diet for 31 months (equivalent to 9 human years). Compared to animals fed a Western diet, those fed the Mediterranean diet exhibited lower sympathetic activity, brisker and more overt heart rate responses to acute stress, more rapid recovery and lower cortisol responses to acute psychological stress and adrenocorticotropin challenge (45). This exciting study raises the possibility that a Mediterranean diet could potentially improve stress resilience and thus reduce the longer-term risk of stress-related psychiatric disorders.

Tryptophan Metabolism

Although little is known about the effect of a Mediterranean diet on tryptophan metabolism in the context of mental health, it is worth mentioning as a possible mechanism of relevance. Tryptophan is an amino acid derived from dietary ingestion which plays an important role as a precursor to serotonin. However, the majority is metabolised through the alternative kynurenine pathway, resulting in the production of several metabolites, including neurotoxic quinolinic acid and neuroprotective kynurenic acid. The tryptophan-kynurenine pathway can be induced by inflammation as well as by stress and glucocorticoids, and has been implicated in a wide variety of psychiatric disorders. Dietary factors can have important influences on tryptophan availability. A diet high in protein increases the pool of tryptophan available for metabolism peripherally, while carbohydrates can increase the amount of free unbound tryptophan which can cross the blood–brain barrier. Interestingly, a Mediterranean diet moderated the association between several kynurenine-related metabolites and heart failure (46), suggesting that nutritional changes have the potential to reduce the negative effects of these metabolites. It remains to be seen whether such an effect could take place in psychiatric disorders.

Vagus Nerve and Heart Rate Variability

The vagus nerve is the main parasympathetic nerve in the body and is involved in an enormous array of bodily functions including digestion, cardiovascular regulation, metabolic homeostasis and immune response. Heart rate variability (HRV) refers to the normal variation in the time interval between consecutive heartbeats and reflects the balance between parasympathetic and sympathetic influences. An attenuation of HRV reflects a reduction in vagally mediated parasympathetic innervation to the heart and is a useful non-invasive tool to explore autonomic dysfunction. Lower HRV is associated with worsening depressive symptoms over time, suggesting that autonomic dysregulation is more likely to be a risk factor for depression rather than a sequela (47). Thus, interventions increasing HRV and modulating autonomic influence may be useful for the prevention and treatment of depression. Indeed, vagal nerve stimulation is effective in treatment-resistant depression and may also be beneficial in treatment-resistant anxiety disorders. Interestingly, consumption of a Mediterranean diet is associated with increased HRV (48). There are numerous components of the Mediterranean diet pattern which could account for this, as several have been shown to individually positively impact HRV, including fatty fish, nuts and wine.

Microglia

Microglia are the resident macrophages in the brain and exist as two phenotypes: M1 which are proinflammatory and M2 which are anti-inflammatory. Microglia and neuroinflammation are of major interest in the pathogenesis of cognitive decline and neurodegenerative disorders such as Alzheimer's disease, Parkinson's disease and multiple sclerosis. Microglial dysfunction is also implicated in the aetiology of depression. Although very much limited to the pre-clinical domain at present, components of the Mediterranean diet appear to reduce neuroinflammation. Docosahexaenoic acid (DHA) and eicosapentaenoic acid (EPA), the two main forms of omega-3 PUFAs in the brain, inhibit microglia-mediated neuroinflammation through a variety of mechanisms, including the inhibition of cytokine gene expression and a shift in microglial polarisation towards the beneficial M2 phenotype both in vitro and in vivo (49). Polyphenols have a similar effect. Hydroxytyrosol, a polyphenol present in significant amounts in EVOO, also reduces microglial activation in vitro (50). Translating these findings to human subjects remains a challenge.

Practical Considerations When Using a Mediterranean Diet Intervention in Clinical Settings

There is keen public interest in the area of nutrition and mental health at present. People have become far more food-conscious over the past decade and are increasingly likely to ask their mental health providers for advice on nutritional strategies to improve mood, energy, anxiety and stress. For mental health professionals, who generally receive little or no nutritional training (51), this can be an intimidating area of discussion. Even for those who are interested, the field of nutritional psychiatry is growing rapidly and it is difficult to keep abreast of new advances involving various aspects of nutrition, from probiotics to micronutrients to herbal supplements. There are several whole-dietary patterns under scrutiny for a range of health problems including gluten-free, ketogenic and vegetarian diets, as well as alternative dietary strategies such as intermittent fasting. While hugely interesting, none of these approaches currently have the robust evidence base of the Mediterranean diet for mental health. This is important for mental health professionals who want to provide patients with safe, well-informed advice.

An important consideration when using lifestyle measures for mental health is the likelihood that the person is willing and able to undertake and maintain the behavioural change inherent in the intervention. It is notoriously difficult to change behavioural patterns, in particular when it comes to food. This can be even more of a challenge for patients who are suffering with depression or another psychiatric condition. Although there is early evidence suggesting that the ketogenic diet may have some therapeutic value in mental illness (52), it is a diet that is difficult to sustain, which will likely limit its use to highly motivated individuals. In contrast, the Mediterranean diet is more varied and far less restrictive and thus may have higher chances of success in the long term. It is possible to gradually integrate Mediterranean diet principles into one's existing diet, leaving room for flexibility and individually determined progression. In addition, the Mediterranean diet is relatively safe and does not require the extensive education and monitoring that the ketogenic diet, for example, would involve, given the potential risks of prolonged ketosis.

However, there are a number of things clinicians should be aware of if recommending the Mediterranean diet. While the Mediterranean diet is associated with improved metabolic health, the increased fat intake due to olive oil and nuts may be off-putting for patients who are concerned about weight gain. Additionally, the emphasis on grains, fruit and vegetables means that meals can be quite high in carbohydrates, which may require some adjusting for patients with diabetes. While the Mediterranean diet is still suitable for such patients, it may be wise to refer them to a dietician to explore the specifics of the diet in more detail. Because of the minimal red meat intake, patients may be concerned about low iron levels but can be reassured that other foods such as fish, poultry and beans should be adequate sources. Switching to a Mediterranean diet may mean eating fewer dairy products for many people with resulting lower calcium intake. Indeed, it has been suggested that supplementing the Mediterranean diet with extra dairy is necessary to meet recommended calcium requirements (53). For a clinician, calcium levels can easily be monitored with consideration of a calcium supplement or increased dairy if needed. Finally, the regular wine consumption may, of course, not be suitable for some patients and any recommendations should be individualised to take this into account.

An important consideration for mental health professionals is that Mediterranean diet principles are straightforward and easy to explain. There are many resources which a clinician can use to explain the principles of the Mediterranean diet to patients, including freely available food pyramids and recipes (54). This could be done relatively quickly within existing psychiatric consultations. As mentioned in the aforesaid clinical studies in depression, some interventions were very limited – in one case a 13-minute dietary video – but they nonetheless yielded beneficial results. Additionally, it appears to be feasible to offer this dietary intervention remotely to psychiatric patients. A trial investigating the use of a remotely delivered, Mediterranean diet intervention in the secondary prevention of depression in Spain, the PREDIDEP study, is currently ongoing. Researchers have reported that the remote nutritional intervention has successfully increased adherence to the Mediterranean diet among recovered depression patients (55).

Conclusion

There is robust evidence that the Mediterranean diet is an effective strategy for improving mental health at a population level and for reducing the risk of developing depression and cognitive disorders. It can be encouraged as a healthy eating pattern for those keen to optimise their overall physical and mental well-being. Additionally, it is evident that switching to a Mediterranean diet can be an effective adjunctive treatment for those suffering with depression. This dietary strategy should be discussed along with the usual treatment options for depressive disorders. The Mediterranean diet is a safe and sustainable eating pattern. It is clear from the high rates of adherence across many clinical trials that such a dietary change is an achievable goal for people keen to try alternative treatments for depression. For mental health professionals interested in the field of nutritional psychiatry and wishing to incorporate diet-based approaches in their management plans, the Mediterranean diet is a good place to start.

References

1. Keys, A., Menotti, A., Aravanis, C., et al., 1984. The seven countries study: 2,289 deaths in 15 years. *Preventive Medicine, 13* (2), pp. 141–54.

2. Ministry of Health and Welfare, s.s.h.c., 1999. Dietary guidelines for adults in Greece. *Archives of Hellenic Medicine, 16*, pp. 516–24.

3. Bach-Faig, A., Berry, E. M., Lairon, D., et al., 2011. Mediterranean diet pyramid today: science and cultural updates. *Public Health Nutrition, 14*(12A), pp. 2274–84.

4. Estruch, R., Ros, E., Salas-Salvado, J., et al., 2018. Primary prevention of cardiovascular disease with a Mediterranean diet supplemented with extra-virgin olive oil or nuts. *New England Journal of Medicine, 378* (25), p. e34.

5. Sánchez-Villegas, A., Martinez-Gonzalez, M. A., Serra-Majem, L., et al., 2013. Mediterranean dietary pattern and depression: the PREDIMED randomized trial. *BMC Medicine, 11*, p. 208.

6. Valls-Pedret, C., Sala-Vila, A., Serra-Mir, M., et al., 2015. Mediterranean diet and age-related cognitive decline: a randomized clinical trial. *JAMA Internal Medicine, 175*(7), pp. 1094–1103.

7. Martínez-Lapiscina, E. H., Clavero, P., Tolego, E., et al., 2013. Virgin olive oil supplementation and long-term cognition: the PREDIMED-NAVARRA randomized trial. *The Journal of Nutrition, Health and Aging, 17*(6), pp. 544–52.

8. Martínez-Lapiscina, E. H., Clavero, P., Toledo, E., et al., 2013. Mediterranean diet improves cognition: the PREDIMED-NAVARRA randomised trial. *Journal of*

Neurology, Neurosurgery, and Psychiatry, 84(12), pp. 1318–25.

9. Molendijk, M., Molero, P., Sanchez-Pedreno, F. O., et al., 2018. Diet quality and depression risk: a systematic review and dose-response meta-analysis of prospective studies. *Journal of Affective Disorders, 226*, pp. 346–54.

10. Lai, J. S., Hiles, S. M., Bisquera, A., et al.,2014. A systematic review and meta-analysis of dietary patterns and depression in community-dwelling adults. *The American Journal of Clinical Nutrition, 99* (1), pp. 181–97.

11. Lassale, C., Batty, G. D., Baghdadli, A., et al., 2019. Healthy dietary indices and risk of depressive outcomes: a systematic review and meta-analysis of observational studies. *Molecular Psychiatry, 24*, 965–86.

12. Firth, J., Marx, W., Dash, S., et al., 2019. The effects of dietary improvement on symptoms of depression and anxiety: a meta-analysis of randomized controlled trials. *Psychosomatic Medicine, 81*(3), pp. 265–80.

13. Madani, S., Ahmadi, A., Shoaei-Jouneghani, F., et al., 2022. The relationship between the Mediterranean diet and Axis I disorders: a systematic review of observational studies. *Food Science & Nutrition, 10*, 3241–58.

14. Chocano-Bedoya, P. O., O'Reilly, E. J., Lucas, M., et al. 2013. Prospective study on long-term dietary patterns and incident depression in middle-aged and older women. *The American Journal of Clinical Nutrition, 98*(3), pp. 813–20.

15. Okubo, R., Matsuoka, Y. J., Sawada, N., et al., 2019. Diet quality and depression risk in a

Japanese population: the Japan Public Health Center (JPHC)-based Prospective Study. *Scientific Reports*, 9(1), p. 7150.

16. Jacka, F. N., O'Neill, A., Opie, R., et al., 2017. A randomised controlled trial of dietary improvement for adults with major depression (the 'SMILES' trial). *BMC Medicine*, 15(1), p. 23.

17. Parletta, N., Zarnowiecki, D., Cho, J., et al., 2019. A Mediterranean-style dietary intervention supplemented with fish oil improves diet quality and mental health in people with depression: A randomized controlled trial (HELFIMED). *Nutritional Neuroscience*, 22(7), pp. 474–87.

18. Bayes, J., Schloss, J. and Sibbritt, D., 2021. A randomised controlled trial assessing the effect of a Mediterranean diet on the symptoms of depression in young men (the 'AMMEND' study): a study protocol. *British Journal of Nutrition*, 126(5), p. 730–7.

19. Francis, H. M., Stevenson, R., Chambers, J. R., et al., 2019. A brief diet intervention can reduce symptoms of depression in young adults: a randomised controlled trial. *PLoS One*, 14(10), p. e0222768.

20. Lin, K., Li, Y., Du Toit, E., et al., 2021. Effects of polyphenol supplementations on improving depression, anxiety, and quality of life in patients with depression. *Frontiers in Psychiatry*, 12, 765485.

21. Chen, L. R., Ko, N. Y. and Chen, K. H., 2019. Isoflavone supplements for menopausal women: a systematic review. *Nutrients*, 11(11).

22. NHS.2021. Medicines used in mental health – England – quarterly summary statistics April to June 2021. www.nhsbsa.nhs.uk/stat istical-collections/medicines-used-mental-he alth-england/medicines-used-mental-health-england-quarterly-summary-statistics-april-june-2021.

23. Chatterton, M. L., Mihalopoulos, C., O'Neill, A., et al., 2018. Economic evaluation of a dietary intervention for adults with major depression (the 'SMILES' trial). *BMC Public Health*, 18(1), p. 599.

24. Opie, R. S., Itsiopoulos, C., Parletta, N., et al., 2015. Assessing healthy diet affordability in a cohort with major depressive disorders.

Journal of Public Health and Epidemiology, 7 (5), pp. 159–69.

25. Wu, L. and Sun, D., 2017. Adherence to Mediterranean diet and risk of developing cognitive disorders: an updated systematic review and meta-analysis of prospective cohort studies. *Scientific Reports*, 7(1), p. 41317.

26. Liu, X., Morris, M. C. and Barnes, L. L., 2021. Mediterranean-DASH Intervention for Neurodegenerative Delay (MIND) study: rationale, design and baseline characteristics of a randomized control trial of the MIND diet on cognitive decline. *Contemporary Clinical Trials*, 102, p. 106270.

27. Yang, W., Cui, K., Li, X., et al., 2021. Effect of polyphenols on cognitive function: evidence from population-based studies and clinical trials. *The Journal of Nutrition, Health & Aging*, 25(10), pp. 1190–1204.

28. Tsolaki, M., Lazarou, E., Kozori, M., et al., 2020. A randomized clinical trial of Greek high phenolic early harvest extra virgin olive oil in mild cognitive impairment: the MICOIL pilot study. *Journal of Alzheimer's Disease*, 78(2), pp. 801–17.

29. Firth, J., Stubbs, B., Teasdale, S. B., et al., 2018. Diet as a hot topic in psychiatry: a population-scale study of nutritional intake and inflammatory potential in severe mental illness. *World Psychiatry*, 17 (3), pp. 365–7.

30. Esposito, K., Marfeela, R., Ciotola, M., et al., 2004. Effect of a Mediterranean-style diet on endothelial dysfunction and markers of vascular inflammation in the metabolic syndrome: a randomized trial. *Journal of the American Medical Association*, 292(12), pp. 1440–6.

31. Liu, T., Zhong, S., Liao, X., et al., 2015. A meta-analysis of oxidative stress markers in depression. *PLoS One*, 10(10), p. e0138904.

32. Andreazza, A. C., Kauer-Sant'anna, M., Frey, B. N., et al., 2008. Oxidative stress markers in bipolar disorder: a meta-analysis. *Journal of Affective Disorders*, 111 (2), pp. 135–44.

33. Flatow, J., Buckley, P. and Miller, B. J., 2013. Meta-analysis of oxidative stress in

schizophrenia. *Biological Psychiatry*, *74*(6), pp. 400–9.

34. Butler, M. I., Cryan, J. F. and Dinan, T. G., 2019. Man and the microbiome: a new theory of everything? *Annual Review of Clinical Psychology*, 15, pp. 371–98.

35. Ghosh, T. S., Rampelli, S., Jeffrey, I., et al., 2020. Mediterranean diet intervention alters the gut microbiome in older people reducing frailty and improving health status: the NU-AGE 1-year dietary intervention across five European countries. *Gut*, *69*(7), p. 1218.

36. Borkent, J., Ioannouet, M., Sommer, I. E. C., et al., 2022. Role of the gut microbiome in three major psychiatric disorders. *Psychological Medicine*, *52*(7), pp. 1222–42.

37. Valles-Colomer, M., Falony, G., Darzy, Y., et al., 2019. The neuroactive potential of the human gut microbiota in quality of life and depression. *Nature Microbiology*, 4, pp. 623–32.

38. McGuinness, A. J., Davis, J. A., Dawson, S. L., et al., 2022. A systematic review of gut microbiota composition in observational studies of major depressive disorder, bipolar disorder and schizophrenia. *Molecular Psychiatry*, *27*(4), pp. 1920–35.

39. Meslier, V., Laiola, M., Roager, H. M., et al., 2020. Mediterranean diet intervention in overweight and obese subjects lowers plasma cholesterol and causes changes in the gut microbiome and metabolome independently of energy intake. *Gut*, *69*(7), pp. 1258–68.

40. Kishi, T., Yoshimura, R., Ikuta, T., et al., 2017. Brain-derived neurotrophic factor and major depressive disorder: evidence from meta-analyses. *Frontiers in Psychiatry*, 8, p. 308.

41. Sánchez-Villegas, A., et al., 2011. The effect of the Mediterranean diet on plasma brain-derived neurotrophic factor (BDNF) levels: the PREDIMED-NAVARRA randomized trial. *Nutritional Neuroscience*, *14*(5), pp. 195–201.

42. Arjmand, G., Abbas-Zadeh, M. and Eftekhari, M. H., 2022. Effect of MIND diet intervention on cognitive performance and brain structure in healthy obese women: a randomized controlled trial. *Scientific Reports*, *12*(1), p. 2871.

43. Carvalho, K. M. B., Ronca, D. B., Michels, N., et al., 2018. Does the Mediterranean diet protect against stress-induced inflammatory activation in European adolescents? The HELENA study. *Nutrients*, *10*(11).

44. Bonaccio, M., Di Castelnuovo, A., Costanzo, S., et al., 2018. Mediterranean-type diet is associated with higher psychological resilience in a general adult population: findings from the Moli-sani study. *European Journal of Clinical Nutrition*, *72*(1), pp. 154–60.

45. Shively, C. A., Appt, S. E. and Register, T. C., 2020 Mediterranean diet, stress resilience, and aging in nonhuman primates. *Neurobiology of Stress*, 13, p. 100254.

46. Razquin, C., Ruiz-Canela, M., Toledo, E., et al., 2021. Metabolomics of the tryptophan-kynurenine degradation pathway and risk of atrial fibrillation and heart failure: potential modification effect of Mediterranean diet. *The American Journal of Clinical Nutrition*, *114*(5), pp. 1646–54.

47. Huang, M., Shah, A. and Su, S., 2018. Association of depressive symptoms and heart rate variability in Vietnam war-era twins: a longitudinal twin difference study. *JAMA Psychiatry*, *75*(7), pp. 705–12.

48. Dai, J., 2010. Mediterranean dietary pattern is associated with improved cardiac autonomic function among middle-aged men: a twin study. *Circulation: Cardiovascular Quality and Outcomes*, *3*(4), pp. 366–73.

49. Chen, S., Zhang, H., Pu, H., et al., 2014. n-3 PUFA supplementation benefits microglial responses to myelin pathology. *Scientific Reports*, *4*(1), p. 7458.

50. Gallardo-Fernández, M., Hornedo-Ortega, R. and de Pablos, R. M., 2019. Hydroxytyrosol decreases LPS- and α-synuclein-induced microglial activation in vitro. *Antioxidants (Basel)*, *9*(1).

51. Mörkl, S., Stell, L., Buhai, D. V., et al., 2021. 'An apple a day'? Psychiatrists, psychologists and psychotherapists report

poor literacy for nutritional medicine: international survey spanning 52 countries. *Nutrients*, 13(3).

52. Danan, A., Westman, E. C., Saslow, L. R., et al., 2022. The ketogenic diet for refractory mental illness: a retrospective analysis of 31 inpatients. *Frontiers in Psychiatry, 13*.

53. Wade, A. T., Davis, C. R., Dyer, K. A., et al., 2018. A Mediterranean diet supplemented with dairy foods improves markers of cardiovascular risk: results from the MedDairy randomized controlled trial. *The American Journal of Clinical Nutrition, 108* (6), pp. 1166–82.

54. Oldways. Mediterranean diet pyramid. https://oldwayspt.org/resources/oldways-mediterranean-diet-pyramid.

55. Cabrera-Suárez, B., Pla, J., González-Pintoet, A., et al., 2022. Effectiveness of a remote nutritional intervention to increase the adherence to the Mediterranean diet among recovered depression patients. *Nutritional Neuroscience, 10*, 1–10.

Chapter 4

Psychobiotics and Fermented Foods

Ted Dinan

Summary

Psychobiotics are bacteria that have a positive mental health benefit when ingested in adequate amounts. They act through the brain–gut–microbiota axis which is a bidirectional communication system linking gut microbes and the brain. Until relatively recently, gut microbes were viewed as commensal with no major impact on brain function. It is now clear that gut microbes produce an array of molecules which are essential for normal brain function, for example short-chain fatty acids. Over 1,000 strains of bacteria have been identified in the human gut and there is increasing evidence to support the view that psychiatric illnesses are associated with a gut dysbiosis. It is within this context that the field of psychobiotic research has emerged. Given the novel state of the field, it is not surprising that there are far more animal than human studies in the literature. However, there is growing evidence that some psychobiotics can play a role in managing stress-related disorders such as anxiety, depression and irritable bowel syndrome. So far, the major focus of psychobiotic research has been on *Lactobacilli* and *Bifidobacteria*, but there is potential to use a far broader range of bacteria. Psychobiotics have the ability to influence the core stress axis, namely the hypothalamic–pituitary–adrenal axis, reduce inflammatory responses, elevate brain trophic factors and impact positively on a 'leaky gut'. Overall, the field represents a paradigm shift in psychiatry.

Probiotic Background

From ancient times, humans have used fermented foods and drinks to maintain physical and mental health, even though there was no understanding as to how fermented food produced such effects (1). *Douchi*, a fermented soybean, is described in the *Yellow Emperor's Classic of Internal Medicine* dating back as far as 475 BC. It was used to relieve psychiatric symptoms such as fatigue and insomnia (2). A 'yellow dragon soup' or 'golden syrup' made of fermented or dry stool was traditionally used to treat abdominal discomfort in ancient China (3). Louis Pasteur is regarded as the father of fermentation science, but he never associated the microbes involved in fermentation with significant health benefits. However, Elie Metchnikoff, who for a time worked with Pasteur, observed that villagers living in the Caucasus mountains drank fermented yogurt on a regular basis (4). Studying the drink, he found it contained *Lactobacillus bulgaricus* and speculated that this type of bacteria improved the villagers' well-being and resulted in an extended lifespan. Although popular immediately after publication, the theory was largely ignored by the medical and scientific community until a recent resurgence in interest over the past 20 years. The gut microbiome is now recognised to play a critical role in health and disease. Several definitions of probiotics have been put forward over the decades. Fuller defined a probiotic as 'A live microbial feed supplement which beneficially affects the host animal by improving its intestinal microbial balance' (5, 6).

On 26 April 1910, George Porter Philips read a paper in the UK at the Spring Meeting of the South East Division in Hanwell. The paper, which was never published in full, was entitled 'The Treatment of Melancholia by the Lactic Acid Bacillus'. His observations seem to have gone largely ignored. Subsequent decades saw no overlap between psychiatry and microbiology but did witness developments in psychopharmacology and psychological treatments such as psychoanalysis. Over 100 years after Philips' paper, Dinan and colleagues at APC Microbiome Ireland introduced the concept of a psychobiotic (7). They defined a psychobiotic as a type of bacteria that produced a positive mental health benefit when ingested in adequate amounts. They proposed that such bacteria can have psychotropic effects. However, prebiotics, usually fibres that promote the growth of beneficial bacteria, can also have psychobiotic properties. As a result, the definition of psychobiotics has been expanded to cover prebiotics (8).

Definitions

Gut microbiota is the range of microorganisms found in the gut, including bacteria, archaea, fungi and viruses.

Probiotics are characterised as living bacteria which, in adequate amounts, are beneficial for health (9). Dosage is described in colony-forming units (CFUs). Most studies use lactic acid bacteria and *Bifidobacteria* but some use probiotic yeast strains such as *Saccharomyces boulardii*. New potential probiotics are arising outside these genera. Probiotics should suppress pathogenic bacteria and contribute to a healthy gut environment by interacting with the host microbiota and the immune system. They can have several effects on host health, including improvements in metabolism, immunity, endocrine and brain function.

Prebiotics are food constituents such as non-digestible carbohydrates and dietary fibre (10). They are selectively fermented in the large intestine and specifically boost the growth of health-promoting bacteria. Prebiotics include resistant starch, inulin, fructooligosaccharides (FOS), galactooligosaccharides (GOS) and soluble dietary fibres. They are found in fruit and vegetables such as asparagus, potatoes, broccoli and chicory and also in nuts and seeds. These compounds are frequently low in the Western-style diet.

Synbiotics are defined as synergistic combinations of probiotics and prebiotics which work to beneficially affect the host (11). They were originally created to counteract difficulties with the survival of probiotics in the gastrointestinal tract and should have a superior impact compared to the activity of a single component. Synbiotics selectively improve the survival and implantation of health-promoting bacteria in the gut. There is little published research on the use of synbiotics in the management of mental illnesses. However, considering the vast number of combinations of prebiotics and probiotics for the modulation of the gut microbiota, this area seems ripe for exploitation.

The term *postbiotics* comprises bioactive substances such as short-chain fatty acids (SCFAs) which are produced by probiotics and components of the bacterial cell wall (12). As soluble factors made by probiotics, postbiotics alone are sufficient to elicit the desired response in the host (13). An example of a postbiotic is butyrate,

Table 4.1 Bacteria frequently viewed as possessing psychobiotic activity

Lactobacillus species	Bifidobacterium species	Others
• plantarum	• breve	• Akkermansia muciniphila
• acidophilus	• bifidum	• Streptococcus salivarius (subspecies
• casei (subspecies	• longum	thermophilus)
rhamnosus)	• infantis	• Lactococcus lactis (subspecies lactis)
• casei Shirota	• adolescentis	• Lactococcus lactis (subspecies cremoris)
• bulgaricus	• lactis	• Enterococcus faecium
• johnsonii	• animalis	• Leuconostocmesenterioides (subspecies
• reuteri		dextranium)
• rhamnosus		• Proprionibacterium freudenreichii
• brevis		• Pediococcus acidilactici
• fermentum		• Saccharomyces boulardii
• lactis		• Escherichia coli Nissle 1917
• salivarius		• Bacteroides thetaiotaomicron
		• Clostridium Butyricum
		• Blautia stercoris

which exerts neuropharmacological effects and influences the brain indirectly via immune and vagal nerve regulation, as well as possible epigenetic modulation (14). Initial studies suggest that postbiotics exert a positive impact on inflammatory markers (13). In addition, we have found that certain postbiotics exhibit promising test-specific antidepressant and anxiolytic effects in animal models (15).

Psychobiotics, as described earlier, are probiotics or prebiotics with a positive impact on mental health (7). Psychobiotic action can be delivered either as ingestion of a single strain of a bacterium or a multiple-strain probiotic cocktail, termed a polybiotic. Furthermore, even dead probiotic microorganisms can induce immune and antidepressant-like effects. Such dead strains are termed parabiotics (7, 16). For example, oxytocin-mediated effects of Lactobacillus reuteri were achievable when using a lysed sterile Lactobacillus reuteri preparation alone (17), and dead Lactobacillus strains have been shown to reduce glucocorticoid levels (18) (see Table 4.1).

Psychobiotic Characteristics

What are the desirable characteristics of an ideal psychobiotic? We have previously characterised the ideal psychobiotic as possessing the following features (1, 14, 19–22):

- Resistance against stomach acids and bile, enabling it to reach the large intestine in adequate quantities. If the bacteria are unduly acid or bile sensitive, they will be destroyed in the upper gastrointestinal tract and have little or no impact.
- Sufficient attachment to the intestinal mucosa. In the absence of such attachment, even transient, it is likely the bacteria will pass from mouth to anus without adequate activity. It should be noted that probiotic bacteria, as a general rule, do not colonise the intestine.
- Metabolic activity in the gastrointestinal tract, such as the production of neurotransmitters and SCFAs. Metabolic activity is considered by many researchers as

the key to functionality, but this ignores the fact that in certain circumstances dead bacteria can produce significant effects.

- Antimicrobial activity against pathogens. This is probably more important in treating infections such as *C. difficile* than in establishing psychobiotic activity.
- Reduction of the pH value in the colon.
- Easy application and palatability. A formulation with low palatability is likely to be poorly received by patients.
- Resistance against the antimicrobial effects of concomitant (psychotropic) medication.
- Anti-inflammatory and immune-modulating effects. There is increasing evidence to indicate that in disorders such as depression, these characteristics are fundamental.
- Ability to strengthen the intestinal barrier. Altered gut barrier function is increasingly viewed as a characteristic of stress-related disorders. The ability to impact a 'leaky gut' is seen by many as essential in psychobiotic development.
- Ability to act directly or indirectly as epigenetic modulators and thus alter gene expression. SCFAs such as butyrate, by acting as histone deacetylase (HDAC) inhibitors, bring about epigenetic modulation.

Key Bacterial Genes

Just as certain genes render bacteria pathogenic, it is likely that clusters of genes provide mental health benefits. The essential genes for effective psychobiotics have yet to be identified. It may be that at some stage in the future, the ideal psychobiotic will be a genetically modified organism containing genes from several different bacteria. Until then, cocktails of bacteria may be more effective than single strains in producing health benefits. A strategy for identifying psychobiotic bacteria was outlined by Bambury and colleagues (23).

Psychobiotics and Stress

Much of the animal and human studies have focussed on stress, which is a risk factor for mental illness but not an illness in its own right. As a result, much of the focus has been on stress in healthy subjects. Allen and colleagues tested whether psychobiotic consumption could alter the stress response, cognition and brain activity patterns (24). In a within-subjects design, healthy volunteers completed cognitive assessments and resting electroencephalography and were exposed to a socially evaluated cold pressor test at baseline, post-placebo and post-psychobiotic. Increases in cortisol output and subjective anxiety in response to the socially evaluated cold pressor test were attenuated by the psychobiotics. Furthermore, daily reported stress was reduced by psychobiotic consumption, and there was a significant correlation between the reduction in perceived stress and the reduction in cortisol. The authors also observed subtle improvements in hippocampus-dependent visuospatial memory performance, as well as enhanced frontal midline electroencephalographic mobility following psychobiotic consumption. These subtle but clear benefits are in line with the predicted impact from pre-clinical screening studies. The results indicate that consumption of *B. longum 1714* is associated with reduced stress and improved memory.

The same bacterial strain was used in a sleep study. A randomised, placebo-controlled, repeated measures, cross-over intervention was conducted to examine the effects of a psychobiotic. Twenty male students participated in this study. Post-intervention assessments took place during the university exam period, which was used as a naturalistic chronic stressor. Self-reported measures of stress, depression, sleep quality, physical activity, gastrointestinal symptoms, cognition and mood were assessed by questionnaire. In addition, tests from the Cambridge Neuropsychological Test Automated Battery (CANTAB) were administered to all participants. Stress and depression scores increased in both placebo- and probiotic-treated groups during the exam period. While overall sleep quality and duration of sleep improved significantly in the psychobiotic-treated group during exam stress compared with the placebo-treated group, *B. longum 1714*, similar to placebo treatment, showed no efficacy in improving measures of working memory, visual memory, sustained attention or perception. Overall, *B. longum 1714* shows promise in improving sleep quality and duration.

Not all psychobiotic studies on stress have proved positive. Kelly and colleagues determined the impact of *L. rhamnosus* (JB1) on stress-related behaviours, physiology, inflammatory response, cognitive performance and brain activity patterns in healthy male participants. A randomised, placebo-controlled, cross-over design was employed. There was no significant effect of psychobiotic treatment on measures of mood, anxiety, stress or sleep quality and no significant effect of psychobiotic over placebo on subjective stress measures or the hypothalamic–pituitary–adrenal (HPA) response. The results sharply contrast with the positive findings in rodent studies (see Figure 4.1).

Stress
Studies show that many psychobiotics reduce stress levels e.g. *Bifidobacterium longum* 1714

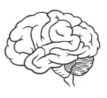

Consequences of dysbiosis
↑inflammatory cytokines
↑cortisol
Altered short-chain fatty acids
Altered gut barrier
↓BDNF

Anxiety
Strong link with dysbiosis
Bifidobacterium infantis effective in IBS

Depression
↓ microbial diversity
Lactobacillus helveticus and *Bifidobacterium longum* strains may be effective in treatment

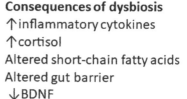

Dysbiosis

Figure 4.1 Changes induced by a gut dysbiosis in stress-related disorders. Examples of psychobiotics used to treat stress, anxiety and depression are provided.

Psychobiotics and Anxiety

Anxiety disorders such as panic disorder and generalised anxiety disorder are very common and seem to be on the increase. A major epidemiological study by Bruch and colleagues found that intestinal infection was associated with a significantly increased odds ratio of an anxiety disorder (25), thus strengthening the link between intestinal dysbiosis and anxiety. That the gut microbiome is altered in some anxiety states has been demonstrated in a recent study of social anxiety disorder. However, so far there is only limited evidence for anxiolytic effects of psychobiotics in humans (26, 27) as most studies in humans have focussed on stress rather than anxiety disorders. In animal models of obsessive-compulsive disorder, *Lactobacillus rhamnosus* has been found effective, and in a single-case report on *Saccharomyces boulardi*, the yeast was reported as beneficial. There is now a large literature on the use of psychobiotics in the treatment of irritable bowel syndrome (IBS), which is frequently comorbid with anxiety. The general consensus is that certain bacterial strains are effective in treating IBS. *Bifidobacterium infantis 35624* has been extensively studied and demonstrated as effective.

Psychobiotics and Depression

Depression is the most common mood disorder and globally is the most important of all psychiatric conditions. In a study of patients with major depression, we found significant differences in the microbiota when compared with healthy controls (28). In a large-scale study, Valles-Colomer and colleagues studied the relationship between gut bacteria and quality of life and depression (29). They combined faecal microbiome data with primary care physician diagnoses of depression from 1,054 individuals enrolled in the Flemish Gut Flora Project. They found specific groups of bacteria that positively or negatively correlated with quality of life. Two bacterial genera, *Coprococcus* and *Dialister*, were depleted in patients with depression, whether or not they were taking antidepressants. Butyrate-producing bacteria were consistently associated with better quality-of-life measures. The findings were replicated in an independent cohort of 1,063 individuals from the Dutch LifeLinesDEEP cohort and in a sample of clinically depressed patients at the University Hospitals Leuven, Belgium. The results provide the first population-based evidence for microbiome links with mental health. Given these findings, it is worth remembering that the first antidepressants were anti-tuberculous drugs and that current antidepressants also act on the gut microbiota.

Currently, patients are treated either with pharmacotherapy or psychological interventions. Many patients are unwilling to accept pharmacological interventions but would accept a natural alternative such as a psychobiotic. In a national cross-sectional study, Kim and colleagues found that fermented food consumption was associated with lower severity and prevalence of depression (30). Akkasheh and colleagues (31) demonstrated a significant amelioration of depressive symptoms after psychobiotics using the Beck Depression Inventory (BDI-II) in 40 patients diagnosed with major depression. Furthermore, they provided evidence for other physiological changes; not only were psychobiotics capable of significantly decreasing serum insulin but they also demonstrated a positive effect on the increase of glutathione, a relevant antioxidant. Also observed was a decrease in the C-reactive protein (CRP), the acute phase protein. Similar conclusions were drawn by Kazemi and colleagues (32), who administered *Lactobacillus helveticus* and *Bifidobacterium longum* for 8 weeks to patients with mild to moderate depression. They found significant decreases in the BDI scores. Moreover, they reported a decrease in the kynurenine to tryptophan ratio and an increase in the tryptophan to isoleucine ratio after psychobiotic administration, a further indication of an interaction between psychobiotics and the underlying pathophysiology of depression (33).

Mohammadi and colleagues (34) compared the effects of probiotic yogurt and freeze-dried capsule probiotics with those of a placebo. Both probiotic forms of administration attained a diminution of the Depression, Anxiety and Stress (DASS)-42 score in comparison with the placebo group, with the yogurt and the capsule group being equally successful. However, it must be stressed that Mohammadi and colleagues did not focus on patients with a diagnosis of major depression, as they examined the effects of probiotics on the mental health of petrochemical workers, though a significant number of these workers had increased DASS-42 scores at baseline and might be considered as stressed and/or in a depressed mood.

In marked contrast to the latter findings, neither Rudzki and colleagues nor Rao and colleagues could provide clear evidence for direct antidepressant effects of psychobiotics (35, 36). Interestingly Rudzki and colleagues did show that an 8-week application of *Lactobacillus plantarum LP299 v* led to a significant improvement of cognitive functions in depressive patients (35).

Schaub and colleagues (37) conducted the first randomised controlled trial to determine whether short-term, high-dose probiotic supplementation reduces depressive symptoms and gut-microbial and neural changes in depressed patients. Patients with major depression took either a multi-strain probiotic supplement or placebo over 31 days in addition to treatment as usual. Assessments occurred at baseline, immediately after and again 4 weeks after the intervention. The Hamilton Depression Rating Scale (HAM-D) was used as the primary outcome measure. Quantitative microbiome profiling and neuroimaging were used to detect changes along the brain–gut–microbiota axis. In the sample that completed the intervention (probiotics N = 21, placebo N = 26), HAM-D scores decreased over time and interactions between time and group indicated a stronger decrease in the probiotics relative to the placebo group. Probiotics maintained microbial diversity and increased the abundance of the genus *Lactobacillus*, indicating the effectivity of the probiotics in increasing specific taxa. The increase of *Lactobacillus* was associated with decreased depressive symptoms in the probiotics group. Finally, putamen activation in response to neutral faces was significantly decreased after the probiotic intervention.

Musazadeh and colleagues (38) published a recent umbrella meta-analysis of psychobiotics in treating depression. They proposed a decisive impact of probiotics on depressive symptoms. The multiple international databases were searched up to July 2021. The pooled data indicated that probiotic supplementation significantly reduced depression symptoms. Subgroup analysis of studies with intervention duration of more than 8 weeks and dosage greater than 10×10^9 CFUs demonstrated a more robust effect of probiotics on decreasing depression symptoms. They noted significant between-study heterogeneity in which dosage was a major issue.

A lack of appropriate dose–response studies is undoubtedly a limitation in all psychobiotic studies to date.

How Do Psychobiotics Work?

Although the connections between gut microbes and the brain have been likened to a 'black box' (39), the mechanisms of psychobiotic action are gradually being unravelled, as is their influence on psychiatric symptoms. The architecture of psychobiotic–gut–brain-communication is complex and includes metabolic, neural, endocrine and immunological pathways. A considerable amount of research has described the influence of psychobiotics on a wide range of central processes such as neurogenesis, neuropeptide expression, inflammation and neurotransmission (40). Nonetheless, it has to be borne in mind that the majority of published studies on this topic describe pathways in rodent models (41), and major clinical conclusions from rodent studies cannot always be drawn. Some important studies have failed to replicate rodent data in humans (42) and it is clear that far more human research is required in the field.

The following mechanisms of psychobiotic action via the gut–brain axis have been proposed:

- Suppression of the HPA axis
- Production of neurotransmitters
- Modulation of brain-derived neurotrophic factor (BDNF) and oxytocin
- Adjustment of vagal tone
- Production of postbiotics (SCFAs)
- Continuity of the intestinal barrier
- Modification of the immune system
- Interaction with gut hormones

From an evolutionary perspective, bacteria enabled the development of the human nervous system via a close symbiotic bacterial host mutualism (43). Therefore, these mechanisms are not to be seen separately or in parallel. They share a complex interconnectivity. Ongoing research is attempting to fully unravel the mechanisms through which gut bacteria can have such a distinct effect on the brain and behaviour.

Hypothalamic–Pituitary–Adrenal Axis

The HPA axis is an essential player in psychobiotic action. It is the core stress axis in humans and rodents. The inability to raise cortisol levels in response to stress is incompatible with life, as is the case in untreated Addison's disease. In 2004, Sudo and colleagues published a seminal paper showing that *Bifidobacterium infantis* reversed an exaggerated stress response with high corticosterone in rodents (44). Messaoudi and colleagues found that in healthy volunteers, the stress hormone cortisol in urine was significantly reduced following the administration of *Lactobacillus helveticus* and *Bifidobacterium longum* (21). In line with this, Desbonnet and colleagues demonstrated that *Bifidobacterium longum 35624* normalised corticosterone levels in a maternal separation model in rodents (45). More recently, *Lactobacillus kefiranofaciens ZW3* isolated from Tibetan kefir was found to regulate the HPA axis and subsequently improve depression-like behaviour in mice (46).

The HPA axis and the gut microbiota are intertwined; each system can impact the other in a regulatory manner. This can be seen in animal models of stress, where HPA-axis alterations lead to changes in microbiota composition and vice versa (47, 48). High glucocorticoid levels in humans directly and significantly impact the gut microbiota. Psychobiotics have been shown to influence cortisol levels. For example, Bimuno®-galactooligosaccharides (B-GOS) administration significantly lowered salivary cortisol awakening responses in healthy subjects. In a dot-probe task B-GOS also increased attentional vigilance to positive information, while no effects were found following FOS (49). Allen and colleagues in a placebo-controlled study found that *Bifidobacterium longum 1714* reduced salivary cortisol levels. The reduction in cortisol was significantly correlated with a perceived reduction in stress. Another strain of *Bifidobacterium longum 1472* has also been found to reduce salivary cortisol levels in a placebo-controlled study (50).

Neurotransmitters

Interestingly, there seems to be a shared chemical lexicon between the human host and the gut microbiota. Most major neurotransmitters (glutamate, serotonin, gamma-aminobutyric acid (GABA), noradrenaline, acetylcholine) are produced in the gut and are in continuous interaction with the gut–brain axis. The same neurotransmitters are involved centrally in regulating mood, behaviour and cognition. It is highly unlikely that neurotransmitters produced by psychobiotic bacteria reach the brain. Even if they did, it is certain they would not cross the blood–brain barrier. However, such neurotransmitters may influence the brain indirectly through the enteric nervous system or the vagus nerve.

Examples of neurotransmitter-generating bacteria are: *Lactobacillus*, *Escherichia* and *Bifidobacterium spp.* that produce GABA (51, 52); *Escherichia*, *Bacillus* and *Saccharomyces spp.* that produce noradrenaline (53, 54); *Candida*, *Streptococcus*, *Escherichia* and *Enterococcus spp.* that produce serotonin; *Bacillus* that produce dopamine (54); and *Lactobacillus* that produce acetylcholine (55, 56).

For example, in rodents, *Lactobacillus rhamnosus* (JB1 strain) has potent anti-anxiety effects mediated by GABA. The vagal nerve is an important modulator of GABA receptors and following vagotomy no alteration of GABA receptors is seen after *Lactobacillus rhamnosus* administration (57, 58). Interestingly, certain *Lactobacillus spp.* are also able to synthesise glutamic acid (59). Both host and bacteria (such as *Lactobacillus spp.* and *Bifidobacterium spp.*) can subsequently convert glutamate to GABA (60–62). The Human Microbiome Project recently confirmed these findings: the gut microbiome encodes glutamate decarboxylase, the enzyme that converts glutamic acid into GABA (63).

Over 95% of the body's serotonin production takes place in the enterochromaffin (EC) cells in the gastrointestinal tract (64). The brain accounts for less than 5% of the body's serotonin. The first description of a probiotic (named *C. perfringens*) modulating the production of serotonin in the gut was in 1962 (65). Some spore-forming *Clostridia* taxa can increase serotonin-biosynthesis and intestinal transit (66, 67). In addition to the direct production of serotonin, probiotics influence serotonin metabolism through a decrease in kynurenine, anthranilic acid and the 3-hydroxykynurenine to kynurenine ratio (32, 35, 68). *Bifidobacterium longum 35624* has been shown to impact on serotonin levels by increasing plasma tryptophan (45). As tryptophan is the essential precursor of serotonin and the brain has a limited storage capacity, tryptophan is acquired from dietary sources and bacterial synthesis.

Another mediator is histamine. For example, *Morganella morganii* and *E. coli* have been shown to produce biogenic amines (69), including histamine (70, 71), and *L. reuteri* was shown to modulate host gut immune function (72), as well as intestinal inflammation via the histamine H2 receptor (73).

Gut-originated neurotransmitters cross the mucosal layer of the intestine. However, as mentioned earlier, they are unlikely to have a direct effect on the brain as most of them cannot pass the blood–brain barrier (74). Nevertheless, they indirectly impact brain function (75, 76).

Brain-Derived Neurotrophic Factor

Prebiotics and probiotics have been shown to enhance molecules in the brain responsible for learning and memory, such as the trophic factor BDNF and the excitatory neurotransmitter glutamate. Research in rodent models shows that hippocampal BDNF increases after prebiotic and probiotic intake (77–80). While germ-free mice (who lack gut microbiota) have reduced BDNF levels, ingestion of a prebiotic (oligosaccharide 2-fucosyllactose) leads to increased BDNF concentrations and enhanced performance on learning and memory tests.

Even more interesting are the results from human studies. In elderly patients, *Lactobacillus helveticus* improved sustained attention and working memory (81). Allen and colleagues found that *Bifidobacterium longum 1714* produced a small but definite improvement in paired-associate learning (82). In contrast, an 8-week placebo-controlled intervention in 79 participants with *Lactobacillus helveticus* and *Bifidobacterium longum* did not produce significant alterations in peripheral BDNF (83).

Oxytocin

Oxytocin is a peptide made in the hypothalamus that influences the limbic system and the cortex (84), as well as being released as a hormone from the posterior pituitary. It has been shown to contribute to social bonding, energy metabolism and wound healing. It has a positive impact on social behaviours and improves learning and memory (85–87). It further enhances the salience of social events, while stressful events can influence oxytocin release and the connectivity of oxytocin-receptor rich areas of the brain (88).

The probiotic bacterium *Lactobacillus reuteri* was found to upregulate oxytocin (89). Additionally, the microbial lysate of *Lactobacillus reuteri* was found to upregulate endogenous oxytocin levels and improve wound healing in rodent models and humans (17). Oxytocin is considered a peptide with potential in treating some cases of autism and depression, and perhaps psychobiotics can be used to mediate such activity.

Modulation of Vagal Tone

The vagus nerve, the long, meandering nerve linking the brain and other organs, provides bidirectional communication between the gut and the brain. Gut bacteria, such as *Bifidobacterium longum*, signal directly from the gut to the brain using vagal pathways. If the vagal nerve is cut, the central behavioural effects of *Lactobacillus rhamnosus* are no longer evident (57). Furthermore, the prebiotic 2'-fucosyllactose does not enhance associative learning or hippocampal long-term potentiation (LPT) following vagotomy (79) and *Lactobacillus reuteri* no longer had an effect on social behaviour in vagotomised mice (90).

In humans, earlier reports show that vagotomy (which was done to treat peptic ulcer disease) correlated with an increase of psychiatric disorders. Vagal afferents are polymodal and therefore respond to mechanical, chemical or hormonal signals (91, 92). For example, the microbial metabolite indole can activate the vagal nerve. Also, *Lactobacillus rhamnosus* increases the firing rate of the mesenteric nerve bundle. Different bacterial strains seem to differentially influence vagal activity. Epidemiological studies in elderly patients who underwent complete rather than partial vagotomy show a reduced prevalence of Parkinson's disease, which supports the view that this disease originates in the gut.

Production of Postbiotics: Short-Chain Fatty Acids and Vitamins

SCFAs, such as butyrate and acetate, are metabolites of microbial fermentation. Many different phyla produce SCFAs, emphasising that SCFA production has been a consistent requirement for the co-evolution of host and microbe. The primary source of SCFAs is indigestible dietary fibre; other sources include the microbial breakdown of proteins and, to a minor degree, the consumption of fermented food. Three compounds, acetate, propionate and butyrate, account for 95% of SCFAs.

SCFAs work peripherally and centrally: in the periphery, they are an energy source for colonocytes; centrally, they affect G-protein-coupled receptors and behave as epigenetic modulators by histone deacetylase inhibition (93). SCFAs have psychobiotic action. For example, *Faecalibacterium prausnitzii* (ATCC 27766) increases SCFA levels and has demonstrated anxiolytic and antidepressant-like effects (94).

SCFAs can affect the permeability of the blood–brain barrier in concentrations as low as 1 μM. Consequently, the type of bacteria present and the quantity of SCFAs produced are likely to be of major importance. As well as impacting the blood–brain barrier, SCFAs also affect the permeability of the gut lining. The intestinal barrier is an enormous interface where the majority of host–microbe interactions take place with the exchange of molecules and the priming of the immune system to recognise self and non-self antigens.

An altered barrier function may lead to a 'leaky gut', allowing the passage of antigens and bacterial lipopolysaccharides (LPS) into the bloodstream. This leads to an increase of proinflammatory cytokines and immune activation. This may be relevant in psychiatric disorders such as major depression, which often show low-grade inflammation and are viewed as having a proinflammatory phenotype.

To date, there are no published human trials on the direct effects of SCFAs on psychiatric disorders. However, research involving animal models has shown that SCFAs demonstrate antidepressant-like effects as well as promoting an increase in mitochondrial function, making them a promising target for future research.

Immune Activation

The gut microbiome has been shown to regulate immune function across the lifespan. Cytokines, a group of proteins that enable intercellular communication, are set free into the bloodstream, where they may travel to the brain (95). Usually, cytokines do not cross the blood–brain barrier but signal across it. Elevated cytokines such as IL-1 and IL-6 also activate the HPA axis and lead to cortisol release. These pathways may be of particular relevance in depression (96).

One of the main psychobiotic effects is a reduction of proinflammatory cytokines and an increase in anti-inflammatory cytokines (97). Psychobiotics such as *Bifidobacteria* were shown to switch the cytokine response to an anti-inflammatory state (98). Furthermore, *Bifidobacteria* increased anti-inflammatory cytokine IL-10 and reduced proinflammatory IL-12, and these findings have also been confirmed with another psychobiotic, *Lactobacillus acidophilus* (99). In addition, *Lactobacillus rhamnosus* and *Lactobacillus helveticus* ameliorated cognition deficits and anxiety-like behaviour in a mouse model with an impairment in the adaptive immune system (100).

The vagal anti-inflammatory loop modulates circulating levels of proinflammatory cytokines. When the vagal reflex is stimulated, macrophages are activated. The gut microbiome influences T helper cells, regulatory T cells, phagocytes and innate lymphoid cells. Recently, it was demonstrated that the gut microbiome influences the immune microglia cells in the brain (101). With reduced bacterial diversity, defects in microglia maturation and microglia morphology occur together with a compromised immune response to bacterial or viral infections. An intervention with a probiotic mixture (VSL#3) led to decreased traffic of monocytes to the brain and subsequently reduced sickness behaviour (102).

Gut Hormones

As the vagus nerve does not project directly into the gut lumen, its activation is dependent on chemical signals originating from peptide hormones produced by enteroendocrine cells (EECs), including peptide YY (PYY), glucagon-like peptide 1 (GLP-1) and cholecystokinin (CCK). EECs line the gut and sense luminal contents. In response, they release peptides which act on receptors and vagal afferent fibres connected to the brain. Gut microbes can modulate the secretion of GLP-1 and PYY, thus regulating the control of food intake. A dietary supplementation of prebiotics (inulin, GOS and FOS) and psychobiotics (*Lactobacillus* strains) was shown to decrease food intake, body weight and glucose tolerance (50). Inulin, as well as FOS and GOS, increase the production of both GLP-1 and PYY, and certain *Lactobacillus* strains stimulate GLP-1 production both in vitro and in vivo.

Conclusions

The field of psychobiotic research is in its infancy. However, over the past 20 years, numerous animal studies have been published supporting the potential role of psychobiotics in treating stress-related psychiatric disorders. Several human intervention studies have been published replicating many of the animal findings, and it is established that those on a Mediterranean diet who consume fermented foods have lower rates of depression. To move the field forward, large-scale, well-powered psychobiotic studies are required at this stage. If these studies fulfil their promise, it will result in a paradigm shift in psychiatry with psychobiotics as a potential therapy, especially in milder forms of depression and anxiety.

References

1. Mörkl, S., Butler, M. I., Holl, A., Cryan, J. F. and Dinan, T. G., 2020. Probiotics and the microbiota-gut-brain axis: focus on psychiatry. *Current Nutrition Reports*, 9(3), pp. 171–82.

2. Zhang, F., Luo, W., Shi, Y., Fan, Z. and Ji, G., 2012. Should we standardize the 1,700-year-old fecal microbiota transplantation? *The American Journal of Gastroenterology*, 107 (11), p. 1755 (author reply on p. 6).

3. Zhang, F., Luo, W., Shi, Y., Fan, Z. and Ji, G., 2012. Should we standardize the 1,700-year-old fecal microbiota transplantation? *The American Journal of Gastroenterology*, 107 (11), pp. 1755.

4. McFarland, L. V., 2015. From yaks to yogurt: the history, development, and current use of probiotics. *Clinical Infectious Diseases*, 60 (suppl. 2), pp. S85–90.

5. Fuller, R., 1989. Probiotics in man and animals. *Journal of Applied Microbiology*, 66 (5), 365–78.

6. Fuller, R., 1991. Probiotics in human medicine. *Gut*, 32(4), pp. 439–42.

7. Dinan, T. G., Stanton, C. and Cryan, J. F., 2013. Psychobiotics: a novel class of psychotropic. *Biological Psychiatry*, 74(10), pp. 720–6.

8. Sarkar, A., Lehto, S. M., Harty, S., et al., 2016. Psychobiotics and the manipulation of bacteria-gut-brain signals. *Trends in Neurosciences*, 39(11), pp. 763–81.

9. Jeżewska-Frąckowiak, J., Łubkowska, B., Sobolewski, I. and Skowron, P. M., 2021. Probiotics in the times of COVID-19. *Acta Biochimica Polonica*, 68(3), pp. 393–8.

10. Gibson, G. R., 2022. Commentary on: prebiotic effects: metabolic and health benefits. *British Journal of Nutrition*, 127 (4), pp. 554–5.

11. Gomez Quintero, D. F., Kok, C. R. and Hutkins, R., 2022. The future of synbiotics: rational formulation and design. *Frontiers in Microbiology*, 13, p. 919725.

12. Batista, V. L., De Jesus, L. C. L., Tavares, L. M., et al., 2022. Paraprobiotics and postbiotics of Lactobacillus delbrueckii CIDCA 133 mitigate 5-FU-induced

intestinal inflammation. *Microorganisms*, *10*(7), p. 1418.

13. Tsilingiri, K. and Rescigno, M., 2012. Postbiotics: what else? *Beneficial Microbes*, *4* (1), pp. 101–7.

14. Stilling, R. M., van de Wouw, M., Clarke, G., et al., 2016. The neuropharmacology of butyrate: the bread and butter of the microbiota-gut-brain axis? *Neurochemistry International*, *99*, pp. 110–32.

15. van de Wouw, M., Boehme, M., Lyte, J. M., et al., 2018. Short-chain fatty acids: microbial metabolites that alleviate stress-induced brain–gut axis alterations. *The Journal of Physiology*, *596*(20), pp. 4923–44.

16. Wei, C.-L., Wang, S., Yen, J.-T., et al., 2019. Antidepressant-like activities of live and heat-killed Lactobacillus paracasei PS23 in chronic corticosterone-treated mice and possible mechanisms. *Brain Research*, *1711*, pp. 202–13.

17. Varian, B. J., Poutahidis, T., DiBenedictis, B. T., et al., 2017. Microbial lysate upregulates host oxytocin. *Brain, Behavior, and Immunity*, *61*, pp. 36–49.

18. Warda, A. K., Rea, K., Fitzgerald, P., et al., 2019. Heat-killed lactobacilli alter both microbiota composition and behaviour. *Behavioural Brain Research*, *362*, pp. 213–23.

19. Drisko, J. A., Giles, C. K. and Bischoff, B. J., 2003. Probiotics in health maintenance and disease prevention. *Alternative Medicine Review*, *8*(2), pp. 143–56.

20. Bambury, A., Sandhu, K., Cryan, J. F. and Dinan, T. G., 2018. Finding the needle in the haystack: systematic identification of psychobiotics. *British Journal of Pharmacology*, *175*(24), pp. 4430–8.

21. Messaoudi, M., Violle, N., Bisson, J. F., et al., 2011. Beneficial psychological effects of a probiotic formulation (Lactobacillus helveticus R0052 and Bifidobacterium longum R0175) in healthy human volunteers. *Gut Microbes*, *2*(4), pp. 256–61.

22. Cussotto, S., Clarke, G., Dinan, T. G. and Cryan, J. F., 2019. Psychotropics and the

microbiome: a chamber of secrets . . . *Psychopharmacology*, *236*(5), pp. 1411–32.

23. Bambury, A., Sandhu, K., Cryan, J. F. and Dinan, T. G., 2018. Finding the needle in the haystack: systematic identification of psychobiotics. *British Journal of Pharmacology*, *175*(24), pp. 4430–8.

24. Allen, A. P., Hutch, W., Borre, Y. E., et al., 2016. Bifidobacterium longum 1714 as a translational psychobiotic: modulation of stress, electrophysiology and neurocognition in healthy volunteers. *Translational Psychiatry*, *6*(11), p. e939.

25. Bruch, J. D., 2016. Intestinal infection associated with future onset of an anxiety disorder: results of a nationally representative study. *Brain, Behavior, and Immunity*, *57*, pp. 222–6.

26. Reis, D. J., Ilardi, S. S. and Punt, S. E. W., 2018. The anxiolytic effect of probiotics: a systematic review and meta-analysis of the clinical and preclinical literature. *Plos One*, *13*(6), p. e0199041.

27. Liu, R. T., Walsh, R. F. and Sheehan, A. E., 2019. Prebiotics and probiotics for depression and anxiety: a systematic review and meta-analysis of controlled clinical trials. *Neuroscience & Biobehavioral Reviews*, *102*, pp. 13–23.

28. Kelly, J. R., Borre, Y., Patterson, E., et al., 2016. Transferring the blues: depression-associated gut microbiota induces neurobehavioural changes in the rat. *Journal of Psychiatric Research*, *82*, pp. 109–18.

29. Valles-Colomer, M., Falony, G., Darzi, Y., et al., 2019. The neuroactive potential of the human gut microbiota in quality of life and depression. *Nature Microbiology*, *4*(4), pp. 623–32.

30. Kim, C. S. and Shin, D. M., 2019. Probiotic food consumption is associated with lower severity and prevalence of depression: a nationwide cross-sectional study. *Nutrition*, *63–4*, pp. 169–74.

31. Akkasheh, G., Kashani-Poor, Z., Tajabadi-Ebrahimi, M., et al., 2016. Clinical and metabolic response to probiotic administration in patients with major depressive disorder: a randomized,

double-blind, placebo-controlled trial. *Nutrition*, 32(3), pp. 315–20.

32. Kazemi, A., Noorbala, A. A., Azam, K., Eskandari, M. H. and Djafarian, K., 2018. Effect of probiotic and prebiotic vs placebo on psychological outcomes in patients with major depressive disorder: a randomized clinical trial. *Clinical Nutrition*, 38(2), pp. 522–8.

33. Kazemi, A., Noorbala, A. A. and Djafarian, K., 2020. Effect of probiotic and prebiotic versus placebo on appetite in patients with major depressive disorder: post hoc analysis of a randomised clinical trial. *Journal of Human Nutrition and Dietetics*, 33(1), pp. 56–65.

34. Mohammadi, A. A., Jazayeri, S., Khosravi-Darani, K., et al., 2016. The effects of probiotics on mental health and hypothalamic-pituitary-adrenal axis: a randomized, double-blind, placebo-controlled trial in petrochemical workers. *Nutritional Neuroscience*, 19(9), pp. 387–95.

35. Rudzki, L., Ostrowska, L., Pawlak, D., et al., 2019. Probiotic Lactobacillus plantarum 299 v decreases kynurenine concentration and improves cognitive functions in patients with major depression: a double-blind, randomized, placebo controlled study. *Psychoneuroendocrinology*, 100, pp. 213–22.

36. Rao, A. V., Bested, A. C., Beaulne, T. M., et al., 2009. A randomized, double-blind, placebo-controlled pilot study of a probiotic in emotional symptoms of chronic fatigue syndrome. *Gut Pathogens*, 1(1), p. 6.

37. Schaub, A. C., Schneider, E., Vazquez-Castellanos, J. F., et al., 2022. Clinical, gut microbial and neural effects of a probiotic add-on therapy in depressed patients: a randomized controlled trial. *Translational Psychiatry*, 12(1), p. 227.

38. Musazadeh, V., Zarezadeh, M., Faghfouri, A. H., et al., 2022. Probiotics as an effective therapeutic approach in alleviating depression symptoms: an umbrella meta-analysis. *Critical Reviews in Food Science and Nutrition*, 29, pp. 1–9.

39. Dinan, T. G., Cryan, J. F. and Stanton, C., 2018. Gut microbes and brain development

have black box connectivity. *Biological Psychiatry*, 83(2), pp. 97–9.

40. Sherwin, E., Sandhu, K. V., Dinan, T. G. and Cryan, J. F., 2016. May the force be with you: the light and dark sides of the microbiota-gut-brain axis in neuropsychiatry. *CNS Drugs*, 30(11), pp. 1019–41.

41. Dinan, T. G. and Cryan, J. F., 2017. Brain-gut-microbiota axis and mental health. *Psychosomatic Medicine*, 79(8), pp. 920–6.

42. Kelly, J. R., Allen, A. P., Temko, A., et al., 2017. Lost in translation? The potential psychobiotic Lactobacillus rhamnosus (JB-1) fails to modulate stress or cognitive performance in healthy male subjects. *Brain, Behavior, and Immunity*, 61, pp. 50–9.

43. Allen, A. P., Dinan, T. G., Clarke, G. and Cryan, J. F., 2017. A psychology of the human brain–gut–microbiome axis. *Social and Personality Psychology Compass*, 11(4), p. e12309.

44. Sudo, N., Chida, Y., Aiba, Y., et al., 2004. Postnatal microbial colonization programs the hypothalamic–pituitary–adrenal system for stress response in mice. *The Journal of Physiology*, 558(1), pp. 263–75.

45. Desbonnet, L., Garrett, L., Clarke, G., et al., 2010. Effects of the probiotic Bifidobacterium infantis in the maternal separation model of depression. *Neuroscience*, 170(4), pp. 1179–88.

46. Sun, Y., Geng, W., Pan, Y., et al., 2019. Supplementation with Lactobacillus kefiranofaciens ZW3 from Tibetan Kefir improves depression-like behavior in stressed mice by modulating the gut microbiota. *Food & Function*, 10(2), pp. 925–37.

47. Grenham, S., Clarke, G., Cryan, J. F. and Dinan, T. G., 2011. Brain-gut-microbe communication in health and disease. *Frontiers in Physiology*, 2, p. 94.

48. Eisenstein, M., 2016. Microbiome: bacterial broadband. *Nature*, 533(7603), pp. S104–6.

49. Schmidt, K., Cowen, P. J., Harmer, C. J., et al., 2015. Prebiotic intake reduces the waking cortisol response and alters emotional bias in

healthy volunteers. *Psychopharmacology (Berl.)*, 232(10), pp. 1793–801.

50. Schellekens, H., Torres-Fuentes, C., van de Wouw, M., et al., 2021. Bifidobacterium longum counters the effects of obesity: partial successful translation from rodent to human. *EBioMedicine*, 63, p. 103176.

51. Richard, H. T. and Foster, J. W., 2003. Acid resistance in Escherichia coli. *Advances in Applied Microbiology*, 52, pp. 167–86.

52. Siragusa, S., De Angelis, M., Di Cagno, R., et al., 2007. Synthesis of gamma-aminobutyric acid by lactic acid bacteria isolated from a variety of Italian cheeses. *Applied and Environmental Microbiology*, 73(22), pp. 7283–90.

53. Shishov, V. A., Kirovskaia, T. A., Kudrin, V. S. and Oleskin, A. V., 2009. Amine neuromediators, their precursors, and oxidation products in the culture of Escherichia coli K-12. *Prikladnaia Biokhimiia i Mikrobiologiia*, 45(5), pp. 550–4.

54. Tsavkelova, E. A., Botvinko, I. V., Kudrin, V. S. and Oleskin, A. V., 2000. Detection of neurotransmitter amines in microorganisms with the use of high-performance liquid chromatography. *Doklady Biochemistry and Biophysics*, 372 (1–6), pp. 115–17.

55. Lyte, M., 2013. Microbial endocrinology in the microbiome-gut-brain axis: how bacterial production and utilization of neurochemicals influence behavior. *PLoS Pathogens*, 9(11), p. e1003726.

56. Lyte, M., 2014. Microbial endocrinology and the microbiota-gut-brain axis. *Advances in Experimental Medicine and Biology*, 817, pp. 3–24.

57. Bravo, J. A., Forsythe, P., Chew, M. V., et al., 2011. Ingestion of Lactobacillus strain regulates emotional behavior and central GABA receptor expression in a mouse via the vagus nerve. *Proceedings of the National Academy of Sciences of the United States of America*, 108(38), pp. 16050–5.

58. Dhakal, R., Bajpai, V. K. and Baek, K.-H., 2012. Production of GABA (γ-aminobutyric acid) by microorganisms: a review. *Brazilian Journal of Microbiology*, 43(4), pp. 1230–41.

59. Zareian, M., Ebrahimpour, A., Bakar, F. A., et al., 2012. A glutamic acid-producing lactic acid bacteria isolated from Malaysian fermented foods. *International Journal of Molecular Sciences*, 13(5), pp. 5482–97.

60. Smith, K. T., Singh, B. and Elliott, J. F., 1992. Escherichia coli has two homologous glutamate decarboxylase genes that map to distinct loci. *Journal of Bacteriology*, 174 (18), pp. 5820–6.

61. Strandwitz, P., Kim, K. H., Terekhova, D., et al., 2019. GABA-modulating bacteria of the human gut microbiota. *Nature Microbiology*, 4(3), pp. 396–403.

62. Barrett, E., Ross, R. P., O'Toole, P. W., et al., 2012. γ-Aminobutyric acid production by culturable bacteria from the human intestine. *Journal of Applied Microbiology*, 113(2), pp. 411–17.

63. Pokusaeva, K., Johnson, C., Luk, B., et al., 2017. GABA-producing Bifidobacterium dentium modulates visceral sensitivity in the intestine. *Neurogastroenterology and Motility*, 29(1).

64. Foster, J. A., Rinaman, L. and Cryan, J. F., 2017. Stress and the gut-brain axis: regulation by the microbiome. *Neurobiology of Stress*, 7, pp. 124–36.

65. Beaver, M. H. and Wostmann, B. S., 1962. Histamine and 5-hydroxytryptamine in the intestinal tract of germ-free animals, animals harbouring one microbial species and conventional animals. *British Journal of Pharmacology and Chemotherapy*, 19, pp. 385–93.

66. Yano, J. M., Yu, K., Donaldson, G. P., et al., 2015. Indigenous bacteria from the gut microbiota regulate host serotonin biosynthesis. *Cell*, 161(2), pp. 264–76.

67. Reigstad, C. S., Salmonson, C. E., Rainey, J. F., 3rd, et al., 2015. Gut microbes promote colonic serotonin production through an effect of short-chain fatty acids on enterochromaffin cells. *The FASEB Journal*, 29(4), pp. 1395–1403.

68. Mohammadi, A. A., Jazayeri, S., Khosravi-Darani, K., et al., 2016. The effects of probiotics on mental health and hypothalamic–pituitary–adrenal axis: a randomized, double-blind, placebo-

controlled trial in petrochemical workers. *Nutritional Neuroscience*, 19(9), pp. 387–95.

69. Pugin, B., Barcik, W., Westermann, P., et al., 2017. A wide diversity of bacteria from the human gut produces and degrades biogenic amines. *Microbial Ecology in Health and Disease*, 28(1), p. 1353881.

70. Kim, S. H., Ben-Gigirey, B., Barros-Velazquez, J., Price, R. J. and An, H., 2000. Histamine and biogenic amine production by Morganella morganii isolated from temperature-abused albacore. *Journal of Food Protection*, 63(2), pp. 244–51.

71. Behling, A. R. and Taylor, S. L., 1982. Bacterial histamine production as a function of temperature and time of incubation. *Journal of Food Science*, 47(4), pp. 1311–1314.

72. Ferstl, R., Frei, R., Schiavi, E., et al., 2014. Histamine receptor 2 is a key influence in immune responses to intestinal histamine-secreting microbes. *The Journal of Allergy and Clinical Immunology*, 134(3), pp. 744–6.

73. Gao, C., Major, A., Rendon, D., et al., 2015. Histamine H2 Receptor-mediated suppression of intestinal inflammation by probiotic Lactobacillus reuteri. *mBio*, 6(6), pp. e01358–15.

74. Donovan, M. H. and Tecott, L. H., 2013. Serotonin and the regulation of mammalian energy balance. *Frontiers in Neuroscience*, 7, p. 36.

75. Mawe, G. M. and Hoffman, J. M., 2013. Serotonin signalling in the gut: functions, dysfunctions and therapeutic targets. *Nature Reviews Gastroenterology & Hepatology*, 10(8), pp. 473–86.

76. Shajib, M. S., Baranov, A. and Khan, W. I., 2017. Diverse effects of gut-derived serotonin in intestinal inflammation. *ACS Chemical Neuroscience*, 8(5), pp. 920–31.

77. Burokas, A., Arboleya, S., Moloney, R. D., et al., 2017. Targeting the microbiota-gut-brain axis: prebiotics have anxiolytic and antidepressant-like effects and reverse the impact of chronic stress in mice. *Biological Psychiatry*, 82(7), pp. 472–87.

78. Savignac, H. M., Corona, G., Mills, H., et al., 2013. Prebiotic feeding elevates central brain derived neurotrophic factor, N-methyl-D-aspartate receptor subunits and D-serine. *Neurochemistry International*, 63(8), pp. 756–64.

79. Vazquez, E., Barranco, A., Ramirez, M., et al., 2016. Dietary 2'-fucosyllactose enhances operant conditioning and long-term potentiation via gut-brain communication through the vagus nerve in rodents. *Plos One*, 11(11), p. e0166070.

80. Desbonnet, L., Garrett, L., Clarke, G., Bienenstock, J. and Dinan, T. G., 2008. The probiotic Bifidobacteria infantis: an assessment of potential antidepressant properties in the rat. *Journal of Psychiatric Research*, 43(2), pp. 164–74.

81. Chung, Y.-C., Jin, H.-M., Cui, Y., et al., 2014. Fermented milk of Lactobacillus helveticus IDCC3801 improves cognitive functioning during cognitive fatigue tests in healthy older adults. *Journal of Functional Foods*, 10, pp. 465–74.

82. Allen, H. W., Borre, Y. E., Kennedy, P. J., et al., 2016. Bifidobacterium longum 1714 as a translational psychobiotic: modulation of stress, electrophysiology and neurocognition in healthy volunteers. *Translational Psychiatry*, 6(11), p. e939.

83. Romijn, A. R., Rucklidge, J. J., Kuijer, R. G. and Frampton, C., 2017. A double-blind, randomized, placebo-controlled trial of Lactobacillus helveticus and Bifidobacterium longum for the symptoms of depression. *Australian & New Zealand Journal of Psychiatry*, 51(8), pp. 810–21.

84. Nelson, E. E. and Panksepp, J., 1998. Brain substrates of infant–mother attachment: contributions of opioids, oxytocin, and norepinephrine. *Neuroscience & Biobehavioral Reviews*, 22(3), pp. 437–52.

85. Carter, C. S., 2014. Oxytocin pathways and the evolution of human behavior. *Annual Review of Psychology*, 65, pp. 17–39.

86. Donaldson, Z. R. and Young, L. J., 2008. Oxytocin, vasopressin, and the neurogenetics of sociality. *Science*, 322(5903), pp. 900–4.

87. Feldman, R., Monakhov, M., Pratt, M. and Ebstein, R. P., 2016. Oxytocin pathway genes: evolutionary ancient system impacting on human affiliation, sociality, and psychopathology. *Biological Psychiatry, 79*(3), pp. 174–84.

88. Crockford, C., Deschner, T., Ziegler, T. E. and Wittig, R. M., 2014. Endogenous peripheral oxytocin measures can give insight into the dynamics of social relationships: a review. *Frontiers in Behavioral Neuroscience, 8*, p. 68.

89. Erdman, S. and Poutahidis, T., 2016. Microbes and oxytocin: benefits for host physiology and behavior. *International Review of Neurobiology, 131*, pp. 91–126.

90. Sgritta, M., Dooling, S. W., Buffington, S. A., et al., 2019. Mechanisms underlying microbial-mediated changes in social behavior in mouse models of autism spectrum disorder. *Neuron, 101*(2), pp. 246–59.

91. Berthoud, H. R., Blackshaw, L. A., Brookes, S. J. and Grundy, D., 2004. Neuroanatomy of extrinsic afferents supplying the gastrointestinal tract. *Neurogastroenterology and Motility, 16* (suppl. 1), pp. 28–33.

92. Egerod, K. L., Petersen, N., Timshel, P. N., et al., 2018. Profiling of G protein-coupled receptors in vagal afferents reveals novel gut-to-brain sensing mechanisms. *Molecular Metabolism, 12*, pp. 62–75.

93. Stilling, R. M., Dinan, T. G. and Cryan, J. F., 2014. Microbial genes, brain and behaviour: epigenetic regulation of the gut-brain axis. *Genes, Brain and Behavior, 13*(1), pp. 69–86.

94. Hao, Z., Wang, W., Guo, R. and Liu, H., 2019. Faecalibacterium prausnitzii (ATCC 27766) has preventive and therapeutic effects on chronic unpredictable mild stress-induced depression-like and anxiety-like behavior in rats. *Psychoneuroendocrinology, 104*, pp. 132–42.

95. El Aidy, S., Dinan, T. G. and Cryan, J. F., 2014. Immune modulation of the brain-gut-microbe axis. *Frontiers in Microbiology, 5*, p. 146.

96. Dinan, T. G. and Cryan, J. F., 2012. Regulation of the stress response by the gut microbiota: implications for psychoneuroendocrinology. *Psychoneuroendocrinology, 37*(9), pp. 1369–78.

97. Dantzer, R., Cohen, S., Russo, S. J. and Dinan, T. G., 2018. Resilience and immunity. *Brain, Behavior, and Immunity, 74*, pp. 28–42.

98. O'Mahony, L., McCarthy, J., Kelly, P., et al., 2005. Lactobacillus and bifidobacterium in irritable bowel syndrome: symptom responses and relationship to cytokine profiles. *Gastroenterology, 128*(3), pp. 541–51.

99. Torii, A., Torii, S., Fujiwara, S., et al., 2007. Lactobacillus Acidophilus strain L-92 regulates the production of Th1 cytokine as well as Th2 cytokines. *Allergology International: Official Journal of the Japanese Society of Allergology, 56* (3), pp. 293–301.

100. Smith, C. J., Emge, J. R., Berzins, K., et al., 2014. Probiotics normalize the gut-brain-microbiota axis in immunodeficient mice. *American Journal of Physiology-Gastrointestinal and Liver Physiology, 307* (8), pp. G793–802.

101. Erny, D., Hrabe de Angelis, A. L., Jaitin, D., et al., 2015. Host microbiota constantly control maturation and function of microglia in the CNS. *Nature Neuroscience, 18*(7), pp. 965–77.

102. D'Mello, C., Le, T. and Swain, M. G., 2009. Cerebral microglia recruit monocytes into the brain in response to tumor necrosis factoralpha signaling during peripheral organ inflammation. *Journal of Neuroscience, 29*(7), pp. 2089–102.

Diet Interventions for Anxiety and Depression[*]

Heidi M. Staudacher, Scott Teasdale, Caitlin Cowan,
Rachelle Opie, Tetyana Rocks and Felice N. Jacka

Summary

Growing evidence from the field of nutritional psychiatry reveals that diet can play an important role in the prevention and/or treatment of depression and possibly anxiety. Healthy dietary patterns, traditional diets such as the Mediterranean diet and other diets such as the Dietary Approaches to Stop Hypertension (DASH) diet, and diets with anti-inflammatory potential have all been studied, with an overall finding of a reduced risk for depression for those with higher adherence to these dietary measures. However, there are several limitations to the research to date, many of which relate to the inherent challenges of studying diet. The exact interplay of mechanisms by which dietary changes can influence mood is as yet unclear, but the gut microbiome is likely intricately involved. Several other proposed pathways through which diet can modify mood include modulation of inflammatory processes, reduction in oxidative stress and modulation of the hypothalamic–pituitary–adrenal axis function. Finally, and importantly, recommendations are provided for mental health clinicians to enable translation of the evidence into practice. Mental health clinicians are well placed to provide nutrition counselling and to use clinical judgement in choosing the specific approach that reflects the needs of the patient but are encouraged to refer to a specialist dietitian where necessary.

Introduction

Growing evidence from the field of nutritional psychiatry indicates that diet can play a critical role in the prevention and/or treatment of depression and possibly anxiety. The exact interplay of mechanisms by which diet can influence mood is unclear, but the gut microbiome is likely intricately involved. Here we describe the diets and dietary patterns that have been evaluated in research, discuss the range of mechanisms potentially underlying their effect and critically evaluate the studies that test the effects of dietary interventions on mental health. Finally, and importantly, we provide recommendations for mental health clinicians to enable translation of the evidence into practice.

---

[*] Thank you to Chantelle Erwin, research assistant from the Food and Mood Centre, for drafting the figures for this chapter.

Diets Evaluated in Research

A range of specific diets and dietary patterns have been studied for their potential role in the prevention or treatment of depressive (and sometimes anxiety) symptoms. This section presents a description of each diet. Table 5.1 and Figures 5.1 and 5.2 present detailed information about the composition of the three main dietary approaches described in this section and how their composition overlaps.

Healthy Diet Pattern

A healthy diet is usually considered to be one that aligns with the national recommended dietary guidelines. These guidelines are developed based on scientific evidence about nutrients essential to health and the intake required to prevent nutritional deficiency, as well as evidence for the intake of specific dietary constituents and reduced risk of chronic disease. National dietary guidelines evolve over time as scientific nutrition knowledge expands. In terms of current dietary guidelines, the universal key messages from national dietary guidelines across the globe are to include plenty of vegetables, fruit and legumes in the diet and to reduce the intake of foods high in saturated fat, added salt or added sugar (1).

Table 5.1 Major food group serve recommendations for diets that have been evaluated for their role in improving symptoms of anxiety and/or depression

	Food group	Healthy diet	Mediterranean diet	DASH diet
Daily serves	Fruit	2	≥3	4–5
	Vegetables	2.5–6	≥2	3–5
	Wholegrains	3–6	-	6–8
	Dairy	2–3	-	2–3
	Olive oil or unsaturated fats	0.5–2 tbs	2–3 tbs	0.4–0.6 tbs
	Combined protein(e.g. meat, fish, poultry, meat alternatives)	2–3	-	≤2
Weekly serves	Nuts and seeds	-	≥3	3–5
	Legumes	-	≥3	-
	Fish	-	≥3	-
	Poultry	-	2–3	-
	Red meat	-	≤1	-
	Alcohol	≤10–14	≥7	-
	Extras	0–3	≤2	≤5

Data presented for the healthy diet is based on national dietary guidelines for the UK (118), USA (119) and Australia (AUS), for the Mediterranean diet from the seminal PREDIMED trial (120), and for the Dietary Approaches to Stop Hypertension (DASH) diet as outlined in the dietary guidelines for the USA (119). Recommended food group servings vary for a healthy diet due to nutrient needs based on age, gender, activity level and weight. Portion sizes varied across all three diets (e.g. 1 serve fruit = 80 g fresh fruit in UK, 150 g or 1 medium piece in AUS).

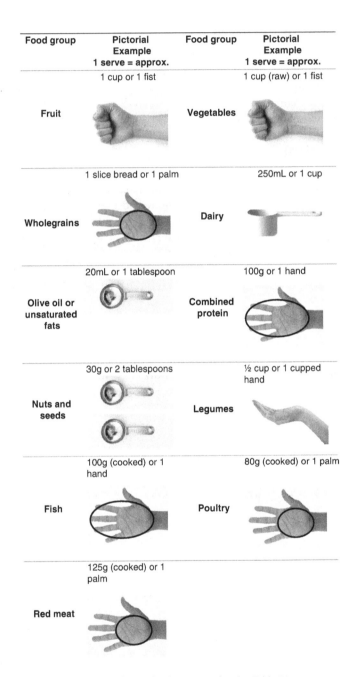

Figure 5.1 Serve size recommendations for key food groups outlined in Table 5.1.

In research, the 'healthiness' of a person's diet is often rated using a specific validated diet quality index, such as the Healthy Eating Index (HEI) (2) or versions thereof (e.g. alternate HEI). Practically speaking, the diet quality score is calculated through diet

Mediterranean Diet

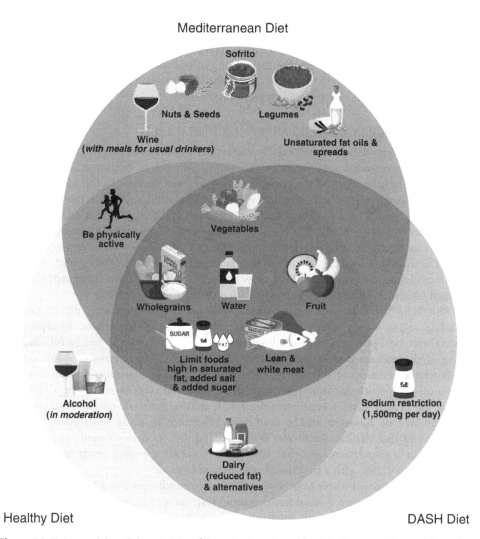

Healthy Diet   DASH Diet

Figure 5.2 Unique and shared characteristics of three diets investigated for their effect on anxiety and depression. This provides a summary of the overlap between the diets that have been investigated. Foods and food groups are presented once each either as 'shared' in the centre of the figure (i.e. recommended in similar quantities across diets) or 'unique' in the periphery (i.e. recommended in higher or lower quantities than the other diets). Alcohol, nuts and seeds and olive oil are among the food groups that differentiate the diets the most.

assessment by a food frequency questionnaire or diet record, followed by numerical scoring of several components according to specific scoring criteria (i.e. food groups and nutrients considered important to health and embedded in dietary guidelines), which are summed to provide a total score. A higher score represents a higher-quality diet. For example, components that positively contribute to the HEI-2015 score are vegetables, greens and beans, total fruit, whole fruit, wholegrains, dairy total protein foods, seafood, and plant proteins. Another method applied in nutrition research is to use statistical methods to identify empirically derived dietary patterns using principal component analysis or cluster analysis.

This is often used in observational research to describe individuals' intakes of particular dietary patterns, often characterised as 'healthy' or 'prudent' and 'Western' (high in saturated fat and sugar). In practice, healthy eating tests are available online and may be useful for mental health clinicians to screen the diet quality of individual diets (3, 4). For research, a diet quality tool validated in the target population or principal component analysis based on comprehensive dietary assessment is recommended (5).

The Mediterranean Diet and Other Traditional Diets

The Mediterranean diet is an extensively researched traditional dietary pattern shown to have wide-ranging health benefits including reducing the risk of cardiovascular outcomes, obesity and diabetes. The dietary pattern originated from nations in the Mediterranean regions including Greece, Cyprus, Spain and southern Italy and, as a result, there are several variants based on the local food availability, preferences and culture within each region (6). The traditional Cretan Mediterranean diet was the first diet variant to be established as protective for health and the basis for the principles of a traditional Mediterranean diet. This diet is characterised by a high intake of vegetables, legumes, fruit, wholegrains, nuts and seeds, a moderate to high intake of fish, a low intake of meat, olive oil as the principal source of added fat and moderate consumption of wine with meals (Figure 5.2).

Other behavioural recommendations are also key to the Mediterranean dietary pattern, including eating slowly without distraction, sharing meals with others, incorporating seasonal and local products and including regular physical activity (7). Successful adoption of the Mediterranean diet by non-Mediterranean populations is possible. Most studies demonstrating take-up of the diet in non-Mediterranean communities use an intensive dietitian-led approach incorporating regular support and written resources. Challenges such as the accessibility of Mediterranean foods, cultural barriers, religion and cost may be prohibitive of adoption and/or long-term adherence in some individuals. Cultural adaptation of the Mediterranean diet while maintaining its core elements may enhance adherence at a population level, but whether a modified approach leads to the disease prevention associated with a traditional version is unknown.

A range of validated scores have been used to measure adherence to a Mediterranean diet in the published literature. Several newer scoring systems recommended for use in research and practice (8) include relatively brief validated questionnaires such as the Mediterranean Diet Serving Score (MDSS) (9) and the Mediterranean Diet Adherence Screener (MEDAS) (10). These scores are calculated by summing individual dietary component scores, with a higher final score representing better adherence to a Mediterranean diet. For example, in the MDSS if an individual consumes at least one to two serves of nuts per day, they are allocated 2 points, if they consume fewer than two serves of red meat per day, they are allocated 1 point, and so on, with a maximum score of 24.

Other traditional dietary patterns with a growing evidence base for their health benefits include the Nordic diet, traditional Brazilian diet and traditional Japanese diet/Okinawa diet. The Nordic diet has similar 'plant-based' principles to the Mediterranean diet but focusses on rapeseed (canola) oil instead of olive oil. The traditional Brazilian diet has soy or corn oil as the predominant oil and includes rice and beans in main meals with small portions of red meat. The traditional Japanese diet is rich in rice, vegetables, soy products (e.g. soybeans and tofu), seafoods and fermented products such as miso and nattō. Similar to the Mediterranean diet, the Nordic and traditional Japanese diets can be evaluated by short tools (indices) created to measure adherence for research and in clinical practice. One example is the Healthy Nordic Food Index, which assigns a total score between 0 and 6 points based on (1 point per category): fish, root vegetables (carrots and swede), cabbage (including broccoli and cauliflower), apples/pears, wholegrain bread and breakfast cereals (oatmeal).

DASH Diet

The Dietary Approaches to Stop Hypertension (DASH) diet is a healthy diet pattern originally developed for the treatment of hypertension. It has demonstrated benefits for reducing the risk of cardiovascular disease (11). It encourages low salt intake and increased intake of foods rich in potassium, calcium and magnesium. It emphasises fruit, vegetables, wholegrains, nuts, seeds, legumes, low- or no-fat dairy products and lean meat. The DASH diet score considers eight components, where fruit, vegetables, legumes and nuts, whole-grain, and low-fat dairy contribute positively and meat, sodium and sweet beverages contribute negatively to the total score.

Anti-Inflammatory Diet

Many chronic, non-communicable diseases, including depression, are associated with chronic, low-grade, systemic inflammation. The exploration of known sources of inflammation including psychosocial stress, poor diet and physical inactivity suggest that inflammation at least partly mediates the risk and progression of these chronic diseases (12). Intake of a range of specific foods, nutrients and dietary constituents has been associated with lower levels of systemic inflammatory markers such as interleukins (IL): IL-1β, IL-4, IL-6 and IL-10, tumour necrosis factor, and C-reactive protein, and have therefore been described as having anti-inflammatory potential. For example, some studies of the Mediterranean-style diet, vegetarian/vegan and DASH diets have been associated with lower levels of inflammation (13). Conversely, increased intake of foods and nutrients characteristic of a Western-style diet, including foods high in sugar or saturated fat, can increase inflammatory markers (14). The Dietary inflammation Index (DII) is a literature-derived tool that attempts to encapsulate these disparate data (15). The DII scores an individual's diet through assessing intake of 45 foods, nutrients and bioactive components in the diet that have been associated with anti- or proinflammatory outcomes. Inflammatory effect scores from the literature are weighted according to study design (i.e. human studies weighted higher than *in vitro* studies). Examples of components that positively contribute to reducing the inflammation score include the macronutrients fat and carbohydrate, bioactive components such as flavanols, and foods such as ginger, garlic and onion.

Mechanisms through which Diet Influences Depression

The relationship between diet and mental health is multifaceted and complex. In part due to this complexity, as well as the relative recency of the field of nutritional psychiatry, studies examining the mechanisms for dietary impacts on mental health are still limited, much of the mechanistic research has been conducted in animal models or is restricted to the examination of specific dietary components in humans. However, there are several strong candidate mechanisms, discussed in the following sections, all of which are likely to interact with each other.

Gut Microbiome

The community of microorganisms that live within the gastrointestinal tract, known as the gut microbiome, is critical to human health. In particular, the gut microbiome plays a vital role in human digestion, extracting nutrients from foods and directly producing or stimulating production of a range of bioactive metabolites in the process (16). These include short-chain fatty acids (SCFAs), vitamins and several neuromodulators (e.g. serotonin, gamma-aminobutyric acid, catecholamines and acetylcholine (17)). Microbial production of neuroactive metabolites represents just one pathway in the complex set of bidirectional lines of communication between the microbiome and the brain, known as the microbiome–gut–brain axis, which also includes the vagus nerve, intestinal barrier and the immune system (Figure 5.3, also discussed in detail in Chapter 2 of this volume).

Gut Microbiome Is Altered in Depression

Several studies have now demonstrated that the microbiome is altered in clinical depression and anxiety, and some show abundances of certain microbiome members (or 'taxa') are correlated with symptom severity (see 18, 19 for systematic reviews). While there is substantial variability in the exact differences reported across studies, there are some consistent patterns. For example, there is consistent upregulation of several taxa with inflammatory properties, such as the opportunistic pathogen *Eggerthella* (18–20). These findings are in keeping with the literature described later on the role of inflammation in mood and anxiety disorders, as well as a growing understanding that the immune system functions as one of the key routes of microbiome–gut–brain communication. Moreover, several reviews have identified downregulation of taxa with anti-inflammatory properties or SCFA-producing capabilities in anxiety and depression (18–20). SCFAs, such as butyrate, are one of the products of microbial fermentation of indigestible carbohydrates (i.e. dietary fibre) and are involved in a range of pathways within the microbiome–gut–brain axis, including modulation of intestinal barrier permeability and immune function (21).

Diet-Induced Microbiome Modulation

The microbiome is highly responsive to changes in diet. For example, with extreme whole-diet alterations, such as switching to an animal-based (high-fat, high-protein, low-fibre) diet, significant changes in the microbiome are possible within a single day (22). Most observational studies of the Mediterranean diet report significant differences in the microbiome compared with controls, although the exact differences are inconsistent across studies (23). Intervention studies have found limited effects of the Mediterranean diet in shifting the microbiome, but this may be partly explained by inconsistent treatment adherence and variability in the initial diet and microbiome (23). Many other studies of whole-diet interventions and restriction of or supplementation with specific dietary components (e.g. fibre, food-based probiotics) have revealed changes in the relative abundance of key microbial taxa (24, 25).

Diet-Induced Microbiome Modulation and Behaviour

In animal studies, whole-diet interventions lead to changes in the microbiome together with altered behavioural outcomes. For example, a study in mice (26) demonstrated that a high-fat diet induces changes in the faecal microbiome that correlated with increased anxiety-like behaviour, supporting the idea that the microbiome may mediate diet-induced

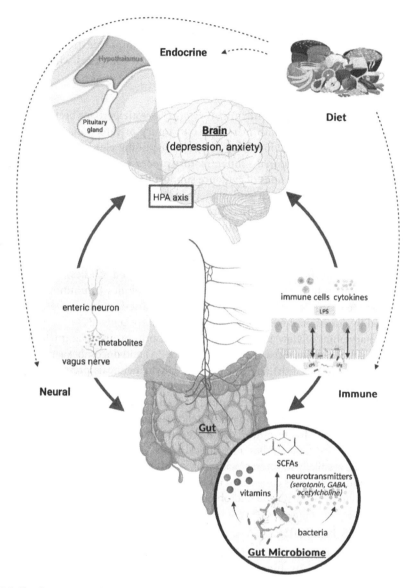

Figure 5.3 The three major pathways through which the microbiome interacts with the brain (endocrine, immune and neural).

changes in behaviour. Studies testing this hypothesis in humans are relatively scarce. A randomised controlled trial (RCT) of participants with obesity found that 16 g/d prebiotic inulin supplementation combined with a high-fibre diet for 3 months had limited effects on mood overall (27), in keeping with the findings of a systematic review of prebiotics for anxiety and depression (28). However, an exploratory analysis showed the treatment improved mood in a subset of participants who had higher baseline depression scores (27). The responders also exhibited an inflammatory profile and elevated levels of

Coprococcus in the faecal microbiome at baseline, supporting the key role of the micro-biome in the mood response to dietary fibre supplementation. However, another study in healthy individuals demonstrated fibre supplementation with polydextrose for 4 weeks did not alter mood, although cognitive flexibility was improved compared with placebo (29).

Inflammation

Immune activation and associated inflammatory processes are perhaps best known for their role in maintaining physical health in response to injury or infection. However, psycho-logical stress also elicits an inflammatory response, including elevation of cytokines (30), and this relationship is bidirectional – inflammatory processes can affect mood and psycho-logical function (12). Multiple lines of evidence support the importance of inflammation in the pathophysiology of depression and anxiety in humans. Inflammatory cytokines are commonly elevated in individuals with depression and anxiety (31, 32). Cytokines are also associated with treatment response in both anxiety and depression, cytokine levels decrease with successful treatment while higher baseline levels predict poorer treatment outcomes (33, 34). Moreover, anti-inflammatory treatments can reduce depressive symptoms (see 35 for a meta-analysis, noting the high risk of bias in reviewed studies), whereas medical treatments involving administration of inflammatory cytokines (immunotherapy) induce depressed mood (e.g. 36). Notably, the onset of such cytokine-induced depressive symptoms can be delayed by concurrent treatment with omega-3 fatty acids (37).

From a dietary point of view, several nutrients have anti- or proinflammatory effects. For example, omega-3 fatty acids eicosapentaenoic acid (EPA) and docosahexaenoic acid (DHA) (naturally occurring in oily fish) and polyphenols (phytochemicals present in many foods, including blueberries, cocoa and curcumin) have anti-inflammatory properties (38, 39). On the other hand, a diet rich in refined carbohydrates and trans-fats but low in plant foods is considered proinflammatory and is also associated with current and future risk of depression (40, 41). Conversely, the Mediterranean diet has been shown to prospectively reduce inflam-mation in both observational studies and clinical trials (42). Such diet-induced changes in inflammatory state are likely to interact with many of the other mechanisms discussed in this section. The immune system is considered a key component of the gut–brain axis, exhibiting a bidirectional relationship with the microbiome, as described earlier (43).

HPA-Axis Stress Response

The hypothalamic–pituitary–adrenal (HPA) axis is better known as the body's main stress response system. In healthy individuals, perceived threats stimulate HPA-axis activity, ultimately leading to the release of glucocorticoids (cortisol in humans, corticosterone in rodents). These stress hormones prepare the body to take action in response to threat. However, chronic stress and persistent glucocorticoid release can have neurotoxic effects, leading to hippocampal atrophy and dysregulation of the HPA axis (44). Such dysregulation is observed in the form of aberrant glucocorticoid responses across a range of psychological conditions, including depression and anxiety (45). Importantly, at least some aspects of HPA-axis function are normalised in patients who respond to pharmacological treatments for anxiety and depression (45).

Diet can impact on the HPA axis in several ways. Firstly, HPA-axis activity is dependent on energy availability, with food restriction shown to dampen HPA-axis responsiveness to acute stress in humans and rodents (46). Secondly, specific nutrients can regulate HPA-axis function. For example, one RCT in healthy adults demonstrated high-dose (3 g/d) ascorbic acid (vitamin C) reduces subjective stress ratings and leads to faster cortisol recovery after an acute stressor compared to placebo (47), while animal studies and small studies of healthy humans have found that omega-3 fatty acid supplementation dampens HPA activity compared with baseline or placebo (48–51). How diet might alter HPA-axis signalling remains unclear, but the HPA-axis involvement in gut–brain signalling has led to hypotheses that there may again be a microbial involvement in this process.

Oxidative Stress

Chronic psychological stress not only disrupts HPA-axis function but also promotes oxidative damage, which is linked to a variety of disease states. Indeed, elevated markers of oxidative stress have consistently been reported in anxiety and depression (52, 53). Successful antidepressant treatment is associated with a reduction in oxidative stress markers (serum and red blood cell malondialdehyde) (53), suggesting oxidative stress is important in the pathophysiology of depression.

With regards to diet, specific nutrients with antioxidant properties (e.g. ascorbic acid, selenium, zinc, cysteine, polyphenols) have been associated with reductions in oxidative stress in cell culture and animal studies (54, 55). In contrast, a high-fat Western-style diet increases oxidative stress markers in serum and rodent brains (56, 57). In humans, dietary antioxidant intake has been associated with reduced depression (e.g. 58). There is also some emerging evidence that antioxidant compounds can have antidepressant and anxiolytic properties in different clinical populations (e.g. major depression, obsessive-compulsive disorder and generalised anxiety disorder (59, 60, 61)).

Tryptophan Metabolism

Tryptophan is an essential amino acid that is synthesised into several important neuroactive catabolites, including serotonin and kynurenine. Kynurenine production is important not only because it occurs at the expense of serotonin production but also because kynurenine is further metabolised into other neuroactive compounds such as the neuroprotective kynurenic acid and the neurotoxic quinolinic acid. A higher kynurenine to tryptophan ratio paired with a decrease in the kynurenic acid to kynurenine ratio in major depression is consistently reported (62), alongside elevation of quinolinic acid levels in untreated depressed patients (63). Tryptophan is derived from a variety of dietary proteins (e.g. meat and fish, seeds, nuts, dairy). However, the relationship between diet and plasma tryptophan is complex and manipulating tryptophan levels via dietary means is difficult (64). Tryptophan metabolism is related to several other mechanisms discussed herein, with the microbiome playing a key role in tryptophan degradation.

Brain-Derived Neurotrophic Factor and Neurogenesis

Brain-derived neurotrophic factor (BDNF), the most abundant neurotrophin in the brain, is essential for the growth, differentiation, maintenance and survival of neurons. Supporting its role in the pathophysiology of depression, lower levels of serum BDNF have been reported in many studies of patients with major depression (65) and increased expression of BDNF has been implicated as one of the mechanisms underlying antidepressant drugs (66). Intriguingly, data from animal and human studies shows that diet has a role in modulating hippocampal volume and influencing circulating BDNF. From animal models it is clear that specific dietary components, including polyphenols, preserve hippocampal neurogenesis, whereas a Western-style diet impairs neurogenesis and lowers hippocampal BDNF levels (67). From human observational data, a healthy diet is associated with a larger hippocampal volume (68). Improvements in BDNF levels have also been reported in individuals with baseline depression after 3 years of dietary intervention. Although only a small sub-group analysis, a Mediterranean-style diet supplemented with 15 g each of walnuts and almonds per day led to higher circulating BDNF concentration compared with controls who followed a standard low-fat diet (69). The mechanisms by which diet influences neurogenesis are likely through direct and indirect pathways (i.e. via the microbiome) (67).

Obesity

The relationship between obesity and anxiety and depression is bidirectional and complex. Individuals with obesity are at higher risk of depression and obesogenic diets in rodents increase anxiety-like behaviour (70). Furthermore, individuals with depression are at higher risk of obesity (71). Obesity and mood disorders also share a series of clinical, neurobiological, genetic characteristics, including higher levels of inflammation and related cytokines. Abnormalities in HPA-axis regulation and reduced concentration of neurotransmitters involved in regulating neurological reward circuitry (e.g. serotonin) in response to diet may also be important (67). However, the nature of the association between obesity and mental disorders remains poorly understood. Importantly, it is possible to reduce depressive symptoms through dietary intervention in the absence of caloric restriction and weight change (72). Negative attitudes about weight can interfere with positive lifestyle change and weight stigma has been shown to contribute to longitudinal weight gain (73). Therefore, the goal of dietary intervention should be to improve diet quality and physical health rather than reducing excess bodyweight.

Overall, it is clear that the mechanisms for diet–mental health interactions are varied, complex and mostly interdependent (Figure 5.4). The data suggests that the association is prospective (i.e. that diet quality predicts depression incidence) rather than the reverse. This should provide hope regarding the potential utility of dietary interventions for treating depression and anxiety.

Evidence for the Efficacy of Diet Interventions in Depression and Anxiety

Healthy Diet

There is a growing body of evidence demonstrating that a healthy diet can reduce the risk or treat symptoms of depression. A 2021 synthesis of prospective observational research identified adherence to a healthy diet (based on the alternate HEI (AHEI) score) or a healthy diet based on diet pattern analysis was associated with a reduced risk of depression. This included evidence from 12 studies and over 150,000 individuals (74). A similar 2019 synthesis that also included cross-sectional studies showed HEI or AHEI diet quality indices were inversely associated with prevalence of depression (75). The strength of the evidence from these studies needs to be interpreted in the light of some challenges. The 'healthy diet' defined in studies using dietary pattern analysis was heterogeneous and

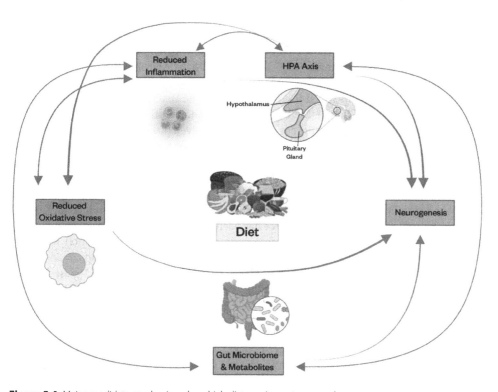

Figure 5.4 Major candidate mechanisms by which diet can impact on mood.

depended on the background culture and preferences of each population. Most studies make appropriate adjustment for confounders (e.g. physical activity, smoking).

Clinical trials in this area have also been conducted, providing important evidence that a healthy diet has a causal role in improving depressive symptomatology. In a 2019 review, 9 trials including a total of nearly 1,000 individuals evaluated the effect of increasing the healthiness of the diet on improving depressive symptoms (76). Most trials included participants with non-clinical depression and comorbidity such as obesity, diabetes or elevated cholesterol, and only one study included a clinically depressed participant group. Generally, participants were provided advice in line with healthy eating principles, some were provided practical advice on meal preparation and developing shopping lists, some used cooking demonstrations and some trials provided food for participants to enhance adherence. Overall, there was a small effect size for the effect of healthy eating interventions on reducing depressive symptoms. Interestingly, across all interventions, those that were delivered by registered dietetic/nutrition professionals were most beneficial for reducing symptoms of depression and anxiety. Because of the totality of the evidence thus far, healthy eating advice is beginning to be incorporated into lifestyle advice in clinical guidelines for mood disorders (77).

Traditional Diets: Mediterranean Diet

The Mediterranean diet has a strong evidence base for the prevention and treatment of depressive disorders. The pooled effect of four longitudinal studies with a mean follow-up period of approximately 10 years found a 33% risk reduction in the development of depression across the studies for the highest compared to the lowest Mediterranean diet adherence categories (75). To test whether modifying a person's diet so that it is more aligned with the Mediterranean diet is effective in preventing the development of a depression disorder, a multicentre, 2×2 factorial 1-year RCT was run with >1,000 people. The intervention groups included food-related behavioural activation therapy, conducted by a psychologist, based on the Mediterranean diet and multi-nutrient supplementation (together and in insolation), and the control groups received placebo and no therapy (78). In the primary analysis there was no difference in incident depression between groups, however, diet adherence scores improved only marginally in the behavioural activation groups, and therefore the role of actual dietary changes in improving depressive symptoms is unclear. After accounting for food-related behavioural activation therapy adherence, there was a significant effect, indicating that further studies should be conducted (78).

Stronger and more consistent evidence has been found for the Mediterranean diet when used adjunctive to usual care (pharmacological and psychological treatments) in people with clinical depression (79–83). The 2017 'SMILES' 12-week parallel group (n=56 adults) trial found a dietitian-delivered, modified Mediterranean diet intervention – based on the dietary guidelines for adults in Greece and the principles from the PREDIMED study but using the Australian dietary guidelines for relevance to the Australian population – was superior to a social support group in reducing depressive symptoms, with remission being achieved in 32% of the Mediterranean diet group compared to 8% in the social support group (79). The 'HELFIMED' trial (n=152 adults) found very similar results in a 6-month study with a social group control (80), whereby intervention participants received a nutrition education workshop and then six group cooking classes supplemented with take-home food hampers over the first 3 months, and fish oil capsules (900 mg DHA and 200 mg EPA per day) over the entire 6-month period (80). In both trials, improvements in Mediterranean diet adherence scores aligned with reductions in depressive symptoms (80, 81) and were found to be cost effective (82, 83). These results have translated to younger population groups as well. A 12-week (n=72) parallel group trial (Mediterranean diet vs. befriending therapy control) in young males (18–25 years) (84), and a brief 3-week trial of diet modification (focussed on national dietary guidelines with additional recommendations in line with the Mediterranean diet) in young adults (17–35 years) (85), both found a greater reduction in depressive symptoms in the Mediterranean diet group.

Other studies are now evaluating other cost-effective, scalable options using technology to reach a larger population, including those who can be difficult to reach and at times when face-to-face intervention is not possible. A single-arm cohort design study demonstrated it was feasible and acceptable to deliver an 8-week smartphone intervention to people with elevated depressive symptoms and increased adherence to the Mediterranean diet correlated with reduced depressive symptoms (86). Further, a 2-year, multicentre, RCT using remote intervention (phone call and web-based intervention) demonstrated increased adherence to the Mediterranean diet in people with depression (87).

There is reasonable consistency in the observational evidence (seven of nine studies assessed in a 2022 review) for the Mediterranean diet being protective against anxiety (88), but intervention studies in people with anxiety disorders are lacking.

Other Traditional Diets

The beneficial effect of traditional diets on depression may not be limited to the Mediterranean diet, but there is less evidence for other traditional dietary patterns. For example, a cross-sectional study of 521 Japanese men and women aged 21–67 years found a 56% risk reduction for depressive symptoms in the highest tertile of Japanese diet adherence compared to the lowest tertile (89). In a 12-week randomised trial, 149 people with severe obesity in Brazil were randomised to one of three groups: (i) 52 ml/day of extra virgin olive oil (EVOO), (ii) traditional Brazilian diet or (iii) traditional Brazilian diet with 52 ml/day of EVOO. There was a significant reduction in the depression and anxiety scores in all three groups from baseline to the end of the study and, again, bodyweight change did not influence the results (90). A small (n=16) randomised trial found that the Nordic diet as a treatment for depression is feasible and well accepted (91), providing a platform for larger efficacy trials.

DASH Diet

The DASH diet has predominantly been studied for its clinical benefits for hypertension and cardiovascular disease and is recommended in clinical practice guidelines for cardiovascular disease reduction (11). The overlapping pathophysiologies of hypertension and depression (e.g. hyperactivation of the HPA axis, oxidative stress, low-grade inflammation) spurred interest in examining whether the DASH diet might have a protective role for mood disorders. Several cross-sectional studies have investigated whether adherence to a DASH-style diet is associated with lower odds of depression and anxiety (92, 93). After controlling for potential confounders, this association was significant for anxiety but not for depression in individuals who were overweight or obese in one study of Iranian adults (92). Others only found a positive association between DASH diet adherence and a World Health Organization-developed well-being score (93). A large prospective study of the Spanish Seguimiento University of Navarra (SUN) cohort showed a moderate relationship between four DASH diet indices and depression risk over 8 years of follow-up (94), in contrast with their clearer inverse relationship between the Mediterranean dietary pattern and depression in the same cohort (95). Adding to the relative limited evidence in the observational research, only one RCT to date has studied the DASH diet and its effect on depressive symptoms. The 14-week study in 111 postmenopausal women failed to show an effect of the DASH diet on depressive scores compared with a healthy diet that had lower targets for fruit and vegetable intake (96). Overall, to date there is insufficient evidence that the DASH diet has a role in the prevention or treatment of depression.

Anti-Inflammatory Diet

People with depressive disorders appear to have dietary intakes with higher inflammatory potential based on DII scoring. An analysis of 68,879 people from the baseline phase (2007–10) of the UK Biobank study found DII scores were significantly higher for people with major depression compared to people without a serious mental illness after adjusting for a range of confounders (41). Evidence from 11 observational studies including >100,000 people demonstrated that a proinflammatory diet was associated with 1.4 times higher odds of having/developing depression in the future (97).

Similar to other dietary patterns or approaches, data for the role of dietary inflammation in anxiety disorders is limited. A study of 2,047 adults found that a proinflammatory diet is associated with 1.6 higher odds of having/developing anxiety (98). However, the direction of effect is unclear given the cross-sectional nature of the study.

The DII scoring requires measurement of an individual's intake of 45 specific foods (e.g. garlic, turmeric), nutrients (e.g. fat) and bioactive compounds (e.g. quercetin). Together these foods and nutrients would not constitute a nutritionally adequate diet, meaning it is impractical to translate this into guidance on how to follow an 'anti-inflammatory diet' (and hence why this approach is not included in Table 5.1 or Figure 5.2). This contrasts with other dietary approaches (e.g. Mediterranean and DASH diets) in which specific portion recommendations for foods and beverages are made. Evidence on anti-inflammatory diets to date has therefore relied on post hoc analysis of individuals' diets and exploring associations with health outcomes.

Limitations to the Research

There are a range of limitations to the research to date that evaluates the role of diet in treating or preventing depressive symptoms. A considerable proportion of intervention research has been conducted either in general-population samples or clinical samples with a primary physical health condition rather than in samples of people with a diagnosis of a depressive or anxiety disorder. Where individuals with a depression diagnosis are included, depression screening tools are generally used for participant selection rather than psychiatrist assessment, meaning findings cannot always be assumed to be generalisable to those with a clinical diagnosis. Additionally, response bias due to recruited participants having a high level of motivation and interest in lifestyle means that research may not represent findings relevant to a broader population group. Therefore, interventions that appear feasible and effective in initial trials may be less promising when scaled up to reach a larger proportion of the clinical population.

Other factors challenge synthesis and interpretation of studies. There is large heterogeneity of the instruments used to measure depressive symptoms and methods used to measure dietary intake or adherence to specific dietary patterns. Particularly relevant for observational studies, many studies measure dietary intake at a single timepoint, which is unlikely to truly reflect individuals' variability in eating behaviour over time. Diet intervention trials differ in the mode of delivery (e.g. verbal vs. written advice, who provides advice, use of food hampers) and intensity (frequency and number of appointments) of the diet interventions, blinding and controls used, hence there is a possibility of expectation bias. Finally, many intervention studies are short term (e.g. 12 weeks) and lack longer-term follow-up. Therefore, the ability of individuals to maintain adherence to diet interventions and their long-term effectiveness remain unclear.

Research Recommendations

Enhancing diet quality is one of a suite of lifestyle changes that can improve symptoms of depression. Future trials need to not only disentangle the effects of individual lifestyle components but also explore whether a combined intervention model (e.g. diet plus exercise intervention) is superior. Further, the efficacy of dietary modification as a sole intervention, given published studies rarely restrict the use of psychotropic medications, is still to be confirmed. The literature is also biased towards participants coming from high-income countries. The role of dietary modification is less clear in low- and middle-income countries where the rates of food insecurity can be considerably high and access to more traditional mental health care is already strained.

Symptoms central to depressive and anxiety disorders can often challenge recruitment to studies as well as engagement and adherence to behavioural interventions. Recruitment strategies should therefore aim to include a diverse range of participants, or at least clearly define the sample group when publishing findings.

The heterogeneity and generalisability of diet intervention delivery require consideration. Some elements, such as the provision of food hampers, are unlikely to be feasible when scaled to real-world implementation. Further, a better understanding of the intensity/frequency of counselling and efficacy of different delivery modes (e.g. face-to-face individualised, group, combination, telehealth or online delivery) is needed. Ideally, future trials should evaluate modes of delivery that are easily adopted and delivered at scale, and the mode of delivery and diet composition should be clearly specified.

Individuals with depression and anxiety are a heterogeneous population. Patients experience a variety of symptoms and levels of acuity, with the potential for differing triggers, different treatment approaches and associated comorbidities. This is an important consideration as the efficacy of different treatment approaches may not be equal across all people, for example, reducing inflammation may only be beneficial to the sub-group of people with depression and/or anxiety who have elevated inflammatory markers. Identification of specific biopsychosocial predictors for diet intervention will be an important step forward. Future long-term trials (6–12+ months) are needed to evaluate the intensity of longer-term intervention required to sustain clinically meaningful improvements.

Application to Practice

In the previous sections, we have reviewed various diets and dietary styles, including what constitutes a 'healthy diet', Mediterranean-style diet, DASH diet and low-inflammatory diet. In this section, we will review the two main modes for delivering dietary advice (face to face and virtually), discussing various aspects and considerations of these in practice. We will also unpack the main factors that should be considered for successful engagement with an individual with regards to diet. However, we encourage application of clinical judgement in choosing a specific approach that reflects the needs of a patient and available resources.

Practical Recommendations for Dietary Assessment and Counselling

Dietitians consider a range of clinical, physical, mental and social factors throughout the nutrition care process, and many of these are important for successful patient engagement. Commonly, the nutrition care process comprises several steps including assessment of dietary intake and behaviour, discussion and identification of the issues to be addressed, provision of information (counselling) and evaluating dietary changes that have been implemented (Figure 5.5). Although many individuals will benefit from dietary counselling by their mental health clinician, there are some groups of individuals that should be referred to a dietitian. For example, those with eating disorders and disordered eating should be referred to a specialist dietitian. The prevalence of disordered eating is up to 32% in younger individuals and is more prevalent in those with mental health problems (99). Individuals

Timing is important. Consider when and how to deliver the advice as fluctuation in symptoms might correspond with responsiveness to messages of change (e.g. what to focus on, how long the discussion should be, what are the goals, when to review and evaluate).

Consumer as the centre of attention. Be guided by the need of the person in front of you. Try not to make assumptions or force your treatment agenda. Listen to what is important to the person seeking your advice and let them know that you appreciate their wishes.

Small steps = sustainable change. Work together to set SMART goals. Build self-efficacy, capacity and self-esteem. Support motivation and help find resolutions for barriers. Help plan short- and long-term reasonable and achievable actions.

Become the biggest believer. Changes are a challenging process that requires continuous authentic positivity. It is important for practitioners to remain motivated and to believe that changes are possible.

Address concerns and barriers. Explore what changes are possible and build capacity for these changes. Ask questions, listen to answers and support finding clear and simple solutions. Consider and respect cultural and individual differences.

Plan for the future. Discuss and schedule sessions and reminders. Provide flexibility but ensure consistency in approach and follow-up (e.g. on SMART goals, barriers or achievements). Engage in a long-term commitment to improvement.

Figure 5.5 Recommendations for the dietary counselling process to facilitate dietary change.

who are young, pregnant or elderly, and those with additional nutrition needs (e.g. comorbid disorders such as gastrointestinal disorders or type 2 diabetes), should also be referred to a dietitian for their nutrition care (Figure 5.6).

An important first step in the nutrition care process for any clinician seeing individuals with anxiety or depression is the assessment of dietary intake and dietary behaviour. For a clinician not trained in nutritional assessment techniques, this conversation could start with simple questions, such as 'How many meals and snacks do you usually eat per day?',

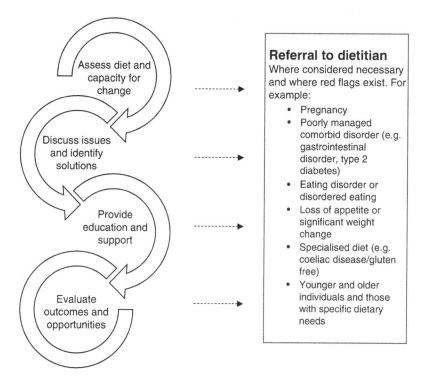

Figure 5.6 Stages in the nutrition care process for mental health clinicians. Referral to a dietitian can occur at any of the four stages.

'What do you usually eat for breakfast/lunch/dinner?', 'Do you cook and eat at home?' or 'How would you describe your usual food intake?'. Initiating a discussion around food and eating will also help to provide some understanding about an individual's knowledge of nutrition and its importance to the individual.

Second, identifying the main barriers for healthy eating is needed to construct a patient-centred plan and to identify the support the individual needs to achieve their nutrition goals. An understanding of the typical side effects of common mental disorders is integral (e.g. altered appetite (reduced or cravings), apathy, low motivation, impaired concentration and memory) to ensuring that recommendations are provided in a sensitive manner and are respectful of individual needs.

Third, to facilitate dietary behaviour change, psychoeducation and evidence-based resources should be provided. Dietary information should be given in bite-size format and take into consideration the individual's learning styles, baseline knowledge and beliefs and motivations, and readiness to receive education. Importantly, motivation and readiness to change can be highly variable and should be assessed in each session. When the individual is ready, focussing on small, attainable and value-based goals will build motivation and self-capacity for change. For example, providing practical tips for cooking and preparing meals and snacks may be warranted, with a large emphasis on forward planning (e.g. developing shopping lists, stocking the home and preparing meals in advance) for times when a patient may experience further lowered mood. Moreover, to support dietary adherence, recommendations should align with common cravings. For example, nutritious foods can be encouraged that address cravings for sugary foods such as Greek natural yoghurt with walnuts, honey and fruits (frozen, fresh, tinned and/or dried), salty and fatty foods such as nuts, olives and feta cheese, and liberal use of EVOO as a main source of added fat.

Lastly, through reflective practice, evaluating outcomes and identifying helpful strategies that facilitated change will assist the clinician in fine-tuning their dietary assessment and counselling skills (100).

Clinical Considerations in Dietary Counselling

Individuals with anxiety and depression commonly present with other forms of mental illness and behaviours. Adding to this, exposure to traumatic events is ubiquitous worldwide and has a well-established deleterious impact on health. For example, globally it is estimated that over 70% of adults have experienced a traumatic event at some point in their life (101). Hence, clinicians should consider using a trauma-informed care approach among patients with mental illness. Trauma-informed care builds awareness and increases clinician confidence in supporting patients who have experienced trauma and/or are experiencing high levels of stress, to enable them to respond in an effective, patient-centred manner (102). Additionally, trauma-informed care involves the clinician being in tune with their own nervous system so that the clinician can work safely within their own capacities.

Moreover, depression and anxiety often co-occur with a variety of other clinical conditions (e.g. cardiovascular disease, metabolic syndrome, type 2 diabetes). Many of these are also responsive to specific dietary intervention. There is strong evidence that diet interventions for depression (i.e. the Mediterranean and DASH diets) also achieve improved health outcomes, at least for cardiovascular disease and diabetes (103), and therefore there is potential for dietary counselling to address both mental and physical health conditions in the same individual.

Importantly, where other comorbidities are present, a weight-neutral approach is critical (i.e. a focus on health behaviour change rather than weight loss) (104), and evidence demonstrates that improvements in depressive symptoms (and physiological health) can occur without weight loss (105). Weight stigma and negative attitudes about one's bodyweight hinder positive changes, create unnecessary pressure and can promote unhelpful lifestyle behaviours, such as poor eating behaviour and low motivation (106), and can essentially exacerbate mental disorders Moreover, for people who live in larger bodies, weight stigma has been suggested to contribute to an increase in BMI over time (73).

Social Considerations in Dietary Counselling

Individuals living with mental illness commonly experience high rates of unemployment or missed days at work and therefore may lack adequate finances to access food or nutrition services. Food insecurity relates to limited or uncertain access to sufficient, safe and nutritious food for normal growth and development and an active and healthy life (107). This may include lack of resources (including finances and transport), lack of access to nutritious food at an affordable price, lack of access due to geographical isolation, lack of cooking facilities and lack of knowledge or skills to make appropriate choices. The clinician should ascertain the degree of food insecurity experienced by the individual and modify dietary recommendations accordingly, for example, strategies for preparing meals with minimal storage and/or cooking utensils and facilities, ready-made meals, food delivery, free community meals, community cooking classes, and so on. For individuals requiring dietetic assessment and counselling, clinicians should explore the potential subsidised dietetic services available and how they may access them. Interestingly, a cost analysis of a healthy Mediterranean-style diet found it to be affordable for individuals with clinical depression whose habitual diet was poor quality (Mediterranean-style diet AUD$112/week vs. habitual diet AUD$138/week). These cost savings were mainly attributed to purchasing cheaper products from the Mediterranean diet (e.g. pulses, tinned fish) and less alcohol and sweets (108).

Service/Delivery Considerations

Dietary consultations should be delivered using an evidence-based approach underpinned by peer-reviewed scientific research, while considering the therapeutic relationship with the patient (109). With regards to the intensity and frequency of nutrition care for efficacy in depression, evidence from the SMILES trial shows that seven individualised face-to-face sessions with a dietitian delivered over 3 months (weekly to fortnightly sessions) can achieve reductions in depressive symptoms (105, 110). In a best-case scenario, initial dietetic appointments usually extend to 60 minutes while review appointments may be shorter (30–60 minutes), determined on a case-by-case basis (111). Other research suggests fewer nutrition appointments are also efficacious for reducing depressive symptoms (112, 113). The complex nature of common mental disorders and the many facets of the individual and their multiple health concerns often necessitate more frequent sessions. Furthermore, some individuals may require stepped care or a gradual increase in the intensity of dietary intervention. Those with lower readiness to change or limited food-related knowledge or skills may benefit from a greater number of diet-focussed sessions, longer period of extensive support and/or 'restart' opportunities. Moreover, for long-term effectiveness, diet interventions should be flexible with continuous motivational support and broad multifaceted strategies for change (114). Limited data is currently available regarding whether sustainable dietary change is possible in individuals with depression, however, dietary patterns, such as the Mediterranean diet, often use a weight-neutral/ad libitum approach, which can help promote adherence and longevity of changes (115).

Delivery Mode

Face to Face

Developing a meaningful and effective therapeutic relationship (e.g. 'connection', 'rapport', 'partnership') is considered crucial in nutrition practice – it is pivotal to how effectively the patient and professional engage and work together (109). Dietary advice can be delivered in several ways, but the most effective delivery mode is one which promotes a patient-centred approach and the development of a therapeutic relationship. Face-to-face consultation allows for tailoring or personalisation of nutrition information to the individual's requirements and lifestyle with the aim of facilitating behaviour change. Evidence from RCTs of personalised nutrition interventions demonstrates that compared to web-based interventions, face-to-face nutrition interventions can achieve significantly greater dietary change and are also more likely to produce long-term benefits (116). Additionally, supporting a patient to attend in-person appointments can play an important role in working through motivation, encouraging forward planning and routine. However, face-to-face nutrition services can be expensive and time-consuming and may not be accessible to everyone (116).

Telehealth, Web-Based and Apps

Following technological advances, web-based and mobile methods of dietary advice are increasingly replacing or supplementing face-to-face consultations. Telehealth offers a convenient service that can be especially desirable for individuals with mood disorders who commonly experience amotivation and/or agoraphobia. Additionally, telehealth can help reduce the burden associated with regular attendance at appointments and potential financial concerns (e.g. transport costs).

Web applications, websites and telehealth can reach a larger population (including individuals living in rural and remote locations or internationally) and allow patients with mobility issues to access high-quality services. Importantly, web-based nutrition interventions should be personalised in order to support dietary change, but there is currently insufficient evidence to suggest that web-based interventions are as effective as face-to-face interventions (116).

Hybrid Approaches

It is worth considering the possible use of multiple delivery modes (e.g. initial face-to-face consultation and review appointments via videoconference and/or telephone), which fosters the development of a therapeutic alliance in the initial phases, while allowing for a convenient service with reduced patient–clinician burden in the latter phase. Finally, group consultations should be considered in the context of providing a valuable opportunity for peer support, in particular for allowing individuals to connect with others with lived experience (117).

Additional Recommendations for Psychiatrists, Psychologists and Other Mental Health Clinicians

Diet interventions can lead to impressive reductions in depressive symptoms, particularly when advice is dietitian-delivered and with sufficient session frequency. However, psychologists, psychiatrists and other mental health clinicians can play an important role in the assessment and counselling of individuals with regards to diet and at a minimum raising patient awareness of the role of diet in mental health. For example, clinicians could discuss with patients the current evidence that healthy dietary patterns containing fish, legumes, fruits, vegetables, nuts and wholegrains can be instrumental in managing symptoms of depression. Conversely, a high intake of discretionary items such as sweets, highly processed cereals, crisps, fast food and sugar-sweetened beverages increases the risk of poor mental health.

Moreover, psychologists and psychiatrists can play a part in working a patient up for a referral to a mental health dietitian. This work-up involves establishing an individual's interest in dietary change, their motivation levels and their readiness to change. As alluded to earlier, awareness of potential 'red flags', which would indicate a referral to a dietitian, is necessary, including eating disorders, disordered eating, poorly managed comorbid medical health conditions, loss of appetite, significant weight change, the need for a specialised diet or pregnancy.

While nutritional care should be delivered by a trained professional, broader mental health teams could routinely raise diet and nutrition as an important issue and encourage changes to improve dietary intake. This must be delivered in a highly sensitive, non-stigmatising fashion, as patients commonly experience shame around food, eating and bodyweight. Support should focus on behavioural changes (e.g. increasing intake of legumes by one serve per week) rather than outcome-focussed goals (e.g. cholesterol) and should be weight-neutral. Raising the profile of nutrition is highly relevant and in accordance with the recent Royal Australian New Zealand College of Psychiatrists' clinical practice guidelines stating that lifestyle approaches (including nutrition) should form the foundation of treatment for mood disorders (77).

Conclusion

The large burden of early mortality due to cardiometabolic illness, alongside the more recent evidence for diet quality as a risk factor and treatment target for mental health problems, support the imperative for the use of dietary interventions to treat depression and anxiety.

There is particularly compelling data to support the use of a Mediterranean diet to improve symptoms of depression. Given the high rates of cardiometabolic comorbidity in individuals with depression, this is a favourable approach because of its protective effects for metabolic syndrome and cardiovascular disease. Recommendations are provided to guide mental health clinicians through the nutrition care process. Clinical judgement should be applied in the timing of nutrition counselling as well as the choice of dietary approach, which should reflect the needs of the patient and available resources.

References

1. Herforth, A., Arimond, M., Álvarez-Sánchez, C., et al., 2019. A global review of food-based dietary guidelines. *Advances in Nutrition*, 10(4), pp. 590–605.

2. Reedy, J., Lerman, J. L., Krebs-Smith, S. M., et al., 2018. Evaluation of the Healthy Eating Index-2015. *Journal of the Academy of Nutrition and Dietetics*, 118(9), pp. 1622–33.

3. Organisation CSaIR. CSIRO Healthy Diet Score, 2021. Available from: www.csiro.au/en/research/health-medical/diets/csiro-healthy-diet-score.

4. Newcastle Uo. Healthy Eating Quiz. Available from: https://healthyeatingquiz.com.au.

5. Institute NNC. Register of Validated Short Dietary Assessment Instruments. Available from: https://epi.grants.cancer.gov/diet/shortreg.

6. Trichopoulou, A. and Lagiou, P., 1997. Healthy traditional Mediterranean diet: an expression of culture, history, and lifestyle. *Nutrition Reviews*, 55(11 Pt 1), pp. 383–9.

7. Mediterranean FD. What is the Mediterranean diet? Available from: https://dietamediterranea.com/en/nutrition.

8. Hutchins-Wiese, H. L., Bales, C. W. and Porter Starr, K. N., 2021. Mediterranean diet scoring systems: understanding the evolution and applications for Mediterranean and non-Mediterranean countries. *British Journal of Nutrition*, 128 (7), pp. 1–22.

9. Monteagudo, C., Mariscal-Arcas, M., Rivas, A., et al., 2015. Proposal of a Mediterranean diet serving score. *PLoS One*, 10(6), p. e0128594.

10. Schroder, H., Fito, M., Estruch, R., et al., 2011. A short screener is valid for assessing Mediterranean diet adherence among older Spanish men and women. *Journal of Nutrition*, 141(6), pp. 1140–5.

11. Chiavaroli, L., Viguiliouk, E., Nishi, S. K., et al., 2019. DASH dietary pattern and cardiometabolic outcomes: an umbrella

review of systematic reviews and meta-analyses. *Nutrients*, *11*(2).

12. Berk, M., Williams, L. J., Jacka, F. N., et al., 2013. So depression is an inflammatory disease, but where does the inflammation come from? *BMC Medicine*, *11*(1), p. 200.

13. Koelman, L., Egea Rodrigues, C. and Aleksandrova, K., 2022. effects of dietary patterns on biomarkers of inflammation and immune responses: a systematic review and meta-analysis of randomized controlled trials. *Advances in Nutrition*, *13*(1), pp. 101–15.

14. Christ, A., Lauterbach, M. and Latz, E., 2019. Western diet and the immune system: an inflammatory connection. *Immunity*, *51*(5), pp. 794–811.

15. Shivappa, N., Steck, S. E., Hurley, T. G., Hussey, J. R. and Hebert, J. R., 2014. Designing and developing a literature-derived, population-based dietary inflammatory index. *Public Health Nutrition*, *17*(8), pp. 1689–96.

16. Rowland, I., Gibson, G., Heinken, A., et al., 2018. Gut microbiota functions: metabolism of nutrients and other food components. *European Journal of Nutrition*, *57*(1), pp. 1–24.

17. Wiley, N., Cryan, J. F., Dinan, T. G., Ross, R. P. and Stanton, C., 2020. Production of psychoactive metabolites by gut bacteria. In C. S. M. Cowan and B. E. Leonard *(eds.), Microbes and the mind: the microbiome-gut-brain axis in neuropsychiatry*. Modern Trends in Pharmacopsychiatry. Karger.

18. Simpson, C. A., Diaz-Arteche, C., Eliby, D., et al., 2021. The gut microbiota in anxiety and depression: a systematic review. *Clinical Psychology Review*, *83*, p. 101943.

19. McGuinness, A. J., Davis, J. A., Dawson, S. L., et al., 2022. A systematic review of gut microbiota composition in observational studies of major depressive disorder, bipolar disorder and schizophrenia. *Molecular Psychiatry*, *27*(4), pp. 1920–35.

20. Nikolova, V. L., Hall, M. R. B., Hall, L. J., et al., 2021. Perturbations in gut microbiota composition in psychiatric disorders: a review and meta-analysis. *JAMA Psychiatry*, *78*(12), pp. 1343–54.

21. O'Riordan, K. J., Collins, M. K., Moloney, G. M., et al., 2022. Short chain fatty acids: microbial metabolites for gut-brain axis signalling. *Molecular and Cellular Endocrinology*, *546*, p. 111572.

22. David, L. A., Maurice, C. F., Carmody, R. N., et al., 2014. Diet rapidly and reproducibly alters the human gut microbiome. *Nature*, *505*(7484), pp. 559–63.

23. Kimble, R., Gouinguenet, P., Ashor, A., et al., 2022. Effects of a Mediterranean diet on the gut microbiota and microbial metabolites: a systematic review of randomized controlled trials and observational studies. *Critical Reviews in Food Science and Nutrition*, *10*, pp. 1–22.

24. Singh, R. K., Chang, H.-W., Yan, D., et al., 2017. Influence of diet on the gut microbiome and implications for human health. *Journal of Translational Medicine*, *15*(1), p. 73.

25. Armet, A. M., Deehan, E. C., O'Sullivan, A. F., et al., 2022. Rethinking healthy eating in light of the gut microbiome. *Cell Host & Microbe*, *30*(6), pp. 764–85.

26. Kang, S. S., Jeraldo, P. R., Kurti, A., et al., 2014. Diet and exercise orthogonally alter the gut microbiome and reveal independent associations with anxiety and cognition. *Molecular Neurodegeneration*, *9*(1), p. 36.

27. Leyrolle, Q., Cserjesi, R., Mulders, M. D. G. H., et al., 2021. Prebiotic effect on mood in obese patients is determined by the initial gut microbiota composition: a randomized, controlled trial. *Brain, Behavior, and Immunity*, *94*, pp. 289–98.

28. Liu, R. T., Walsh, R. F. L. and Sheehan, A. E., 2019. Prebiotics and probiotics for depression and anxiety: a systematic review and meta-analysis of controlled clinical trials. *Neuroscience & Biobehavioral Reviews*, *102*, pp. 3–23.

29. Berding, K., Long-Smith, C. M., Carbia, C., et al., 2021. A specific dietary fibre supplementation improves cognitive performance: an exploratory

randomised, placebo-controlled, crossover study. *Psychopharmacology (Berl).*, *238*(1), pp. 149–63.

30. Steptoe, A., Hamer, M. and Chida, Y., 2007. The effects of acute psychological stress on circulating inflammatory factors in humans: a review and meta-analysis. *Brain, Behavior, and Immunity*, *21*(7), pp. 901–12.

31. Costello, H., Gould, R. L., Abrol, E. and Howard, R., 2019. Systematic review and meta-analysis of the association between peripheral inflammatory cytokines and generalised anxiety disorder. *BMJ Open*, *9* (7), p. e027925.

32. Osimo, E. F., Pillinger, T., Rodriguez, I. M., et al., 2020. Inflammatory markers in depression: a meta-analysis of mean differences and variability in 5,166 patients and 5,083 controls. *Brain, Behavior, and Immunity*, *87*, pp. 901–9.

33. Hou, R., Ye, G., Liu, Y., et al., 2019. Effects of SSRIs on peripheral inflammatory cytokines in patients with Generalized Anxiety Disorder. *Brain, Behavior, and Immunity*, *81*, pp. 105–10.

34. Strawbridge, R., Arnone, D., Danese, A., et al., 2015. Inflammation and clinical response to treatment in depression: a meta-analysis. *European Neuropsychopharmacology*, *25*(10), pp. 1532–43.

35. Köhler-Forsberg, O., Hjorthøj, C., Nordentoft, M., Mors, O. and Benros, M. E., 2019. Efficacy of anti-inflammatory treatment on major depressive disorder or depressive symptoms: *meta*-analysis of clinical trials. *Acta Psychiatrica Scandinavica*, *139*(5), pp. 404–19.

36. Capuron, L., Ravaud, A., Neveu, P. J., et al., 2002. Association between decreased serum tryptophan concentrations and depressive symptoms in cancer patients undergoing cytokine therapy. *Molecular Psychiatry*, *7*(5), pp. 468–73.

37. Su, K. P., Lai, H. C., Yang, H. T., et al., 2014. Omega-3 fatty acids in the prevention of interferon-alpha-induced depression: results from a randomized, controlled trial. *Biological Psychiatry*, *76* (7), pp. 559–66.

38. Yahfoufi, N., Alsadi, N., Jambi, M. and Matar, C., 2018. The immunomodulatory and anti-inflammatory role of polyphenols. *Nutrients*, *10*(11).

39. Giacobbe, J., Benoiton, B., Zunszain, P., Pariante, C. M. and Borsini, A., 2020. The anti-inflammatory role of omega-3 polyunsaturated fatty acids metabolites in pre-clinical models of psychiatric, neurodegenerative, and neurological disorders. *Frontiers in Psychiatry*, *11*.

40. Lassale, C., Batty, G. D., Baghdadli, A., et al., 2019. Healthy dietary indices and risk of depressive outcomes: a systematic review and meta-analysis of observational studies. *Molecular Psychiatry*, *24*(7), pp. 965–86.

41. Firth, J., Stubbs, B., Teasdale, S. B., et al., 2018. Diet as a hot topic in psychiatry: a population-scale study of nutritional intake and inflammatory potential in severe mental illness. *World Psychiatry: Official Journal of the World Psychiatric Association (WPA)*, *17*(3), pp. 365–7.

42. Itsiopoulos, C., Mayr, H. L. and Thomas, C. J., 2022. The anti-inflammatory effects of a Mediterranean diet: a review. *Current Opinion in Clinical Nutrition & Metabolic Care*, *25*(6), pp. 415–22.

43. Dantzer, R., O'Connor, J. C., Freund, G. G., Johnson, R. W. and Kelley, K. W., 2008. From inflammation to sickness and depression: when the immune system subjugates the brain. *Nature Reviews Neuroscience*, *9*(1), pp. 46–56.

44. Sapolsky, R. M., 2000. Glucocorticoids and hippocampal atrophy in neuropsychiatric disorders. *Archives of General Psychiatry*, *57*(10), pp. 925–35.

45. Tafet, G. E. and Nemeroff, C. B., 2020. Pharmacological treatment of anxiety disorders: the role of the HPA axis. *Frontiers in Psychiatry*, *11*.

46. Rohleder, N. and Kirschbaum, C., 2007. Effects of nutrition on neuro-endocrine stress responses. *Current Opinion in Clinical Nutrition & Metabolic Care*, *10*(4).

47. Brody, S., Preut, R., Schommer, K. and Schürmeyer, T. H., 2002. A randomized

controlled trial of high dose ascorbic acid for reduction of blood pressure, cortisol, and subjective responses to psychological stress. *Psychopharmacology, 159*(3), pp. 319–24.

48. Delarue, J., Matzinger, O., Binnert, C., et al., 2003. Fish oil prevents the adrenal activation elicited by mental stress in healthy men. *Diabetes & Metabolism, 29*(3), pp. 289–95.

49. Robertson, R. C., Seira Oriach, C., Murphy, K., et al., 2017. Omega-3 polyunsaturated fatty acids critically regulate behaviour and gut microbiota development in adolescence and adulthood. *Brain, Behavior, and Immunity, 59*, pp. 21–37.

50. Larrieu, T., Hilal, L. M., Fourrier, C., et al., 2014. Nutritional omega-3 modulates neuronal morphology in the prefrontal cortex along with depression-related behaviour through corticosterone secretion. *Translational Psychiatry, 4*(9), p. e437–e.

51. Jahangard, L., Hedayati, M., Abbasalipourkabir, R., et al., 2019. Omega-3-polyunsatured fatty acids (O3PUFAs), compared to placebo, reduced symptoms of occupational burnout and lowered morning cortisol secretion. *Psychoneuroendocrinology, 109*, p. 104384.

52. Hovatta, I., Juhila, J. and Donner, J., 2010. Oxidative stress in anxiety and comorbid disorders. *Journal of Neuroscience Research, 68*(4), pp. 261–75.

53. Liu, T., Zhong, S., Liao, X., et al., 2015. A meta-analysis of oxidative stress markers in depression. *PLoS One, 10*(10), p. e0138904.

54. Machlin, L. J. and Bendich, A., 1987. Free radical tissue damage: protective role of antioxidant nutrients. *The FASEB Journal, 1*(6), pp. 441–5.

55. Zhang, H. and Tsao, R., 2016. Dietary polyphenols, oxidative stress and antioxidant and anti-inflammatory effects. *Current Opinion in Food Science, 8*, pp. 33–42.

56. Matsuzawa-Nagata, N., Takamura, T., Ando, H., et al., 2008. Increased oxidative stress precedes the onset of high-fat diet-induced insulin resistance and obesity. *Metabolism, 57*(8), pp. 1071–7.

57. Studzinski, C. M., Li, F., Bruce-Keller, A. J., et al., 2009. Effects of short-term Western diet on cerebral oxidative stress and diabetes related factors in APP x PS1 knock-in mice. *Journal of Neurochemistry, 108*(4), pp. 860–6.

58. Ferriani, L. O., Silva, D. A., Molina, M. D. C. B., et al., 2022. Associations of depression and intake of antioxidants and vitamin B complex: results of the Brazilian Longitudinal Study of Adult Health (ELSA-Brasil). *Journal of Affective Disorders, 297*, pp. 259–68.

59. Fernandes, B. S., Dean, O. M., Dodd, S., Malhi, G. S. and Berk, M., 2016. N-acetylcysteine in depressive symptoms and functionality: a systematic review and meta-analysis. *The Journal of Clinical Psychiatry, 77*(4), pp. e457–66.

60. Lafleur, D. L., Pittenger, C., Kelmendi, B., et al., 2006. N-acetylcysteine augmentation in serotonin reuptake inhibitor refractory obsessive-compulsive disorder. *Psychopharmacology, 184*(2), pp. 254–6.

61. Gautam, M., Agrawal, M., Gautam, M., et al., 2012. Role of antioxidants in generalised anxiety disorder and depression. *Indian Journal of Psychiatry, 54*(3), pp. 244–7.

62. Marx, W., McGuinness, A. J., Rocks, T., et al., 2021. The kynurenine pathway in major depressive disorder, bipolar disorder, and schizophrenia: a meta-analysis of 101 studies. *Molecular Psychiatry, 26*(8), pp. 4158–78.

63. Ogyu, K., Kubo, K., Noda, Y., et al., 2018. Kynurenine pathway in depression: a systematic review and meta-analysis. *Neuroscience & Biobehavioral Reviews, 90*, pp. 16–25.

64. Soh, N. L. and Walter, G., 2014. Tryptophan and depression: can diet alone be the answer? *Acta Neuropsychiatrica, 23*(1), pp. 3–11.

65. Çakici, N., Sutterland, A. L., Penninx, B. W. J. H., et al., 2020. Altered peripheral blood compounds in drug-naïve first-episode patients with either schizophrenia or major depressive disorder: a meta-analysis. *Brain, Behavior, and Immunity, 88*, pp. 547–58.

66. Castrén, E. and Monteggia, L. M., 2021. Brain-derived neurotrophic factor signaling in depression and antidepressant action. *Biological Psychiatry*, *90*(2), pp. 128–36.

67. Marx, W., Lane, M., Hockey, M., et al., 2020. Diet and depression: exploring the biological mechanisms of action. *Molecular Psychiatry*, *26*(1), pp. 134–50.

68. Jacka, F. N., Cherbuin, N., Anstey, K. J., Sachdev, P. and Butterworth, P., 2015. Western diet is associated with a smaller hippocampus: a longitudinal investigation. *BMC Medicine*, *13*, p. 215.

69. Sanchez-Villegas, A., Galbete, C., Martinez-Gonzalez, M. A., et al., 2011. The effect of the Mediterranean diet on plasma brain-derived neurotrophic factor (BDNF) levels: the PREDIMED-NAVARRA randomized trial. *Nutritional Neuroscience*, *14*(5), pp. 195–201.

70. Clark, T. D., Crean, A. J. and Senior, A. M., 2022. Obesogenic diets induce anxiety in rodents: a systematic review and meta-analysis. *Obesity Reviews*, *23*(3), p. e13399.

71. Luppino, F. S., de Wit, L. M., Bouvy, P. F., et al., 2010. Overweight, obesity, and depression: a systematic review and meta-analysis of longitudinal studies. *Archives of General Psychiatry*, *67*(3), pp. 220–9.

72. Jacka, F. N., O'Neil, A., Opie, R., et al., 2017. A randomised controlled trial of dietary improvement for adults with major depression (the 'SMILES' trial). *BMC Medicine*, *15*(1), p. 23.

73. Lambert, E. R., Koutoukidis, D. A. and Jackson, S. E., 2019. Effects of weight stigma in news media on physical activity, dietary and weight loss intentions and behaviour. *Obesity Research & Clinical Practice*, *13*(6), pp. 571–8.

74. Xu, Y., Zeng, L., Zou, K., et al., 2021. Role of dietary factors in the prevention and treatment for depression: an umbrella review of meta-analyses of prospective studies. *Translational Psychiatry*, *11*(1), p. 478.

75. Lassale, C., Batty, G. D., Baghdadli, A., et al., 2018. Healthy dietary indices and risk of depressive outcomes: a systematic review and meta-analysis of observational studies. *Molecular Psychiatry*, *24*(7), pp. 965–86.

76. Firth, J., Marx, W., Dash, S., et al., 2019. The effects of dietary improvement on symptoms of depression and anxiety: a meta-analysis of randomised controlled trials. *Psychosomatic Medicine*, *81*, pp. 265–80.

77. Malhi, G. S., Outhred, T., Hamilton, A., et al., 2018. Royal Australian and New Zealand College of Psychiatrists clinical practice guidelines for mood disorders: major depression summary. *Medical Journal of Australia*, *208*(4), pp. 175–80.

78. Bot, M., Brouwer, I. A., Roca, M., et al., 2019. Effect of multinutrient supplementation and food-related behavioral activation therapy on prevention of major depressive disorder among overweight or obese adults with subsyndromal depressive symptoms: the MooDFOOD randomized clinical trial. *JAMA*, *321*(9), pp. 858–68.

79. Jacka, F. N., O'Neil, A., Opie, R., et al., 2017. A randomised controlled trial of dietary improvement for adults with major depression (the 'SMILES' trial). *BMC Medicine*, *15*(1), pp. 1–13.

80. Parletta, N., Zarnowiecki, D., Cho, J., et al., 2019. A Mediterranean-style dietary intervention supplemented with fish oil improves diet quality and mental health in people with depression: a randomized controlled trial (HELFIMED). *Nutritional Neuroscience*, *22*(7), pp. 474–87.

81. Opie, R. S., O'Neil, A., Jacka, F. N., Pizzinga, J. and Itsiopoulos, C., 2018. A modified Mediterranean dietary intervention for adults with major depression: dietary protocol and feasibility data from the SMILES trial. *Nutritional Neuroscience*, *21*(7), pp. 487–501.

82. Chatterton, M. L., Mihalopoulos, C., O'Neil, A., et al., 2018. Economic evaluation of a dietary intervention for adults with major depression (the 'SMILES' trial). *BMC Public Health*, *18*(1), pp. 1–11.

83. Segal, L., Twizeyemariya, A., Zarnowiecki, D., et al., 2020. Cost effectiveness and cost-utility analysis of a group-based diet intervention for treating major depression: the HELFIMED trial. *Nutritional Neuroscience*, 23(10), pp. 770–8.

84. Bayes, J., Schloss, J. and Sibbritt, D., 2022. The effect of a Mediterranean diet on the symptoms of depression in young males (the 'AMMEND: A Mediterranean Diet in MEN with Depression' study): a randomized controlled trial. *The American Journal of Clinical Nutrition*, 116(2), pp. 572–80.

85. Francis, H. M., Stevenson, R. J., Chambers, J. R., et al., 2019. A brief diet intervention can reduce symptoms of depression in young adults: a randomised controlled trial. *PloS One*, 14(10), p. e0222768.

86. Young, C. L., Mohebbi, M., Staudacher, H., et al., 2021. Assessing the feasibility of an m-Health intervention for changing diet quality and mood in individuals with depression: the My Food & Mood program. *International Review of Psychiatry*, 33(3), pp. 266–79.

87. Cabrera-Suárez, B., Pla, J., González-Pinto, A., et al., 2022. Effectiveness of a remote nutritional intervention to increase the adherence to the Mediterranean diet among recovered depression patients. *Nutritional Neuroscience*, 18, pp. 1–10.

88. Madani, S., Ahmadi, A., Shoaei-Jouneghani, F., Moazen, M. and Sasani, N., 2022. The relationship between the Mediterranean diet and Axis I disorders: a systematic review of observational studies. *Food Science & Nutrition*, 10(10), pp. 3241–58.

89. Nanri, A., Kimura, Y., Matsushita, Y., et al., 2010. Dietary patterns and depressive symptoms among Japanese men and women. *European Journal of Clinical Nutrition*, 64(8), pp. 832–9.

90. Canheta, A. B. S., Santos, A., Souza, J. D. and Silveira, E. A., 2021. Traditional Brazilian diet and extra virgin olive oil reduce symptoms of anxiety and depression in individuals with severe obesity: randomized clinical trial. *Clinical Nutrition*, 40(2), pp. 404–11.

91. Sabet, J. A., Ekman, M. S., Lundvall, A. S., et al., 2021. Feasibility and acceptability of a healthy Nordic diet intervention for the treatment of depression: a randomized controlled pilot trial. *Nutrients*, 13(3).

92. Valipour, G., Esmaillzadeh, A., Azadbakht, L., et al., 2017. Adherence to the DASH diet in relation to psychological profile of Iranian adults. *European Journal of Nutrition*, 56(1), pp. 309–20.

93. Meegan, A. P., Perry, I. J. and Phillips, C. M., 2017. The association between dietary quality and dietary guideline adherence with mental health outcomes in adults: a cross-sectional analysis. *Nutrients*, 9(3).

94. Perez-Cornago, A., Sanchez-Villegas, A., Bes-Rastrollo, M., et al., 2017. Relationship between adherence to Dietary Approaches to Stop Hypertension (DASH) diet indices and incidence of depression during up to 8 years of follow-up. *Public Health Nutrition*, 20(13), pp. 2383–92.

95. Sanchez-Villegas, A., Delgado-Rodriguez, M., Alonso, A., et al., 2009. Association of the Mediterranean dietary pattern with the incidence of depression: the Seguimiento Universidad de Navarra/University of Navarra follow-up (SUN) cohort. *Archives of General Psychiatry*, 66 (10), pp. 1090–8.

96. Torres, S. J. and Nowson, C. A., 2012. A moderate-sodium DASH-type diet improves mood in postmenopausal women. *Nutrition*, 28(9), pp. 896 900.

97. Tolkien, K., Bradburn, S. and Murgatroyd, C., 2019. An anti-inflammatory diet as a potential intervention for depressive disorders: a systematic review and meta-analysis. *Clinical Nutrition*, 38(5), pp. 2045–52.

98. Phillips, C. M., Shivappa, N., Hébert, J. R. and Perry, I. J., 2018. Dietary inflammatory index and mental health: a cross-sectional analysis of the relationship with depressive symptoms, anxiety and well-being in adults. *Clinical Nutrition*, 37(5), pp. 1485–91.

99. Sparti, C., Santomauro, D., Cruwys, T., Burgess, P. and Harris, M., 2019. Disordered eating among Australian adolescents: prevalence, functioning, and help received. *International Journal of Eating Disorders*, 52(3), pp. 246–54.

100. Koshy, K., Limb, C., Gundogan, B., Whitehurst, K. and Jafree, D. J., 2017. Reflective practice in health care and how to reflect effectively. *International Journal of Surgical Oncology*, 2(6), p. e20.

101. Benjet, C., Bromet, E., Karam, E. G., et al., 2016. The epidemiology of traumatic event exposure worldwide: results from the World Mental Health Survey Consortium. *Psychological Medicine*, 46 (2), pp. 327–43.

102. Gerber, M. and Gerber, M., 2019. An introduction to trauma and health. In M. R. Gerber (ed.),*Trauma-informed healthcare approaches*. Springer Nature.

103. Martinez-Lacoba, R., Pardo-Garcia, I., Amo-Saus, E. and Escribano-Sotos, F., 2018. Mediterranean diet and health outcomes: a systematic meta-review. *European Journal of Public Health*, 28(5), pp. 1–6.

104. Hunger, J., Smith, J. and Tomiyama, J., 2020. An evidence-based rationale for adopting weight-inclusive health policy. *Social Issues and Policy Review*, 14(1), pp. 73–107.

105. Jacka, F. N., O'Neil, A., Opie, R., et al., 2017. A randomised controlled trial of dietary improvement for adults with major depression (the 'SMILES' trial). *BMC Medicine*, 15(1).

106. Vartanian, L. R. and Porter, A. M., 2016. Weight stigma and eating behavior: a review of the literature. *Appetite*, 102, pp. 3–14.

107. FAO. Hunger and food insecurity, 2022. Available from: www.fao.org/hunger/en.

108. Opie, R., Segal, L., Jacka, F., et al., 2015. Assessing healthy diet affordability in a cohort with major depressive disorders. *Journal of Epidemiology and Public Health*, 7(5), pp. 159–69.

109. Nagy, A., McMahon, A., Tapsell, L. and Deane, F., 2022. The therapeutic relationship between a client and dietitian: a systematic integrative review of empirical literature.*Nutrition & Dietetics*, 79(3), pp. 303–48.

110. Opie, R. S., O'Neil, A., Jacka, F. N., Pizzinga, J. and Itsiopoulos, C., 2018. A modified Mediterranean dietary intervention for adults with major depression: dietary protocol and feasibility data from the SMILES trial. *Nutritional Neuroscience*, 21(7), pp. 487–501.

111. Employees Assistance Programme Administration, 2019. *The social and economic benefits of improving mental health*. Melbourne: EAPAssist.

112. Francis, H. M., Stevenson, R. J., Chambers, J. R., et al., 2019. A brief diet intervention can reduce symptoms of depression in young adults: a randomised controlled trial. *PLoS One*, 14(10), p. e0222768.

113. Bayes, J., Schloss, J. and Sibbritt, D., 2021. A randomised controlled trial assessing the effect of a Mediterranean diet on the symptoms of depression in young men (the 'AMMEND' study): a study protocol. *British Journal of Nutrition*, 126(5), pp. 730–7.

114. Firth, J., Siddiqi, N., Koyanagi, A., et al., 2019. The Lancet Psychiatry Commission: a blueprint for protecting physical health in people with mental illness. *Lancet Psychiatry*, 6(8), pp. 675–712.

115. Franquesa, M., Pujol-Busquets, G., García-Fernández, E., et al., 2019. Mediterranean diet and cardiodiabesity: a systematic review through evidence-based answers to key clinical questions. *Nutrients*, 11(3).

116. Al-Awadhi, B., Fallaize, R., Franco, R. F. H. and Lovegrove, J., 2021. Insights into the delivery of personalised nutrition: evidence from face-to-face and web-based dietary interventions. *Frontiers in Nutrition*, 7, pp. 1–14.

117. Watkins, A., Denney-Wilson, E., Curtis, J., et al., 2020. Keeping the body in mind: a qualitative analysis of the experiences of people experiencing first-episode psychosis participating in a lifestyle intervention programme. *International Journal of Mental Health Nursing*, 29(2), pp. 278–89.

118. British Nutrition Foundation. Your balanced diet, 2015. Available from: www .nutrition.org.uk/media/ohunys2u/your-balanced-diet_16pp_final_web.pdf.

119. USDoA. Dietary Guidelines for Americans, 2020–2025, 2020. Available from: www.dietaryguidelines.gov/sites/de fault/files/202012/Dietary_Guidelines_fo r_mericans_2020-2025.pdf.

120. Estruch, R., Ros, E. and Martínez-González, M. A., 2013. Mediterranean diet for primary prevention of cardiovascular disease. *The New England Journal of Medicine*, 369(7), pp. 676–7.

Schizophrenia, Microbiota and Nutrition

John R. Kelly

Summary

Schizophrenia is a complex heterogeneous neurodevelopmental disorder involving the intricate interplay of genetic susceptibilities and the accumulation of prenatal and postnatal environmental stressors. At the interface between the individual and the environment, the diverse microbial ecosystem in the gut (microbiota) plays an important role in the regulation of homeostasis, particularly immune, metabolic and endocrine pathways. Pre-clinical studies show that the signalling pathways of the microbiome–gut–brain (MGB) axis influence brain development and function, including modulation of stress sensitivity, social interaction and cognitive function. Human studies in infants indicate associations between the gut microbiota and components of cognition and behaviour. Preliminary clinical studies demonstrate that schizophrenia is associated with altered gut microbiota signatures compared to healthy controls. Faecal microbiota transplantation studies from people with schizophrenia induce changes in brain neurochemistry and behaviour, which suggests a physiologically relevant role. Microbial-based interventions in schizophrenia are at an early stage of development, but a deeper understanding of the overlapping and complementary interaction between the MGB axis and diet and exercise and their relationship to other lifestyle factors could open avenues to modify susceptibility to, or exacerbation of, components of schizophrenia. This chapter will review the MGB axis and its interaction with diet, exercise, stress and antipsychotics in the hope that this will provide mental health professionals with an understanding of the MGB axis as an additional modifiable system that could be harnessed to improve health outcomes in schizophrenia.

Introduction

Schizophrenia is a highly complex heterogeneous neurodevelopmental disorder involving the intricate interplay of genetic susceptibilities and the accumulation of prenatal and postnatal environmental stressors. The disorder presents with varying degrees of positive symptoms (delusions and hallucinations), negative symptoms (poverty of speech, diminished emotional expression/pleasure, motivation, sociality) and cognitive deficits. It is associated with a 13–15-year premature mortality rate (1), primarily driven by cardiometabolic and respiratory disease, compounded by poor-quality diet, low physical activity and high levels of smoking, alcohol and substance use. Metabolic dysregulation, such as persistently high fasting insulin levels (2) and lipid dysregulation during childhood (3), together with subtle aberrations in immune signalling pathways (4), is associated with an increased susceptibility to the development of schizophrenia.

An integrative multi-systems approach to schizophrenia that encompasses central–peripheral interactions and wider environmental influences may expand opportunities to understand this disorder and improve health outcomes. At the interface between the individual and the environment, the complex and diverse microbial ecosystem in the gut (microbiota) plays an important role in the regulation of homeostasis, particularly immune, metabolic and endocrine pathways.

Over the last two decades, animal studies using different but complementary approaches, such as germ-free (GF) rodents (born and raised without microbes), antibiotics, probiotics, gastrointestinal infection studies and faecal microbiota transplantation (FMT) studies, have elucidated the pathways by which the gut microbiota acting via the gut–brain axis contributes to the regulation of brain and behaviour (5). These microbiome–gut–brain (MGB) axis signalling pathways operate throughout life but are especially important during early development in shaping aspects of the stress response (6), cognition (7) and social (8–10) and emotional domains (11).

Perturbations in the MGB axis are associated with a diverse range of disorders in adults. Preliminary clinical studies, though limited in sample size and consistent methodologies, suggest that schizophrenia is associated with altered gut microbiota profiles (Table 6.1). The translational FMT components of these studies, which induce changes in brain neurochemistry and behaviour, hint at a possible pathophysiological role of the MGB axis in overlapping domains of relevance to the trajectory of schizophrenia. However, it remains an open question as to whether subtle deviations in MGB-axis signalling, in conjunction with other factors, play a causative role in neurodevelopmental disorders (12, 13).

Identification of a schizophrenia-specific gut microbiota signature remains elusive and will require large longitudinal studies. Meta-analyses suggest that there may be general gut microbiota patterns that signify suboptimal homeostasis across psychiatric disorders (14–18). These trends include alterations in beta diversity (variation between communities/samples) with depletion of certain anti-inflammatory butyrate-producing bacteria (e.g. *Faecalibacterium* and *Coprococcus*) and higher levels of proinflammatory bacteria (e.g. *Eggerthella*) (14), lactic acid-producing bacteria and bacteria associated with glutamate and gamma-aminobutyric acid (GABA) metabolism (16).

While the MGB axis offers a tractable therapeutic target, perhaps via promotion of gut microbiota diversification, definitive microbial-based therapeutics specifically targeting schizophrenia are at an early stage of development (19–21). Given the role of the MGB axis in the regulation of glucose homeostasis (22), insulin sensitivity (23, 24) and lipid variability (25), it may mediate antipsychotic (AP)-induced metabolic side effects (26–29) and even play a subtle role in response (or non-response) to APs (30).

Against this background, a deeper understanding of the overlapping and complementary relationship between the MGB axis and diet and exercise and their relationship to other lifestyle factors could open avenues to modify susceptibility to, or exacerbation of, components of schizophrenia. This chapter will review the MGB axis and its interaction with diet, exercise, stress and APs in the hope that this will provide mental health professionals with an understanding of the MGB axis as an additional modifiable system that could be integrated into a multifaceted systems-based paradigm to potentially improve health outcomes in schizophrenia.

Table 6.1 Schizophrenia and gut microbiota

Design, number	Results	Ref
Amisulpride treatment for 4 weeks 33 SCZ	*Dorea*, *Desulfovibrio* and *Butyricicoccus* significantly increased *Actinomyces* and *Porphyromonas* significantly decreased elevated blood levels of IL-4 and decreased IL-6	(26)
Cross-sectional 132 SCZ 132 HCs 132 metabolic syndrome	SCZ: *Flavonifractor plautii*, *Collinsella aerofaciens*, *Bilophila wadsworthia* and *Sellimonas intestinalis* increased *Faecalibacterium prausnitzii*, *Ruminococcus lactaris*, *Ruminococcus biciruclans* and *Veillonella rogosae* Reduced diversity and richness The bacterial functional module for synthesising tyrosine, a precursor for dopamine, was in SCZ cases positively associated with cognitive score	(125)
Cross-sectional 82 SZ patients 80 HCs	SCZ: phylum: *Actinobacteria* increased, *Firmicutes* decreased genus: *Collinsella*, *Lactobacillus*, *Succinivibrio*, *Mogibacterium*, *Corynebacterium*, undefined *Ruminococcus* and undefined *Eubacterium* increased *Adlercreutzia*, *Anaerostipes*,*Ruminococcus* and *Faecalibacterium* decreased *Succinivibrio* was positively correlated with the total PANSS scores and the general PANSS scores *Corynebacterium* negatively related to the negative scores of PANSS	(126)
29 SCZ over two different periods (remission and onset period) 29 HCs	aSCZ vs HCs; f_Ruminococcaceae, c_Deltaproteobacteria, o_Desulfovibrionales, f_Desulfovibrionaceae, g_Turicibacter, g_Anaerotruncus, g_Bilophila, g_Intestinibacter, g_Ruminococcaceae_UCG_004, g__Flavonifractor, g_Ruminiclostridium_9, o_Actinomycetales, f_Actinomycetaceae, g_Actinomyces and g_Acetanaerobacterium rSCZ vs HCs; Clostridium_sensu_stricto_1, Intestinibacter, Parabacteroides, Turicibacter, norank_-f_Ruminococcaceae, Bilophila, Anaerotruncus, Ruminococcaceae_UCG_004, Flavonifractor, Epulopiscium, Lactonifactor, Anaerofustis, Comamonas, norank_f_Christensenellaceae, Solobacterium, Prevotella, Holdemania, Atopobium, and Actinomyces were increased	(127)

Table 6.1 (cont.)

Design, number	Results	Ref
Cross-sectional 84 SCZ 84 HCs	19 gut microbiota taxonomies were associated with schizophrenia Found that MD index was positively correlated with ME diversity and gut IgA levels and negatively correlated with gut microbiota richness Glutamate synthase (GOGAT) was more active in the guts of patients with schizophrenia than in those of healthy controls, and high GOGAT activity was associated with altered gut microbiota taxonomies associated with gut IgA levels	(66)
Cross-sectional 90 medication-free SCZ 81 HCs	SCZ: increase in *Lactobacillus fermentum*, *Enterococcus faecium*, *Alkaliphilus oremlandii* and *Cronobacter sakazakii/turicensis*, *Veillonella atypica*, *Veillonella dispar*, *Bifidobacterium dentium*, *Dialister invisus*, *Lactobacillus oris* and *Streptococcus salivarius* FMT of a schizophrenia-enriched bacterium, *Streptococcus vestibularis* induced deficits in social behaviours and hyperactivity in mice and altered neurotransmitter levels in peripheral tissues in recipient mice	(85)
Cross-sectional First episode drug-naive SCZ (n=40) Antipsychotic-treated SCZ (n=85) HC (n=69)	Lower alpha-diversity in antipsychotic-treated SCZ compared to HCs No difference between FEP compared to HCs Both FEP and antipsychotic-treated SCZ had altered composition including *Christensenellaceae*, *Enterobacteriaceae*, *Pasteurellaceae*, *Turicibacteraceae* at the family level and *Escherichia* at genus level compared to HCs Positive correlation of genus *Actinobacillus* and family *Veillonellaceae* with right middle frontal gyrus volume in FEP	(128)
Cross-sectional 25 chronic SCZ, 25 HCs	SCZ: At the phylum level, *Proteobacteria*. At the genus level, Anaerococcus increased; *Haemophilus*, *Sutterella* and *Clostridium* decreased. *Ruminococcaceae* correlated with lower severity of negative symptoms	(129)
Translational Antibiotic-treated male mice FMT: 11 drug-free SCZ, and 10 HC	SCZ FMT: psychomotor hyperactivity, impaired learning and elevation of the kynurenine–kynurenic acid pathway of tryptophan degradation in both periphery and brain, and increased basal extracellular dopamine in prefrontal cortex and 5-hydroxytryptamine in hippocampus compared to HC FMT	(68)

Table 6.1 (cont.)

Design, number	Results	Ref
Open-label single-arm trial of 4 weeks of *Bifidobacterium breve A-1*. 29 SCZ	At 4 weeks: HADS total score and PANSS anxiety/depression score were significantly improved (12 responders and 17 non-responders)	(19)
Translational SCZ (n=63), 58 antipsychotics HC (n=69), sex, age, BMI matched FMT: from 5 randomly selected SCZ and 5 matched controls Male GF mice	SCZ: decreased α-diversity index, *Veillonellaceae* and *Lachnospiraceae* associated with SCZ severity, *Aerococcaceae*, *Bifidobacteriaceae*, *Brucellaceae*, *Pasteurellaceae* and *Rikenellaceae* discriminated SCZ from HCs with 0.769 area under the curve GF SCZ FMT: elevated glutamine in serum and hippocampus, decreased glutamate (glutamic acid) in stool and hippocampus, GABA increased in hippocampus, altered lipid profile in serum and hippocampus Behaviour: increased startle responses, locomotor hyperactivity, decreased anxiety and depressive-like behaviours	(80)
Longitudinal (24 weeks of risperidone treatment) First episode SCZ (n=41 patients completed 24 weeks) 41 matched HC (baseline only)	Lower numbers of faecal *Bifidobacterium* spp., *Escherichia coli*, *Lactobacillus* spp. and higher number of *Clostridium coccoides* compared to HC After 24 weeks of risperidone treatment, increase in weight, BMI, fasting glucose, triglycerides, LDL, hs-CRP Changes in faecal *Bifidobacterium* spp remained stable after controlling for confounding variables	(88)
Cross-sectional High-risk (HR) subjects (n=81) All drug naive Ultra-high-risk (UHR) subjects (n=19) 69 HC	Increased *Clostridiales*, *Prevotella* and *Lactobacillus ruminis* in faecal samples Increased level of choline in ACC in UHR No sig. differences between HR and HC groups	(130)
Cross-sectional SCZ (n=64) HC (n=53)	SCZ: Phylum level: relative abundance of *Proteobacteria* was significantly increased vs. HC At the genus level: *Succinivibrio*, *Megasphaera*, *Collinsella*, *Clostridium*, *Klebsiella* and *Methanobrevibacter* were significantly higher vs. HC *Blautia*, *Coprococcus*, *Roseburia* was decreased vs. HC	(131)
Longitudinal (12 months) FEP (n=28), 26 antipsychotics HC (n=16)	FEP: family level; *Lactobacillaceae*, *Halothiobacillaceae*, *Brucellaceae* and *Micrococcineae* increased *Veillonellaceae* decreased	(132)

Table 6.1 (cont.)

Design, number	Results	Ref
	FEP: genus level; *Lactobacillus*, *Tropheryma*, *Halothiobacillus*, *Saccharophagus*, *Ochrobactrum*, *Deferribacter* and *Halorubrum* increased *Anabaena*, *Nitrosospira* and *Gallionella* decreased *Lactobacillus* group bacterial numbers correlated positively with severity of psychotic symptoms measured by BPRS and negatively with GAF scale No sig. differences in serum markers	
14-week, double-blind, placebo-controlled *L. rhamnosus* strain GG and *B. animalis* subsp. *lactis Bb12* SCZ (n=56) Probiotic (n=30) Placebo (n=26) (same cohort as Dickerson et al. 2014)	SCZ: in males – reduced *C. albicans* antibodies, *S. cerevisiae* were not altered Trends towards improvement in the PANSS positive symptom subset score in males treated with probiotics who were seronegative for *C. albicans*	(98)
Two case-control cohorts (n=947) SCZ (n=261), including: FEP (n=139, 78 antipsychotic naive) Bipolar (n=270) HC (n=277)	No differences in *C. albicans* exposures until diagnostic groups stratified by sex SCZ: males; *C. albicans* seropositivity conferred increased odds (OR 2.04–9.53) for SCZ SCZ: females; *C. albicans* seropositivity conferred increased odds (OR 1.12) for lower cognitive scores on RBANS with significant decreases on memory modules *C. albicans* IgG levels were not impacted by antipsychotics. GI disturbances associated with elevated *C. albicans* in SCZ males and bipolar females	(133)
Cross-sectional SCZ (n=16). HCs (n=16) Differences in smoking and BMI between groups	SCZ: higher proportions of *Firmicutes*, *Ascomycota*, *Bifidobacterium* and *Lactobacilli* (largest effect in *L. gasseri*) SCZ: increased *Candida* and *Eubacterium* and reduction of *Neisseria*, *Haemophilus* and *Capnocytophaga* SCZ: increased number of metabolic pathways related to metabolite transport systems including siderophores, glutamate and vitamin B12	(134)
Cross-sectional SCZ (n=41). HC (n=33) Differences in smoking, BMI and age	SCZ: increased *L. phage phiadh* (controlling for age, gender, race, socioeconomic status and smoking)	(135)
14-week, double-blind, placebo-controlled	No sig. differences in the PANSS	(21) (97)

Table 6.1 (cont.)

Design, number	Results	Ref
L. rhamnosus strain GG and *B. animalis* subsp. *lactis* Bb12 SCZ (n=65), 33 probiotic, 32 placebo All on antipsychotic medication	Probiotic: significantly less likely to develop severe bowel difficulty Probiotic: reduced serum levels of von Willebrand factor (vWF), increased MCP-1, BDNF, T-cell-specific protein RANTES	

SCZ: schizophrenia, GF: germ-free, PANSS: Positive and Negative Syndrome Scale, BPRS: Brief Psychiatric Rating Scale, GAF: Global Assessment of Functioning scale, BMI: body mass index, GI: gastrointestinal, RBANS: Repeatable Battery for the Assessment of Neuropsychological Status, FEP: First Episode Psychosis, FMT: Faecal Microbiota Transplantation, GABA: gamma-aminobutyric acid, SANS: Scale for the Assessment of Negative Symptoms, CRP: C-reactive protein, HDL: high-density lipoprotein, LDL: low-density lipoprotein, vWF: von Willebrand factor, MCP-1: monocyte chemotactic protein-1, BDNF: brain-derived neurotrophic factor, QPCR: quantitative polymerase chain reaction, SOD: anti-oxidant superoxide dismutase, HC: healthy controls, ACC: anterior cingulate cortex.

Gut Microbiome

Most of the human body's microbes reside in the gastrointestinal tract (GIT). The vast majority are bacteria, predominately from the phyla *Firmicutes*, *Actinobacteria* and *Bacteroidetes*, with lower relative abundances of *Verrucomicrobia* and *Proteobacteria* (31). Viruses and bacteriophages, protozoa, archaea and fungi are also present but in much smaller proportions. Fungal populations or the mycobiome within the microbiota comprise 0.001–0.1% of the total gut microbiome and are dominated by yeasts including *Saccharomyces*, *Malassezia* and *Candida* and yeasts in the family *Dipodascaceae* (*Galactomyces*, *Geotrichum*, *Saprochaete*) (32). There are also an estimated 10^{12} virus-like particles in the human gut (33). A multitude of environmental factors influence the gut microbiota, including diet (34), exercise (35), medications (36) and to a lesser degree genetics (37). Because of the vast individual differences between the gut microbiomes of healthy people, defining a healthy gut microbiome is a major ongoing challenge (38, 39). Nevertheless, it is generally thought that a more diverse gut microbiome is beneficial for health (40, 41).

Gut Microbiome Acquisition and Maturation

Microbial acquisition occurs during delivery and undergoes reorganisation during the early developmental phase (42). Delivery mode (43), feeding mode (breast or formula) (44), antibiotic usage (45) and nutrition (46) influence the trajectory of gut microbiota acquisition during the early phase of development. Pre-clinical studies indicate that the signalling pathways of the MGB axis play a role in shaping the trajectory of early postnatal brain development and function (47, 48). In humans, the mechanistic pathways are less clear, but studies in infants show associations between the gut microbiota and elements of cognition and behaviour during the early developmental phase (49–55). Maternal malnutrition and infection, obstetric complications and childhood infections increase the risk of schizophrenia, but it is not yet known whether aberrant MGB-axis signalling combines with these risk factors to increase susceptibility to schizophrenia.

Communication Channels: The MGB Axis

The MGB-axis signalling pathways include: stimulation of components of the immune system (56), vagus nerve activation (57), production of circulating microbial metabolites (e.g. short-chain fatty acids (SCFAs) and/or microbial induction of host molecules) (58), amino acid derivatives (catecholamines, other indole derivatives and p-cresol), secondary bile acids, stimulation of enteroendocrine cells and enteric nervous system signalling (59), tryptophan metabolism (60), and the hypothalamic–pituitary–adrenal (HPA) axis (6). Some of these signalling pathways may indirectly influence the trajectory of certain domains in schizophrenia.

The MGB Axis, the Immune System and Schizophrenia

It has been proposed that a genetically programmed subtle alteration in the immune system, in combination with a precisely timed pathogen exposure (particularly during pregnancy or childhood), may amplify susceptibility to schizophrenia (4). Sub-groups of people across all stages of schizophrenia exhibit a low-grade inflammation profile, both peripherally and centrally, including those without medication (4). However, a multitude of factors (e.g. obesity, smoking, APs, stress) influence immune system function, and the source of low-grade inflammation and relevance to underlying pathophysiological processes in schizophrenia are still not fully clear. Regardless of causality, immune system dysregulation, whether primary or secondary, could exacerbate other factors which negatively impact health outcomes in schizophrenia.

It is well established that the gut microbiome modulates immune system homeostasis by maintaining proinflammatory and anti-inflammatory signalling in the GIT. A lack of balanced gut microbiota may contribute to immune dysregulation. *Bifidobacteria* may be of particular importance in immune programming during early development (61, 62). Sub-groups of people with schizophrenia may have altered antibody (IgM/IgA) responses to gut bacteria (63) and altered gut barrier function (64, 65). A recent study showed that people with schizophrenia (n=84) had altered gut microbiota profiles, including reduced gut microbiota richness (total number of species in a sample) and increased faecal IgA levels and glutamate synthase levels compared to healthy controls (66).

The MGB Axis, Serotonin (5-HT) and Tryptophan–Kynurenine Pathway and Schizophrenia

Tryptophan is an essential amino acid and the precursor for serotonin (5-HT). The kynurenine pathway (KP) is an alternative metabolic route for tryptophan. Under normal physiological conditions, approximately 99% of tryptophan is metabolised to kynurenine. The gut microbiome exerts influence over the immune- and stress-sensitive KP enzymes at multiple levels of the gut–brain axis (60). Gut microbiota can metabolise tryptophan directly and shift its accessibility to the KP. Sub-groups of people with schizophrenia exhibit altered tryptophan–kynurenine metabolism (67) and the gut microbiota–immuno–KP pathway may play a contributory role in schizophrenia. A study using antibiotic-treated mice that received FMT from medication-free people with schizophrenia exhibited psychomotor hyperactivity and cognitive deficits associated with elevated kynurenine–kynurenic acid pathway of tryptophan degradation in both periphery and brain, as well as increased basal extracellular dopamine in prefrontal cortex and 5-HT in the hippocampus, compared to mice that received FMT from healthy controls (68).

The MGB Axis, Neuromodulators and Schizophrenia

The gut microbiome is essential for healthy brain development and function. GF rodents display deficits in neuroplasticity (50), neurotransmitter signalling (49), myelination patterns (69) and blood–brain barrier integrity (70). Dopaminergic dysfunction is a key pathophysiological process underpinning the manifestation of psychotic symptoms (hallucinations and delusions). GF and antibiotic-treated mice exhibit altered dopaminergic neurotransmission in certain brain regions (71–73). The gut microbiota also influences glutamatergic (74–76) and GABA pathways in rodents (77–79).

An FMT study showed that gut microbiota transfer from individuals with schizophrenia to GF mice modulated the glutamate–glutamine–GABA cycle associated with increased startle responses and locomotor hyperactivity (80). This study found elevated glutamine in the serum and hippocampus and decreased glutamate (glutamic acid) in the stool and hippocampus in GF mice that received the FMT from patients with schizophrenia compared to healthy controls (80). This study also showed that GABA was increased in the hippocampus in GF mice that received the FMT from schizophrenia patients (80). Collectively, these pre-clinical studies suggest that neurodevelopmental processes of direct and indirect relevance to the neurodevelopmental trajectory of certain features of schizophrenia are under the partial influence of MGB-axis signalling.

The MGB Axis, the Stress Response and Schizophrenia

An accumulation of stressors, particularly during sensitive neurodevelopmental periods, increase the risk of mental health disorders. Early life stress is a risk factor for the development of schizophrenia (81), and stressors can precipitate psychotic relapses or more intense psychotic experiences (82). Pre-clinical studies suggest that the gut microbiota signature acquired and maintained during the pivotal early developmental stage may affect stress sensitivity, in part via the HPA axis, the main neuroendocrine regulator of stress responses (6). This MGB-axis modulation of stress sensitivity may influence multiple aspects of behaviour including social interaction (8–10) and cognitive function (7). Psychosis tends to present to mental health services during adolescence, a period with an additional burden of stress. Indeed, certain gut microbiome configurations or diet–MGB-axis configurations may form part of the resilience system to help counteract the impact of stress (83, 84). Conversely, other gut microbiota configurations, perhaps those including reduced diversity, may reduce stress resilience, which could interact with other factors to alter stress sensitivity thresholds. However, it is not yet known whether microbial signature aberrations in conjunction with stress serve as additional risk factors or mediators in psychotic relapses.

Altered Gut Microbiota Profiles in Schizophrenia

A growing number of clinical studies show that different stages of schizophrenia are associated with altered gut microbiota profiles (Table 6.1). These studies are limited by small sample sizes and confounding factors (e.g. diet and medications) and variable methodologies. A specific gut microbiota signature associated with schizophrenia has yet to emerge. Nonetheless, FMT studies in schizophrenia indicate that altered gut microbiota induce changes in behaviour and brain neurochemistry that overlap with aspects of schizophrenia. Apart from the aforementioned FMT studies suggesting a physiological role of the gut microbiota in the modulation of the glutamate–glutamine–GABA (80) and tryptophan–kynurenine pathways (68), a recent study using a medication-free transplantation of a schizophrenia-enriched bacterium, *Streptococcus vestibularis*, induced deficits in social behaviours and hyperactivity in mice and altered serum and gut neurotransmitter levels (85).

Antipsychotics and the MGB Axis

Pre-clinical (86, 87) and clinical studies (26, 88–90) demonstrate that APs alter the gut microbiota, but the physiological implications have yet to be fully disentangled. There are indicators mainly from pre-clinical studies that the gut microbiota may play a mediating role in the metabolic side effects of APs (27, 28). FMT from risperidone-treated mice to risperidone-naive recipients resulted in a 16% reduction in total resting metabolic rate (91). In an adolescent clinical cohort, chronic risperidone treatment was associated with an increase in body mass index and a significantly lower ratio of *Bacteroidetes* to *Firmicutes* compared to AP-naive psychiatric controls (92). In the first episode, drug-naive patients with schizophrenia, 24 weeks of risperidone altered the gut microbiota profile and resulted in weight gain, increased C-reactive protein and increased fasting lipids and glucose (88).

Similarly, chronic olanzapine treatment altered gut microbiota composition and induced significant bodyweight gain in female rats, while both males and females had olanzapine-induced increases in adiposity (86). Pre-treatment with an antibiotic cocktail attenuated this weight gain (87). Another study using GF mice demonstrated that the gut microbiome is necessary and sufficient for weight gain caused by oral olanzapine, which shifted the microbiota profile towards an 'obesogenic' bacterial profile (93). Weight gain was attenuated when olanzapine was co-administered with prebiotics. The prebiotic B-GOS, known to induce the growth of beneficial bacteria, including *Bifidobacteria*, reduced weight gain in olanzapine-treated rats (94). Although the sample size is too small to draw conclusions, preliminary analyses from 25 chronically treated clozapine patients and 9 healthy controls showed the relative abundance of the phylum *Proteobacteria* and class *Gammaproteobacteria* was increased in schizophrenia patients taking clozapine (29). Larger sample sizes will be required to elucidate the precise MGB-axis configurations needed to mitigate the metabolic burden of APs or conceivably mediate the inter-individual variability in AP response. An interesting avenue of further exploration would be to explore the potential mediating role of the MGB axis on metformin and glucagon-like peptide-1 agonists in AP-induced metabolic dysregulation.

Microbiota Interventional Studies in Schizophrenia

There is a paucity of well-powered, high-quality clinical trials of microbial-based therapeutic interventional studies in schizophrenia. Studies conducted to date show mixed results (95). An open-label, single-arm study (n=29) of *bifidobacterium breve* A-1 suggested a benefit in anxiety and depressive symptoms in schizophrenia, but the lack of placebo precludes definitive conclusions (19). Notwithstanding the recent negative clinical trial of vitamin D augmentation in schizophrenia (96), a smaller study (n=60) showed that administration of a probiotic cocktail (*Lactobacillus acidophilus*, *Bifidobacterium bifidum*, *Lactobacillus reuteri* and *Lactobacillus fermentum*) and vitamin D for 12 weeks to people with chronic schizophrenia had beneficial effects on the general and total Positive and Negative Syndrome Scale (PANSS) score and metabolic profiles compared to placebo (20).

An earlier 14-week, randomised, double-blind, placebo-controlled trial (n=65) of *L. rhamnosus strain GG* and *B. animalis subsp. lactis strain Bb12*, added to AP treatment, improved gastrointestinal symptoms and increased levels of serum brain-derived neuro-trophic factor (BDNF) but did not impact positive or negative symptoms (21, 97, 98). In contrast, a randomised parallel design reported that patients hospitalised for a manic episode (n=66) who received 24 weeks of adjunctive probiotics (*L. rhamnosus strain GG* and *B. animalis subsp. lactis strain Bb12*) had lower rates of re-hospitalisation compared to the group that received the placebo (99). A pilot trial of B-GOS in 39 non-hospitalised adult participants with psychosis reported an improvement in subtests of executive function, though this may have been influenced by learning effects (100). Interestingly, a well-powered (n=207) randomised controlled trial of minocycline augmentation (known to reduce the diversity of gut microbiota) in early stage schizophrenia spectrum disorder did not impact symptoms or biomarkers (101). There are early indicators from open-labelled studies that microbial-based therapies may improve aspects of autism spectrum disorder (102, 103). We await larger trials to determine whether this will translate into tangible clinical benefits for patients.

Nutraceuticals

Despite the poor-quality dietary patterns and nutritional deficits associated with schizophrenia (104), clear benefits of nutraceuticals/supplements have not been demon-strated (96, 105–108). A recent well-powered, double-blind, randomised, placebo-controlled trial found no association between vitamin D supplementation and mental health or metabolic outcomes at 6 months in people with early psychosis, even though participants had low vitamin D levels (96). Similarly, Coenzyme Q10 (106), B-vitamin supplementation (108) and ω-3 polyunsaturated fatty acids (107) have not shown therapeutic benefits in various stages of schizophrenia. Given the complexities, it is perhaps unsurprising that a single intervention would be effective in such a complex heterogeneous neurodevelop-mental disorder. However, there are broad diet–MGB- and exercise–MGB-axis patterns that are optimal for homeostasis that if consistently and rigorously applied could improve health outcomes in schizophrenia.

The MGB Axis, Diet and Schizophrenia

Diet quality is one of the main contributors to human health (109). Maternal nutrition over the early developmental phase is especially important (110). There is increasing recognition that diet, via multiple overlapping biological pathways, may be a modifiable risk factor for mental health disorders. There are dietary patterns that are optimal for mental health, such as plant-based diets with a high content of grains/fibres, fermented foods and fish (111, 112). Conversely, it is established that processed or fried foods, refined grains and sugary products are broadly detrimental to mental health.

Diet is the primary contributing factor to the gut microbiome (34) and can rapidly alter its composition. Certain dietary patterns are associated with gut microbial signatures. The Mediterranean diet, characterised by high amounts of plant-based foods (fruit, vegetables, nuts, beans, seeds and grains), olive oil and dairy products, and low to moderate amounts of fish and poultry, is associated with increased levels of faecal SCFAs, *Prevotella* and some fibre-degrading *Firmicutes* (113), and may have mental health benefits. Lower gut microbiota diversity is associated with low-fibre Western diets (114, 115), whereas high-fermented-food diets may increase microbiota diversity, decrease inflammatory markers (116) and alter tryptophan metabolites (117).

Most of the preliminary clinical studies in schizophrenia (Table 6.1) show reduced gut microbiota diversity, but few studies captured detailed dietary information. People with schizophrenia tend to have diets characterised by a high intake of saturated fat and a low consumption of fibre and fruit, higher dietary energy and sodium intake (104), and a lower adherence to Mediterranean diets (118, 119).

The mechanisms underlying poor diet in schizophrenia are complex, multifaceted and involve interacting central, peripheral and environmental influences. The initiation or re-initiation and maintenance of more optimal diet–MGB patterns is particularly challenging in people with schizophrenia and it is intriguing to consider the role of MGB-axis signalling, not only in homeostatic and energy metabolism in schizophrenia but also in the contribution to the regulation of reward-related feeding behaviour (120). Indeed, obesity-related MGB-axis signatures may be associated with reward processing (121). A recent study in obese but otherwise healthy adults showed that obesity was associated with an increase in the *Prevotella* to *Bacteroides* ratio and a decrease in faecal tryptophan (121). The *Prevotella* to *Bacteroides* ratio was positively correlated with resting state functional connectivity in the nucleus accumbens (a region involved in reward processing) and negatively correlated to faecal tryptophan (121). A recent general-population cohort (n=786) study showed an association between alpha-diversity (variation within a single sample) and another system involved in reward processing – the endocannabinoid system – with measures of anhedonia/amotivation mediated by faecal levels of the palmitoylethanolamide (the endogenous equivalent of cannabidiol) (122).

MGB–Exercise Axis in Schizophrenia

Physical inactivity, potentially compounded by negative symptoms and AP side effects, is a major contributor to poor health in people with schizophrenia. Exercise can enhance (stress) resilience, improve mood and improve cardiorespiratory fitness in schizophrenia, and may play a preventative role in mental health disorders. There is an intersecting relationship between exercise and the MGB axis (35). In addition to influencing glucose (22) and lipid variability (25), the gut microbiota may mediate exercise-induced improvements in glucose homeostasis and insulin sensitivity (123), possibly via modulation of SCFAs (124).

Conclusions and Future Perspectives

As outlined in this chapter, the gut microbiome, at the intersection of immune, metabolic and endocrine pathways, plays a vital role in health. Animal studies have shown that the signalling pathways of the MGB axis partially modulate important processes in brain development and function, including aspects of cognition-, social and stress-related behaviour. Studies in human infants demonstrate associations of gut microbiota patterns with components of cognition and behaviour during the early developmental phase, but the precise relevance to schizophrenia is not yet clear. Some of the risk factors for the development of schizophrenia interact with elements of the MGB axis. However, large longitudinal population-based studies from birth, with extensive follow-up periods, will be required to determine whether subtle deviations of the MGB axis at birth and over the early developmental period combine with other vulnerability factors to increase the risk of schizophrenia.

The emerging clinical studies showing altered gut microbiota signatures in people with schizophrenia compared to healthy controls need to be considered in the context of the heterogeneity of schizophrenia and the extensive inter-individual differences in the gut microbiota of healthy people. Larger studies using consistent methodologies will decipher whether there is a specific gut microbiota signature associated with schizophrenia. However, the dysregulated MGB-axis patterns (and the manifestations in animal models) may signify suboptimal homeostasis, which can be targeted by microbial-based therapeutic approaches. Future well-powered clinical trials of microbial-based therapeutics that harness the synergistic relationship with diet, exercise and other lifestyle factors (perhaps assisted by digital health platforms) may optimise the chances of delivering tangible health benefits for people with schizophrenia.

References

1. Hjorthøj, C., Stürup, A. E., McGrath, J. J. and Nordentoft, M., 2017. Years of potential life lost and life expectancy in schizophrenia: a systematic review and meta-analysis. *Lancet Psychiatry*, 4(4), pp. 295–301.

2. Perry, B. I., Stochl, J., Upthegrove, R., et al., 2021. Longitudinal trends in childhood insulin levels and body mass index and associations with risks of psychosis and depression in young adults. *JAMA Psychiatry*, 78(4), pp. 416–25.

3. Madrid-Gambin, F., Föcking, M., Sabherwal, S., et al., 2019. Integrated lipidomics and proteomics point to early blood-based changes in childhood preceding later development of psychotic experiences: evidence from the Avon longitudinal study of parents and children. *Biological Psychiatry*, 86(1), pp. 25–34.

4. Millerm B. J. and Goldsmith, D. R., 2019. Inflammatory biomarkers in schizophrenia: implications for heterogeneity and neurobiology. *Biomarkers in Neuropsychiatry*, 1, p. 100006.

5. Cryan, J. F., O'Riordan, K. J., Cowan, C. S. M., et al., 2019. The microbiota-gut-brain axis. *Physiological Reviews*, 99(4), pp. 1877–2013.

6. Sudo, N., Chida, Y., Aiba, Y., et al., 2004. Postnatal microbial colonization programs the hypothalamic-pituitary-adrenal system for stress response in mice. *The Journal of Physiology*, 558(pt. 1), pp. 263–75.

7. Desbonnet, L., Clarke, G., Traplin, A., et al., 2015. Gut microbiota depletion from early adolescence in mice: implications for brain and behaviour. *Brain, Behavior, and Immunity*, 48, pp. 165–73.

8. Wu, W.-L., Adame, M. D., Liou, C.-W., et al., 2021. Microbiota regulate social behaviour via stress response neurons in the brain. *Nature*, 595(7867), pp. 409–14.

9. Buffington, S. A., Di Prisco, G. V., Auchtung, T. A., et al., 2016. Microbial reconstitution reverses maternal diet-induced social and synaptic deficits in offspring. *Cell*, 165(7), pp. 1762–75.

10. Desbonnet, L., Clarke, G., Shanahan, F., Dinan, T. G. and Cryan, J. F., 2014. Microbiota is essential for social development in the mouse. *Molecular Psychiatry*, 19(2), pp. 146–8.

11. Cowan, C. S., Callaghan, B. L. and Richardson, R., 2016. The effects of a probiotic formulation (Lactobacillus rhamnosus and L. helveticus) on developmental trajectories of emotional learning in stressed infant rats. *Translational Psychiatry*, 6(5), p. e823.

12. Yap, C. X., Henders, A. K., Alvares, G. A., et al., 2021. Autism-related dietary preferences mediate autism-gut microbiome associations. *Cell*, 184(24), p. 5916-31.e17.

13. Kelly, J. R., Minuto, C., Cryan, J. F., Clarke, G. and Dinan, T. G., 2021. The role

of the gut microbiome in the development of schizophrenia. *Schizophrenia Research*, 234, pp. 4–23.

14. Nikolova, V. L., Smith, M. R. B., Hall, L. J., et al., 2021. Perturbations in gut microbiota composition in psychiatric disorders: a review and meta-analysis. *JAMA Psychiatry*, 78(12), pp. 1343–54.

15. Valles-Colomer, M., Falony, G., Darzi, Y., et al., 2019. The neuroactive potential of the human gut microbiota in quality of life and depression. *Nature Microbiology*, 4(4), pp. 623–32.

16. McGuinness, A. J., Davis, J. A., Dawson, S. L., et al., 2022. A systematic review of gut microbiota composition in observational studies of major depressive disorder, bipolar disorder and schizophrenia. *Molecular Psychiatry*, 27, pp. 1920–35.

17. Nguyen, T. T., Kosciolek, T., Eyler, L. T., Knight, R. and Jeste, D. V., 2018. Overview and systematic review of studies of microbiome in schizophrenia and bipolar disorder. *Journal of Psychiatric Research*, 99, pp. 50–61.

18. Borkent, J., Ioannou, M., Laman, J. D., Haarman, B. C. M. and Sommer, I. E. C., 2022. Role of the gut microbiome in three major psychiatric disorders. *Psychological Medicine*, 52(7), pp. 1222–42.

19. Okubo, R., Koga, M., Katsumata, N., et al., 2019. Effect of bifidobacterium breve A-1 on anxiety and depressive symptoms in schizophrenia: A proof-of-concept study. *Journal of Affective Disorders*, 245, pp. 377–85.

20. Ghaderi, A., Banafshe, H. R., Mirhosseini, N., et al., 2019. Clinical and metabolic response to vitamin D plus probiotic in schizophrenia patients. *BMC Psychiatry*, 19(1), p. 77.

21. Dickerson, F. B., Stallings, C., Origoni, A., et al., 2014. Effect of probiotic supplementation on schizophrenia symptoms and association with gastrointestinal functioning: a randomized, placebo-controlled trial. *Primary Care Companion for CNS Disorders*, 16(1).

22. Zeevi, D., Korem, T., Zmora, N., et al., 2015. Personalized nutrition by prediction of glycemic responses. *Cell*, 163(5), pp. 1079–94.

23. Pedersen, H. K., Gudmundsdottir, V., Nielsen, H. B., et al., 2016. Human gut microbes impact host serum metabolome and insulin sensitivity. *Nature*, 535(7612), pp. 376–81.

24. Schüssler-Fiorenza Rose, S. M., Contrepois, K., Moneghetti, K. J., et al., 2019. A longitudinal big data approach for precision health. *Nature Medicine*, 25(5), pp. 792–804.

25. Fu, J., Bonder, M. J., Cenit, M. C., et al., 2015. The gut microbiome contributes to a substantial proportion of the variation in blood lipids. *Circulation Research*, 117(9), pp. 817–24.

26. Zheng, J., Lin, Z., Ko, C.-Y, et al., 2022. Analysis of gut microbiota in patients with exacerbated symptoms of schizophrenia following therapy with amisulpride: a pilot study. *Behavioural Neurology*, 2022, p. 4262094.

27. Maier, L., Pruteanu, M., Kuhn, M., et al., 2018. Extensive impact of non-antibiotic drugs on human gut bacteria. *Nature*, 555 (7698), pp. 623–8.

28. Nehme, H., Saulnier, P., Ramadan, A. A., et al., 2018. Antibacterial activity of antipsychotic agents, their association with lipid nanocapsules and its impact on the properties of the nanocarriers and on antibacterial activity. *PLoS One*, 13(1), p. e0189950.

29. Liu, J., De Palma, G., Gorbovskaya, I., et al., 2021. The role of the microbiome-gut-brain axis in schizophrenia and clozapine-induced weight gain. *Biological Psychiatry*, 89(9), p. S342.

30. Manchia, M., Fontana, A., Panebianco, C., et al., 2021. Involvement of gut microbiota in schizophrenia and treatment resistance to antipsychotics. *Biomedicines*, 314–318.

31. Zhernakova, A., Kurilshikov, A., Bonder, M. J., et al., 2016. Population-based metagenomics analysis reveals markers for gut microbiome composition and diversity. *Science*, 352(6285), pp. 565–9.

32. Nash, A. K., Auchtung, T. A., Wong, M. C., et al., 2017. The gut mycobiome of the Human Microbiome Project healthy cohort. *Microbiome*, 5(1), p. 153.

33. Shkoporov, A. N., Clooney, A. G., Sutton, T. D. S., et al., 2019. The human gut virome is highly diverse, stable, and individual specific. *Cell Host & Microbe*, 26 (4), pp. 527–41.e5.

34. David, L. A., Maurice, C. F., Carmody, R. N., et al., 2014. Diet rapidly and reproducibly alters the human gut microbiome. *Nature*, 505(7484), pp. 559–63.

35. Clarke, S. F., Murphy, E. F., O'Sullivan, O., et al., 2014. Exercise and associated dietary extremes impact on gut microbial diversity. *Gut*, 63(12), pp. 1913–20.

36. Clarke, G., Sandhu, K. V., Griffin, B. T., 2019. Gut reactions: breaking down xenobiotic-microbiome interactions. *Pharmacological Reviews*, 71(2), pp. 198–224.

37. Rothschild D, Weissbrod O, Barkan E, Kurilshikov A, Korem T, Zeevi D, et al., 2018. Environment dominates over host genetics in shaping human gut microbiota. *Nature*, 555(7695), pp. 210–15.

38. The Human Microbiome Project Consortium, 2012. Structure, function and diversity of the healthy human microbiome. *Nature*, 486, p. 207.

39. Falony, G., Joossens, M., Vieira-Silva, S., et al., 2016. Population-level analysis of gut microbiome variation. *Science (New York, NY)*, 352(6285), pp. 560–4.

40. Lozupone, C. A., Stombaugh, J. I., Gordon, J. I., Jansson, J. K. and Knight, R., 2012. Diversity, stability and resilience of the human gut microbiota. *Nature*, 489 (7415), pp. 220–30.

41. Gacesa, R., Kurilshikov, A., Vich Vila, A., et al., 2022. Environmental factors shaping the gut microbiome in a Dutch population. *Nature*, 604, pp. 732–9.

42. Roswall, J., Olsson, L. M., Kovatcheva-Datchary, P., et al., 2021. Developmental trajectory of the healthy human gut microbiota during the first 5 years of life. *Cell Host & Microbe*, 29(5), pp. 765–76.e3.

43. Chu, D. M., Ma, J., Prince, A. L., et al., 2017. Maturation of the infant microbiome community structure and function across multiple body sites and in relation to mode of delivery. *Nature Medicine*, 23(3), pp. 314–26.

44. Timmerman, H. M., Rutten, N. B. M. M., Boekhorst, J., et al., 2017. Intestinal colonisation patterns in breastfed and formula-fed infants during the first 12 weeks of life reveal sequential microbiota signatures. *Scientific Reports*, 7(1), p. 8327.

45. Reyman, M., van Houten, M. A., Watson, R. L., et al., 2022. Effects of early-life antibiotics on the developing infant gut microbiome and resistome: a randomized trial. *Nature Communications*, 13(1), p. 893.

46. Robertson, R. C., Manges, A. R., Finlay, B. B. and Prendergast, A. J., 2019. The human microbiome and child growth: first 1000 days and beyond. *Trends in Microbiology*, 27(2), pp. 131–47.

47. O'Donnell, M. P., Fox, B. W., Chao, P. H., Schroeder, F. C. and Sengupta, P., 2020. A neurotransmitter produced by gut bacteria modulates host sensory behaviour. *Nature*, 583(7816), pp. 415–20.

48. Heijtz, R. D., Wang, S., Anuar, F., et al., 2011. Normal gut microbiota modulates brain development and behavior. *Proceedings of the National Academy of Sciences*, 108(7), pp. 3047–52.

49. Aatsinki, A.-K., Lahti, L., Uusitupa, H.-M., et al., 2019. Gut microbiota composition is associated with temperament traits in infants. *Brain, Behavior, and Immunity, 80*, pp. 849–58.

50. Loughman, A., Ponsonby, A.-L., O'Hely, M., et al., 2020. Gut microbiota composition during infancy and subsequent behavioural outcomes. *EBioMedicine*, 52, p. 102640.

51. Kelsey, C. M., Prescott, S., McCulloch, J. A., et al., 2021. Gut microbiota composition is associated with newborn functional brain connectivity and behavioral temperament. *Brain, Behavior, and Immunity, 91*, pp. 472–86.

52. Sordillo, J. E., Korrick, S., Laranjo, N., et al., 2019. Association of the infant gut microbiome with early childhood neurodevelopmental outcomes: an ancillary study to the VDAART randomized clinical trial. *JAMA Network Open, 2*(3), p. e190905.

53. Carlson, A. L., Xia, K., Azcarate-Peril, M. A., et al., 2018. Infant gut microbiome associated with cognitive development. *Biological Psychiatry, 83*(2), pp. 148–59.

54. Carlson, A. L., Xia, K., Azcarate-Peril, M. A., et al., 2021. Infant gut microbiome composition is associated with non-social fear behavior in a pilot study. *Nature Communications, 12*(1), p. 3294.

55. Streit, F., Prandovszky, E., Send, T., et al., 2021. Microbiome profiles are associated with cognitive functioning in 45-month-old children. *Brain, Behavior, and Immunity, 98*, pp. 151–60.

56. Erny, D., Hrabe de Angelis, A. L., Jaitin, D., et al., 2015. Host microbiota constantly control maturation and function of microglia in the CNS. *Nature Neuroscience, 18*(7), pp. 965–77.

57. Fülling, C., Dinan, T. G. and Cryan, J. F., 2019. Gut microbe to brain signaling: what happens in vagus . . .. *Neuron, 101*(6), pp. 998–1002.

58. O'Riordan, K. J., Collins, M. K., Moloney, G. M., et al., 2022. Short chain fatty acids: microbial metabolites for gut-brain axis signalling. *Molecular and Cellular Endocrinology, 546*, p. 111572.

59. Ye, L., Bae, M., Cassily, C. D., et al., 2021. Enteroendocrine cells sense bacterial tryptophan catabolites to activate enteric and vagal neuronal pathways. *Cell Host & Microbe, 29*(2), pp. 179–96.e9.

60. O'Mahony, S. M., Clarke, G., Borre, Y. E., Dinan, T. G. and Cryan, J. F., 2015. Serotonin, tryptophan metabolism and the brain-gut-microbiome axis. *Behavioural Brain Research, 277*, pp. 32–48.

61. Henrick, B. M., Rodriguez, L., Lakshmikanth, T., et al., 2021. Bifidobacteria-mediated immune system imprinting early in life. *Cell, 184*(15), pp. 3884–98.e11.

62. Olm, M. R., Dahan, D., Carter, M. M., et al., 2022. Robust variation in infant gut microbiome assembly across a spectrum of lifestyles. *Science, 376*(6598), pp. 1220–3.

63. Maes, M., Kanchanatawan, B., Sirivichayakul, S. and Carvalho, A. F., 2019. In schizophrenia, increased plasma IgM/IgA responses to gut commensal bacteria are associated with negative symptoms, neurocognitive impairments, and the deficit phenotype. *Neurotoxicity Research, 35*(3), pp. 684–98.

64. Maes, M., Sirivichayakul, S., Kanchanatawan, B. and Vodjani, A., 2019. Upregulation of the intestinal paracellular pathway with breakdown of tight and adherens junctions in deficit schizophrenia. *Molecular Neurobiology, 56* (10), pp. 7056–73.

65. Severance, E. G., Gressitt, K. L., Stallings, C. R., et al., 2013. Discordant patterns of bacterial translocation markers and implications for innate immune imbalances in schizophrenia. *Schizophrenia Research, 148*(1–3), pp. 130–7.

66. Xu, R., Wu, B., Liang, J., et al., 2020. Altered gut microbiota and mucosal immunity in patients with schizophrenia. *Brain, Behavior, and Immunity, 85*, pp. 120–7.

67. Marx, W., McGuinness, A. J., Rocks, T., et al., 2021. The kynurenine pathway in major depressive disorder, bipolar disorder, and schizophrenia: a meta-analysis of 101 studies. *Molecular Psychiatry, 26*(8), pp. 4158–78.

68. Zhu, F., Guo, R., Wang, W., et al., 2020. Transplantation of microbiota from drug-free patients with schizophrenia causes schizophrenia-like abnormal behaviors and dysregulated kynurenine metabolism in mice. *Molecular Psychiatry, 25*(11), pp. 2905–18.

69. Hoban, A. E., Stilling, R. M., Ryan, F. J., et al., 2016. Regulation of prefrontal cortex myelination by the microbiota. *Translational Psychiatry, 6*, p. e774.

70. Braniste, V., Al-Asmakh, M., Kowal, C., et al., 2014. The gut microbiota influences

blood-brain barrier permeability in mice. *Science Translational Medicine*, 6(263), 263ra158.

71. Diaz Heijtz, R., Wang, S., Anuar, F., et al., 2011. Normal gut microbiota modulates brain development and behavior. *Proceedings of the National Academy of Sciences of the United States of America*, 108 (21282636), pp. 3047–52.

72. Crumeyrolle-Arias, M., Jaglin, M., Bruneau, A., et al., 2014. Absence of the gut microbiota enhances anxiety-like behavior and neuroendocrine response to acute stress in rats. *Psychoneuroendocrinology*, 42, pp. 207–17.

73. Hoban, A. E., Moloney, R. D., Golubeva, A. V., et al., 2016. Behavioural and neurochemical consequences of chronic gut microbiota depletion during adulthood in the rat. *Neuroscience*, 339, pp. 463–77.

74. Neufeld, K. M., Kang, N., Bienenstock, J. and Foster, J. A., 2011. Reduced anxiety-like behavior and central neurochemical change in germ-free mice. *Neurogastroenterology and Motility: The Official Journal of the European Gastrointestinal Motility Society*, 23(3), pp. 255–64, e119.

75. Savignac, H. M., Corona, G., Mills, H., et al., 2013. Prebiotic feeding elevates central brain derived neurotrophic factor, N-methyl-D-aspartate receptor subunits and D-serine. *Neurochemistry International*, 63(8), pp. 756–64.

76. Gronier, B., Savignac, H. M., Di Miceli, M., et al., 2018. Increased cortical neuronal responses to NMDA and improved attentional set-shifting performance in rats following prebiotic (B-GOS®) ingestion. *European Neuropsychopharmacology: The Journal of the European College of Neuropsychopharmacology*, 28(1), pp. 211–24.

77. Bravo, J. A., Forsythe, P., Chew, M. V., et al., 2011. Ingestion of Lactobacillus strain regulates emotional behavior and central GABA receptor expression in a mouse via the vagus nerve. *Proceedings of the National Academy of Sciences of the United States of America*, 108(38), pp. 16050–5.

78. Janik, R., Thomason, L. A. M., Stanisz, A. M., et al., 2016. Magnetic resonance spectroscopy reveals oral Lactobacillus promotion of increases in brain GABA, N-acetyl aspartate and glutamate. *NeuroImage*, 125, pp. 988–95.

79. Burokas, A., Arboleya, S., Moloney, R. D., et al., 2017. Targeting the microbiota-gut-brain axis: prebiotics have anxiolytic and antidepressant-like effects and reverse the impact of chronic stress in mice. *Biological Psychiatry*, 82(7), pp. 472–87.

80. Zheng, P., Zeng, B., Liu, M., et al., 2019. The gut microbiome from patients with schizophrenia modulates the glutamate-glutamine-GABA cycle and schizophrenia-relevant behaviors in mice. *Science Advances*, 5(2), p. eaau8317.

81. Dragioti, E., Radua, J., Solmi, M., et al., 2022. Global population attributable fraction of potentially modifiable risk factors for mental disorders: a meta-umbrella systematic review. *Molecular Psychiatry*, 27, pp. 3510–19.

82. Martland, N., Martland, R., Cullen, A. E. and Bhattacharyya, S., 2020. Are adult stressful life events associated with psychotic relapse? A systematic review of 23 studies. *Psychological Medicine*, 50(14), pp. 2302–16.

83. Provensi, G., Schmidt, S. D., Boehme, M., et al., 2019. Preventing adolescent stress-induced cognitive and microbiome changes by diet. *Proceedings of the National Academy of Sciences*, 116(19), pp. 9644–51.

84. Johnson, K. V. A., 2020. Gut microbiome composition and diversity are related to human personality traits. *Human Microbiome Journal*, 15, p. 100069.

85. Zhu, F., Ju, Y., Wang, W., et al., 2020. Metagenome-wide association of gut microbiome features for schizophrenia. *Nature Communications*, 11(1), p. 1612.

86. Davey, K. J., O'Mahony, S. M., Schellekens, H., et al., 2012. Gender-dependent consequences of chronic olanzapine in the rat: effects on body weight, inflammatory, metabolic and microbiota parameters. *Psychopharmacology*, 221(1), pp. 155–69.

87. Davey, K. J., Cotter, P. D., O'Sullivan, O., et al., 2013. Antipsychotics and the gut microbiome: olanzapine-induced metabolic dysfunction is attenuated by antibiotic administration in the rat. *Translational Psychiatry*, 3, p. e309.

88. Yuan, X., Zhang, P., Wang, Y., et al., 2018. Changes in metabolism and microbiota after 24-week risperidone treatment in drug naive, normal weight patients with first episode schizophrenia. *Schizophrenia Research*, 201, pp. 299–306.

89. Flowers, S. A., Evans, S. J., Ward, K. M., McInnis, M. G. and Ellingrod, V. L., 2017. Interaction between atypical antipsychotics and the gut microbiome in a bipolar disease cohort. *Pharmacotherapy*, 37(3), pp. 261–7.

90. Flowers, S. A., Baxter, N. T., Ward, K. M., et al., 2019. Effects of atypical antipsychotic treatment and resistant starch supplementation on gut microbiome composition in a cohort of patients with bipolar disorder or schizophrenia. *Pharmacotherapy*, 39(2), pp. 161–70.

91. Bahra, S. M., Weidemann, B. J., Castro, A. N., et al., 2015. Risperidone-induced weight gain is mediated through shifts in the gut microbiome and suppression of energy expenditure. *EBioMedicine*, 2(11), pp. 1725–34.

92. Bahr, S. M., Tyler, B. C., Wooldridge, N., et al., 2015. Use of the second-generation antipsychotic, risperidone, and secondary weight gain are associated with an altered gut microbiota in children. *Translational Psychiatry*, 5, p. e652.

93. Morgan, A. P., Crowley, J. J., Nonneman, R. J., et al., 2014. The antipsychotic olanzapine interacts with the gut microbiome to cause weight gain in mouse. *Plos One*, 9(12), p. e115225.

94. Kao, A. C., Spitzer, S., Anthony, D. C., Lennox, B. and Burnet, P. W. J., 2018. Prebiotic attenuation of olanzapine-induced weight gain in rats: analysis of central and peripheral biomarkers and gut microbiota. *Translational Psychiatry*, 8(1), p. 66.

95. Minichino, A., Brondino, N., Solmi, M., et al., 2021. The gut-microbiome as a target for the treatment of schizophrenia: a systematic review and meta-analysis of randomised controlled trials of add-on strategies. *Schizophrenia Research*, 234, pp. 1–13.

96. Gaughran, F., Stringer, D., Wojewodka, G., et al., 2021. Effect of vitamin D supplementation on outcomes in people with early psychosis: the DFEND randomized clinical trial. *JAMA Network Open*, 4(12), pp. e2140858–e.

97. Tomasik, J., Yolken, R. H., Bahn, S. and Dickerson, F. B., 2015. Immunomodulatory effects of probiotic supplementation in schizophrenia patients: a randomized, placebo-controlled trial. *Biomarker Insights*, 10, pp. 47–54.

98. Severance, E. G., Gressitt, K. L., Stallings, C. R., et al., 2017. Probiotic normalization of Candida albicans in schizophrenia: a randomized, placebo-controlled, longitudinal pilot study. *Brain, Behavior, and Immunity*, 62, pp. 41–5.

99. Dickerson, F., Adamos, M., Katsafanas, E., et al., 2018. Adjunctive probiotic microorganisms to prevent rehospitalization in patients with acute mania: a randomized controlled trial. *Bipolar Disorders*, 20(7), pp. 614–21.

100. Kao, A. C., Safarikova, J., Marquardt, T., et al., 2019. Pro-cognitive effect of a prebiotic in psychosis: a double blind placebo controlled cross-over study. *Schizophrenia Research*, 208, pp. 460–1.

101. Deakin, B., Suckling, J., Barnes, T. R. E., et al., 2018. The benefit of minocycline on negative symptoms of schizophrenia in patients with recent-onset psychosis (BeneMin): a randomised, double-blind, placebo-controlled trial. *The Lancet Psychiatry*, 5(11), pp. 885–94.

102. Kang, D.-W., Adams, J. B., Coleman, D. M., et al., 2019. Long-term benefit of microbiota transfer therapy on autism symptoms and gut microbiota. *Scientific Reports*, 9(1), p. 5821.

103. Stewart Campbell, A., Needham, B. D., Meyer, C. R., et al., 2022. Safety and target engagement of an oral small-molecule

sequestrant in adolescents with autism spectrum disorder: an open-label phase 1b/2a trial. *Nature Medicine, 28*(3), pp. 528–34.

104. Teasdale, S. B., Ward, P. B., Samaras, K., et al., 2019. Dietary intake of people with severe mental illness: systematic review and meta-analysis. *British Journal of Psychiatry, 214*(5), pp. 251–9.

105. Sarris, J., Ravindran, A., Yatham, L. N., et al., 2022. Clinician guidelines for the treatment of psychiatric disorders with nutraceuticals and phytoceuticals: the World Federation of Societies of Biological Psychiatry (WFSBP) and Canadian Network for Mood and Anxiety Treatments (CANMAT) Taskforce. *The World Journal of Biological Psychiatry, 23* (6), pp. 424–55.

106. Maguire, Á., Mooney, C., Flynn, G., et al., 2021. No effect of coenzyme Q10 on cognitive function, psychological symptoms, and health-related outcomes in schizophrenia and schizoaffective disorder: results of a randomized, placebo-controlled trial. *Journal of Clinical Psychopharmacology, 41*(1), pp. 53–7.

107. McGorry, P. D., Nelson, B., Markulev, C., et al., 2017. Effect of ω-3 polyunsaturated fatty acids in young people at ultrahigh risk for psychotic disorders: the NEURAPRO randomized clinical trial. *JAMA Psychiatry, 74*(1), pp. 19–27.

108. Allott, K., McGorry, P. D., Yuen, H. P., et al., 2019. The vitamins in psychosis study: a randomized, double-blind, placebo-controlled trial of the effects of vitamins B(12), B(6), and folic acid on symptoms and neurocognition in first-episode psychosis. *Biological Psychiatry, 86*(1), pp. 35–44.

109. Afshin, A., Sur, P. J., Fay, K. A., et al., 2019. Health effects of dietary risks in 195 countries, 1990–2017: a systematic analysis for the Global Burden of Disease Study 2017. *The Lancet, 393*(10184), pp. 1958–72.

110. Bhutta, Z. A., Das, J. K., Rizvi, A., et al., 2013. Evidence-based interventions for improvement of maternal and child nutrition: what can be done and at what cost? *Lancet, 382*(9890), pp. 452–77.

111. Deehan, E. C., Yang, C., Perez-Muñoz, M. E., et al., 2020. Precision microbiome modulation with discrete dietary fiber structures directs short-chain fatty acid production. *Cell Host & Microbe, 27*(3), pp. 389–404.e6.

112. Dinan, T. G., Stanton, C., Long-Smith, C., et al., 2019. Feeding melancholic microbes: MyNewGut recommendations on diet and mood. *Clinical Nutrition, 38* (5), pp. 1995–2001.

113. De Filippis, F., Pellegrini, N., Vannini, L., et al., 2016. High-level adherence to a Mediterranean diet beneficially impacts the gut microbiota and associated metabolome. *Gut, 65*(11), pp. 1812–21.

114. Vangay, P., Johnson, A. J., Ward, T. L., et al., 2018. US immigration Westernizes the human gut microbiome. *Cell, 175*(4), pp. 962–72.e10.

115. Sonnenburg, E. D. and Sonnenburg, J. L., 2019. The ancestral and industrialized gut microbiota and implications for human health. *Nature Reviews Microbiology, 17* (6), pp. 383–90.

116. Wastyk, H. C., Fragiadakis, G. K., Perelman, D., et al., 2021. Gut-microbiota -targeted diets modulate human immune status. *Cell, 184*(16), pp. 4137–53.e14.

117. Zhu, C., Sawrey-Kubicek, L., Beals, E., et al., 2020. Human gut microbiome composition and tryptophan metabolites were changed differently by fast food and Mediterranean diet in 4 days: a pilot study. *Nutrition Research, 77*, pp. 62–72.

118. Vassilopoulou, E., Efthymiou, D., Tsironis, V., et al., 2022. The benefits of the Mediterranean diet in first episode psychosis patients taking antipsychotics. *Toxicology Reports, 9*, pp. 120–5.

119. Kowalski, K., Bogudzińska, B., Stańczykiewicz, B., et al., 2022. The deficit schizophrenia subtype is associated with low adherence to the Mediterranean diet: findings from a case–control study. *Journal of Clinical Medicine, 11*(3), p. 568.

120. Trevelline, B. K. and Kohl, K. D., 2022. The gut microbiome influences host diet selection behavior. *Proceedings of the National Academy of Sciences of the United States of America*, 119(17), p. e2117537119.

121. Dong, T. S., Guan, M., Mayer, E. A., et al., 2022. Obesity is associated with a distinct brain-gut microbiome signature that connects Prevotella and Bacteroides to the brain's reward center. *Gut Microbes*, 14 (1), p. 2051999.

122. Minichino, A., Jackson, M. A., Francesconi, M., et al., 2021. Endocannabinoid system mediates the association between gut-microbial diversity and anhedonia/amotivation in a general population cohort. *Molecular Psychiatry*, 26(11), pp. 6269–76.

123. Atzeni, A., Bastiaanssen, T. F. S., Cryan, J. F., et al., 2022. Taxonomic and functional fecal microbiota signatures associated with insulin resistance in non-diabetic subjects with overweight/ obesity within the frame of the PREDIMED-Plus study. *Frontiers in Endocrinology*, 13.

124. Liu, Y., Wang, Y., Ni, Y., et al., 2020. Gut microbiome fermentation determines the efficacy of exercise for diabetes prevention. *Cell Metabolism*, 31(1), pp. 77–91.e5.

125. Thirion, F., Speyer, H., Hansen, T. H., et al., in press. Alteration of gut microbiome in patients with schizophrenia indicates links between bacterial tyrosine biosynthesis and cognitive dysfunction. *Biological Psychiatry Global Open Science*.

126. Li, S., Zhuo, M., Huang, X., et al., 2020. Altered gut microbiota associated with symptom severity in schizophrenia. *PeerJ*, 8, p. e9574.

127. Pan, R., Zhang, X., Gao, J., et al., 2020. Analysis of the diversity of intestinal microbiome and its potential value as a biomarker in patients with schizophrenia: a cohort study. *Psychiatry Research*, 291, p. 113260.

128. Ma, X., Asif, H., Dai, L., et al., 2020. Alteration of the gut microbiome in first-episode drug-naive and chronic medicated schizophrenia correlate with regional brain volumes. *Journal of Psychiatric Research*, 123, pp. 136–44.

129. Nguyen, T. T., Kosciolek, T., Maldonado, Y., et al., 2019. Differences in gut microbiome composition between persons with chronic schizophrenia and healthy comparison subjects. *Schizophrenia Research*, 204, pp. 23–9.

130. He, Y., Kosciolek, T., Tang, J., et al., 2018. Gut microbiome and magnetic resonance spectroscopy study of subjects at ultra-high risk for psychosis may support the membrane hypothesis. *European Psychiatry: The Journal of the Association of European Psychiatrists*, 53, pp. 37–45.

131. Shen, Y., Xu, J., Li, Z., et al., 2018. Analysis of gut microbiota diversity and auxiliary diagnosis as a biomarker in patients with schizophrenia: a cross-sectional study. *Schizophrenia Research*, 197, pp. 470–7.

132. Schwarz, E., Maukonen, J., Hyytiainen, T., et al., 2018. Analysis of microbiota in first episode psychosis identifies preliminary associations with symptom severity and treatment response. *Schizophrenia Research*, 192, pp. 398–403.

133. Severance, E. G., Gressitt, K. L., Stallings, C. R., et al., 2016. Candida albicans exposures, sex specificity and cognitive deficits in schizophrenia and bipolar disorder. *NPJ Schizophrenia*, 2, p. 16018.

134. Castro-Nallar, E., Bendall, M. L., Perez-Losada, M., et al., 2015. Composition, taxonomy and functional diversity of the oropharynx microbiome in individuals with schizophrenia and controls. *PeerJ*, 3, p. e1140.

135. Yolken, R. H., Severance, E. G., Sabunciyan, S., et al., 2015. Metagenomic sequencing indicates that the oropharyngeal phageome of individuals with schizophrenia differs from that of controls. *Schizophrenia Bulletin*, 41(5), pp. 1153–61.

Recognising the Importance of Nutrition for Child and Adolescent Mental Health

Kathrin Cohen Kadosh and Nicola Johnstone

Summary

In recognising the importance of nutrition for child and adolescent mental health, we describe how the gut microbiome is a valuable organ that contains a wealth of potential mechanistic explanations for understanding the development of child and adolescent mental health and as a therapeutic target. The gut microbiome contains trillions of microorganisms that are influenced by not only the food we eat but also the environment in which we live, and this has implications for the functional potential of these microorganisms in sustaining the immune system and metabolic homeostasis. Moreover, a decade of research has shown that there are functional bidirectional pathways linking the gut microbiome and the brain. Herein we postulate that understanding child and adolescent mental health may be advanced by situating research within the conceptual framework of the microbiome–gut–brain (MBA) axis.

To illustrate how the MBA axis can enhance our understanding of the development of mental health, we describe how first milks may set the trajectory for later psychological development and how dietary interventions may prove effective across childhood. Critically, we highlight periods of development in which the gut microbiome may be influential. Finally, we discuss how multidimensional research approaches will be invaluable to further understanding and develop effective treatments for child and adolescent mental health.

The transitional period from childhood to adulthood is marked by a multitude of changes in social and cognitive abilities and brain maturation, as well as genetic and hormonal changes (1). One implication of these many changes is that they increase the risk of developing mental health problems, such as anxiety or depression (2–4). Moreover, there is the risk that maladaptive behavioural patterns can become persistent while brain networks mature (5, 6). Supporting adolescents during this transition has important implications not only for an individual's lifelong well-being but also with regards to the significant social and economic burden that mental health problems place on society (7). Despite these implications, little is currently known about how these developmental changes work together to increase the risk of developing mental health problems. One explanation for this lack of progress is that current research approaches have yet to integrate the important role that nutrition, and by extension a healthy gut microbiome, plays during this developmental period.

The gut is dominated by microorganisms including bacteria, archaea, yeasts, viruses and protozoa, and the term 'gut microbiome' refers to the combined genetic material of these organisms (8). The potential of the gut microbiome to influence development is inferred from multiple bidirectional systems connecting to and from the brain, including neural, endocrine and immune pathways (9–12), commonly called the microbiome–gut–brain (MGB) axis. The last decade has seen considerable interest in the MGB axis, with many recognising its therapeutic potential for a wealth of pathologies – not only for physical health but also for mental health.

To date, much of the research on the MGB axis has focussed on understanding the composition of the gut microbiome (which can be thought of as the combination of the presence and balance of groups of trillions of possible microorganisms) and how variations in gut-microbiome composition relate to brain function and responsiveness and, by extension, behaviours in health and disease. The efforts of these endeavours are to identify novel mechanisms that underpin behaviours to stimulate different approaches to treating or even preventing pathologies in physical and mental health. This is particularly exciting for research studying human development, where extended periods of maturation offer increased levels of plasticity and opportunities to shape emerging behaviours and brain networks as they mature. Moreover, children and young people are very interested in using nutrition to shape their own health, particularly adolescents who seek ways to cope with a myriad of changes (13).

It has been suggested that the composition of the gut microbiome influences not only postnatal brain development but also brain responsiveness and function across the lifespan (14, 15), with gut microbiota regulating gene expression and release of metabolites in the brain (16, 17). Critically, there are a number of sensitive periods in childhood and adolescence (18) when the gut–brain axis is fine-tuned and when we can use dietary intervention to change the gut microbiome (19). Yet despite much research effort characterising the effects of gut-microbiome composition on behaviour and mental health (20, 21), research into development is sparse (22–24). More research is now needed to investigate the psychoactive properties of the gut microbiome in development.

Setting the Trajectory of the Developing Gut–Brain Axis

Brain development is most prolific in the first 2 years of life (25), yet little is known about how early infant feeding practices, in terms of first milks (mothers' own breastmilk, donated breastmilk, formula compositions or a combination of each) and the onset of complementary feeding, influence the development of the nervous system (including the brain) in the longer term. The gut microbiome is seeded during birth (26, 27) and subsequently diversifies with the intake of first milks and other environmental factors that reflect interactions with microorganisms (28). Beyond this, the gut-microbiome composition proceeds though a series of stages over several years signified by the introduction of complementary foods (29), the reduction of first milks and the diversification in diet in toddlerhood (30), before reaching an adult-like state of diverse composition around at around 2–3 years (31). Regarding first milks, there are differences in the make-up of the gut-microbiome composition of infants fed breastmilk and those who are not. Primarily, infants fed breastmilk have a less diverse gut-microbiome composition but one that is dominated by probiotic bacteria (32). Strikingly, one of the biggest transition events evident in the composition of the gut microbiome is the cessation of breastmilk (33). Although there is a dearth of evidence in this area, the available research suggests that breastmilk is strongly represented in the gut-microbiome composition for as long as it is provided, including into toddlerhood and beyond. This poses an interesting question about the utility of breastmilk via the gut–brain axis in ongoing brain development, as a significant body of research has shown that gut microorganisms are important in stimulating the building blocks of the nervous system to affect how the brain develops over time (15).

Bioactive Potential of Breastmilk in the Gut Microbiome

The MGB axis is a framework for understanding homeostasis via bidirectional communications between the gut bacteria and host systems. There is a wealth of studies showing how supplementing the diet influences the gut bacteria to induce changes in emotional behaviour (13, 34) and cognition (35, 36), showing that food consumption influences behaviour via the MGB axis. The gut microbiome is an important catalyst in steering developmental trajectories that rapidly occur in early childhood. Studies of the gut-microbiome composition in infants less than 1 year old show distinct differences in gut-microbiome composition depending on the type of milk received (37, 38) and on milk delivery method (e.g. expressed or breast) (39). Breastmilk is thought to contribute to the development of the gut-microbiome composition via transformative effects of bioactive properties rather than direct transfer of milk bacteria to the gut. For example, there are common bacterial strains between human milk and gut microbiota, but this relationship lessens when milk is expressed (40). Further, women of distinct ethnicities have distinct breastmilk microbiota, but these differences are not reflected in their infant's gut microbiome (41). In a similar line, the addition of pro- or prebiotic compounds to formula milks does not replicate a gut microbiome nourished by breastmilk (42). Bioactive components in human milk are therefore critical for shaping the gut-microbiome composition.

Breastmilk has a wealth of bioactive properties that shape the development of multiple body systems including the nervous, endocrine and immune systems (43). For example, breastmilk has antibodies, growth factors, lactoferrin and human milk oligosaccharides (HMOs), in addition to nutrients (44). HMOs are diverse prebiotic bioactive compounds with various functional potentials in the gut microbiome (45). HMOs function as decoys against pathogens (46) and grow specific species and strains of *Bifidobacteria* that are important in developing intestinal homeostasis and immune responses (47). The critical aspect of HMOs is that, to date, the bioactive potential has not been replicated. While prebiotic fortified infant milk formulas can induce a *Bifidobacteria* dominant microbiome, this does not replicate a gut microbiome grown by HMOs, which needs a complex set of enzymes working in harmony to break down HMO chains (48). The abundance of HMOs decreases over time, but this does not correlate to decreases in dominant bacteria in the gut microbiome (49), illustrating a relationship of optimal microbe–host co-evolution (50) (Figure 7.1).

Bioactive Potential of Breastmilk in Psychological Development

Breastmilk has specific bioactive properties that have the potential to shape psychological development via bidirectional communications between the gut microbiome and the brain, which can influence the trajectory of neural development and in turn influence cognition and psychological behaviours. This process has been termed *Lactocrine-programming* (51) and is the epitome of personalised nutrition (52, 53). Breastfeeding has long been linked to improvements in cognitive outcomes (54), but it is not well understood how. There has been considerable debate in the literature about the magnitude of effect on cognition by breast-feeding and confounding with other relevant factors including maternal, paternal, child and

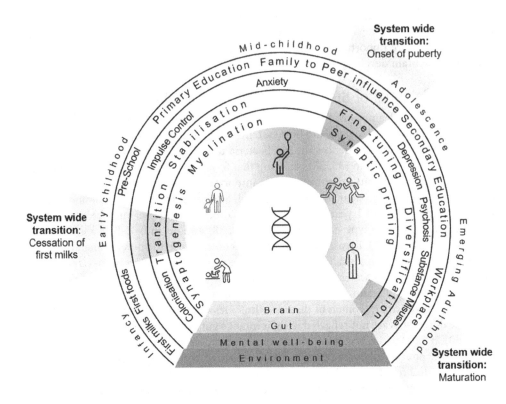

Figure 7.1 Layers of developmental progression from birth to adulthood at the level of the brain, gut microbiome, maladaptive psychological symptoms and external environmental events. Pivotal cross-layer events in development are signified by the cessation of first milks, onset of puberty and brain maturation.

environmental characteristics. However, effects appear persistent into early adolescence after accounting for alternative explanations (55).

With regard to emotional development, there have been several large population cohort studies linking breastfeeding to better emotional outcomes in comparison to those never breastfed in Brazil (56), Australia (57), Ireland (58) and the UK (59, 60). For example, the millennial cohort studies of the UK found longer breastfeeding duration was associated with fewer parental-rated behavioural problems in term-born children aged 3, 5, 7, 11 and 14 years of age. However, similar confounding issues are encountered in emotional development. For example, the 2005–7 Infant Feeding Practices Study II with 6-year follow-up also found at age 6, when compared with children who were never breastfed, those who were breastfed for at least 6 months and exclusively breastfed for at least 3 months had decreased odds of difficulties with emotional symptoms, conduct issues and total difficulties overall. Yet, adjusting for potential confounding factors eliminated the positive associations of breastfeeding (61).

Rather than dismiss the positive associations between breastfeeding and emotional and cognitive development as so small as to be immaterial, or as an additive bonus to desirable characteristics of the environment and parental fortunes, we should remember that breastmilk is a complex, bioactive and *personalised* food that emerging research is only just beginning to understand and that it will be better understood within the context of the gut–brain axis. The gut-microbiome composition has established links to cognitive and emotional development in animal models, with evidence emerging in human studies too. For example, specific gut-microbiome characteristics have been associated with continued breastfeeding at 1 year old and improved cognitive function at 2 years old (22) and reduced fear reactivity in behaviour (62). Critically, the gut-microbiome composition has also been associated with functional connectivity in brain regions that link neural processing to behavioural effects (63) and shows alterations due to early life stress that may alter the trajectory of psychological development (64). Herein, showing how the bioactive property of breastmilk continues to contribute to cognitive and emotional development via the gut microbiome could transform understanding of human developmental trajectories.

Gut-Microbiome Maturation in Early Childhood

The maturation of the gut microbiome co-evolves with host physiology to prime and influence the development of biological processes (48). A multitude of perinatal factors shape the trajectory of gut maturation in early childhood (65), with the gut microbiome of infants considered 'matured' (e.g. in an adult-like state) following a process of bacterial succession from birth to 2–3 years of age (31). The stages of early succession in the first year of life are well documented (66), but recent evidence suggests maturation may be prolonged throughout early childhood. In a longitudinal study with children aged 3 months to 4 years, three distinct phases of the gut-microbiome progression were characterised: (i) a developmental phase (3–14 months), (ii) a transitional phase (15–30 months) and (iii) a stable phase (31–46 months) (67). This extended maturational process is unsurprising considering early childhood is a period of rapid development of many body systems (e.g. nervous system), which the gut microbiota mirrors.

This poses a question about the sensitivity of the gut microbiome to external influence during this extended period, particularly in the transitional phase (aged 15–30 months). The gut-microbiome composition is responsive to external influences with significant effects from breastmilk and environmental factors, including geographical location and household members (e.g. siblings and pets) (67). While the longitudinal study retained a small number of breastfed toddlers at the later testing points (10% at 15 months, dropping to 6% at around 2 years plus), there is otherwise a notable absence of children who are breastfed beyond early infancy in studies of gut-microbiome maturation. This is important because the bioactive components of breastmilk temporally adapt to the needs of the breastfed child to protect against pathogens and support immunological function and brain development, and may be significant in the transitional phase (15–30 months) of gut-microbiome maturation in toddlers. Deeper understanding of the biological mechanisms activated by breastmilk to support optimal development would help clarify the developmental trajectories in health and disease (Box 7.1).

The Gut Microbiome in Mid-Childhood and Adolescence: Implications for Mental Health

The transition from childhood to early adulthood has long been understood to be a period of increased risk for mental health problems, with two-thirds of all mental health problems

Box 7.1 Open Question: Breastfeeding beyond Infancy and Developmental Implications

From around 6 months of age, infants require additional nutrients to first milks in the form of food to support growth and development via processes initiated in the gut microbiome (68). Infants who continue to be breastfed after this time have a different gut-microbiome composition to those not receiving breastmilk (38), showing breastmilk has a persistent influence on the gut microbiome alongside solid foods. Additionally, dietary differences in food types consumed (e.g. plant-based or dairy) by young children have also been found in the gut-microbiome composition (69–71). Yet, no study to date has considered breastmilk in relation to food intake in the gut-microbiome composition of young children. Research on breastmilk composition produced for children beyond their first year illustrates a wealth of protein, fat and vitamin availability (72, 73), and immuno-protective factors (74) to support healthy development. Moreover, studies estimate breastmilk contributes up to one-third of daily calorie intake in toddlers' diets (74, 75), highlighting a substantial energy source. While all mammal milks are comparably rich sources of nutrients (76), only human milk temporally and responsively adapts composition to meet the child's needs (77). Herein, breastmilk has the potential to form a critical part of toddlers' diets. To understand how the bioactive potential of breastmilk shapes gut-microbiome composition in toddlers' diets and subsequent development, nutrient intake from food at this age should be considered.

emerging before the age of 18 (78, 79). However, whereas much work has focussed on describing the contribution of ongoing brain maturation during this period (6, 80–82), as well as the role of changes in the social environment and peer relationships (1, 2, 83), little progress has been made to date in using these findings to improve the outcome for the individual. One possible reason for this lack of progress, in our view, is that we have so far overlooked another important aspect in understanding the complex developmental interplay during this period, namely the gut microbiome and how gut bacteria influence brain function (13). In our opinion, protective or adaptive gut-microbiome function in development is important for three reasons, as we will explain in greater detail in the following sections.

Psychobiotics

Psychobiotics are compounds, such as probiotics and prebiotics, that have the potential to exert antidepressant or anxiolytic effects (84, 85). There is reliable evidence from animal models but also a handful of high-quality human randomised control trials that show that dietary interventions using psychobiotics are effective in changing gut-microbiome composition, leading to robust, reproducible, attenuating effects on anxious and depressive-like behaviours (13, 34, 36). Probiotics have been used most commonly in this approach, with beneficial effects identified in hormones (86), cognitive processing (21) and neural responses in brain regions responsible for emotion processing and regulation (87). Recent reviews and meta-analyses of such studies on probiotic effects for improving mental health outcomes have found modest effects in reducing depressive symptoms (34, 88), although there remains problematic between-study heterogeneity.

Prebiotic compounds have alternatively been deployed as psychobiotics in human randomised control trials because prebiotics are able to circumvent potential issues while adding non-native external probiotic bacteria to the host's gut microbiome. Prebiotics stimulate the growth of probiotic bacteria, allowing adaptation of the gut-microbiome composition to the host's present condition. Human randomised control trials using prebiotics have also shown reductions in indicators of stress and decreased attentional vigilance to negative information in a dot-probe task (20). Given that anxious people routinely exhibit increased biases towards negative information (89), this suggests that probiotics, in this case galacto-oligosaccharide (GOS) intake, may be useful in modifying anxiety-related psychological mechanisms.

This result was replicated in our recent randomised placebo-controlled trial of the effects of GOS on indices of anxiety and well-being in young adult females (23). Here we found that GOS supplementation over 4 weeks reduced trait anxiety and indicators of anxious behaviour in the dot-probe task. These changes were mirrored by a significant shift in gut-microbiome composition driven by relative *Bifidobacterium* abundance increases. Moreover, we found that GOS supplementation influenced nutrient intake, such as a reduction in carbohydrate intake in the GOS group (90). As psychobiotics are safe food compounds with no adverse side effects, they may be effective therapeutic tools for low mood and anxiety. These findings highlight the importance of understanding the interactive relationships between gut-microbiome composition, GOS supplementation and its impact on diet longer term in order to establish directional predictions for interventions.

The Adolescent Gut Microbiome As a Window for Intervention

There is some evidence from animal research that adolescence represents a sensitive period for fine-tuning the MGB axis. Within the context of anxiety in adolescence, animal models have also provided new insights that could allow us to achieve a significant breakthrough in supporting adaptive threat-learning and extinction outcomes in adolescence, and in particular in anxious adolescents. In pathological anxiety, the acquired fear response to a threat becomes persistent and maladaptive, and it has been suggested that a deficiency in extinction learning plays a role in the maintenance of pathological anxiety (91). A recent study showed that a lack of gut microbiota diversity interfered with adapting to threat responses in a mouse model (92). This behavioural deficit was accompanied by changes in gene expression in cells in the brain and alterations in the firing patterns and rewiring ability of neurons (92). Most importantly, however, whereas adult mice regained the ability to adapt threat responses once their microbiome had recovered, adolescent mice continued to exhibit a maladaptive response, indicating that extinction learning did not take place and that this newly acquired fear response persisted.

The behavioural evidence of threat-learning in human adolescence shows a similar pattern (91, 93), which further highlights the importance of obtaining a better understanding of the role of the gut microbiome in development in order to produce gut-microbiome-based interventions. Similarly, there is evidence that the significantly stronger peer-orientation during adolescence aids gut-microbiome diversification (94), which suggests that the increased focus on interacting with peers could serve as a protective factor for both gut-microbiome development and gut–brain axis maturation.

Acceptability

Gut-microbiome-based interventions are met with much interest by children and young people, who welcome the opportunity for low-stigma interventions that can be implemented at the kitchen table, in particular as most traditional diets already contain an abundance of both prebiotic- and probiotic-rich ingredients. As recent focus-group work by our group has shown, two-thirds of young people have tried to use a psychobiotic supplement or dietary intervention to improve their mental health problems (13). It would therefore seem that this approach, if done correctly, is promising.

To conclude, the field of nutrition research holds potential for understanding children and adolescent mental health. In particular, recent progress in the role of the MGB axis in development has highlighted not only the important role the gut microbiome plays in influencing both initial brain maturation and function but also its relationship to behaviour and mental health across the lifespan. In order to build on this research and ensure that the field maintains momentum and that we continue to build a bridge from successful animal research to human models, it will be essential to adopt a multi-disciplinary and multilevel approach, which considers the complex interplay of changes at multiple levels. Such an approach is already being used in the field of developmental cognitive neuroscience (DCN) to date. DCN research investigates how the complex interplay of genetic, environmental and brain maturational factors shapes psychological functioning in development to improve the outcome for the individual. Placed at the intersection of nature and nurture, the DCN research approach always assumes a multilevel and multifactor approach to understanding change which by definition is multi-disciplinary.

Given that the field of microbiome and gut–brain axis research is still emerging and finding its shape, any real progress will depend on the adoption of a similarly comprehensive research approach for pinpointing mechanisms and translation in both animal and human models. Discussion must be given to specifying mechanisms, differentiating correlational from causal explanations and addressing a priori realistic outcomes. Moreover, there needs to be rigorous assessment in human populations coupled with well-defined research questions and appropriate statistical analysis. This is particularly important given that strong public and commercial interests are presently outpacing research efforts. Based on an extensive body of research in the field of DCN, we are aware that even simple changes in behaviour or diet can have long-lasting effects on the brain, mental health and well-being, all of which need to be considered as the ethical implications are significant. Therefore, to maintain current momentum and to future-proof the field of MGB research, a multi-disciplinary research approach such as currently practised in the field of DCN is key if we want to reach our aims of translation and targeted intervention approaches to improve mental health and well-being.

References

1. Burnett, S., Sebastian, C., Cohen Kadosh, K. and Blakemore, S. J., 2011. The social brain in adolescence: evidence from functional magnetic resonance imaging and behavioural studies. *Neuroscience & Biobehavioral Reviews, 35* (8), pp. 1654–64.

2. Haller, S. P. W., Cohen Kadosh, K., Scerif, G. and Lau, J. Y. F., 2015. Social anxiety disorder in adolescence: how developmental cognitive neuroscience findings may shape understanding and interventions for psychopathology. *Developmental Cognitive Neuroscience, 13*, pp. 11–20.

3. Platt, B., Cohen Kadosh, K. and Lau, J. Y. F., 2013. The role of peer rejection in adolescent depression. *Depression and Anxiety, 30*(9), pp. 809–21.

4. Trentacosta, C. J. and Fine, S. E. 2010. Emotion knowledge, social competence, and behavior problems in childhood and adolescence: a meta-analytic review. *Social Development, 19*(1), pp. 1–29.

5. Cohen, A. O., Breiner, K., Steinberg, L., et al., 2016. When is an adolescent an adult? Assessing cognitive control in emotional and nonemotional contexts. *Psychological Science, 27*(4), pp. 549–62.

6. Tamnes, C. K., Herting, M. M., Goddings, A. L., et al., 2017. Development of the cerebral cortex across adolescence: a multisample study of inter-related longitudinal changes in cortical volume, surface area, and thickness. *Journal of Neuroscience*, 37(12), pp. 3402–12.

7. Beddington, J., Cooper, C. L., Field, J., et al., 2008. The mental wealth of nations. *Nature*, 455(7216), pp. 1057–60.

8. Methé, B. A., Nelson, K. E., Pop, M., et al., 2012. A framework for human microbiome research. *Nature*, 486(7402), pp. 215–21.

9. Grenham, S., Clarke, G., Cryan, J. F. and Dinan, T. G., 2011. Brain-gut-microbe communication in health and disease. *Frontiers in Physiology*, 2, p. 94.

10. Grossman, M. I., 2003. Neural and hormonal regulation of gastrointestinal function: an overview. *Annual Review of Physiology*, 41(1), p. 27.

11. Mayer, E. A., 2011. Gut feelings: the emerging biology of gut–brain communication. *Nature Reviews Neuroscience*, 12(8), pp. 453–66.

12. Mayer, E. A., Knight, R., Mazmanian, S. K., Cryan, J. F. and Tillisch, K., 2014. Gut microbes and the brain: paradigm shift in neuroscience. *The Journal of Neuroscience*, 34(46), pp. 15490–6.

13. Cohen Kadosh, K., Basso, M., Knytl, P., et al., 2021. Psychobiotic interventions for anxiety in young people: a systematic review and meta-analysis, with youth consultation. *Translational Psychiatry*, 11(1), p. 352.

14. Diaz Heijtz, R., Wang, S., Anuar, F., et al., 2011. Normal gut microbiota modulates brain development and behavior. *Proceedings of the National Academy of Sciences of the United States of America*, 108 (7), pp. 3047–52.

15. Cohen Kadosh, K., Muhardi, L., Parikh, P., et al., 2021. Nutritional support of neurodevelopment and cognitive function in infants and young children: an update and novel insights. *Nutrients*, 13(1), p. 199.

16. Desbonnet, L., Garrett, L., Clarke, G., Bienenstock, J. and Dinan, T. G., 2008. The probiotic Bifidobacteria infantis: an assessment of potential antidepressant properties in the rat. *Journal of Psychiatric Research*, 43(2), pp. 164–74.

17. Oldham, M. C., Konopka, G., Iwamoto, K., et al., 2008. Functional organisation of the transcriptome in human brain. *Nature Neuroscience*, 11(11).

18. McVey Neufeld, K. A., Luczynski, P., Seira Oriach, C., Dinan, T. G. and Cryan, J. F., 2016. What's bugging your teen? The microbiota and adolescent mental health. *Neuroscience & Biobehavioral Reviews*, 70, 300–12.

19. Ezra-Nevo, G., Henriques, S. F. and Ribeiro, C., 2020. The diet-microbiome tango: how nutrients lead the gut brain axis. *Current Opinion in Neurobiology*, 1(62), 122–32.

20. Schmidt, K., Cowen, P. J., Harmer, C. J., et al., 2015. Prebiotic intake reduces the waking cortisol response and alters emotional bias in healthy volunteers. *Psychopharmacology* (Berl.), 232(10), pp. 1793–1801.

21. Steenbergen, L., Sellaro, R., Hemert, S. van, Bosch, J. A. and Colzato, L. S., 2015. A randomized controlled trial to test the effect of multispecies probiotics on cognitive reactivity to sad mood. *Brain, Behavior, and Immunity*, 48, pp. 258–64.

22. Carlson, A. L., Xia, K., Azcarate-Peril, M. A., et al., 2018. Infant gut microbiome associated with cognitive development. *Biological Psychiatry*, 83(2), pp. 148–59.

23. Johnstone, N., Milesi, C., Burn, O., et al., 2021. Anxiolytic effects of a galacto-oligosaccharides prebiotic in healthy females (18–25 years) with corresponding changes in gut bacterial composition. *Scientific Reports*, 11(1), p. 8302.

24. Johnstone, N. and Cohen Kadosh, K., 2019. Why a developmental cognitive neuroscience approach may be key for future-proofing microbiota-gut-brain research. *Behavioral and Brain Sciences*, 42, p. e73.

25. Bethlehem, R. A. I, Seidlitz, J., White, S. R., et al., 2022. Brain charts for the human lifespan. *Nature*, 604(7906), pp. 525–33.

26. Stinson, L. F., Payne, M. S. and Keelan, J. A., 2017. Planting the seed: origins, composition, and postnatal health significance of the fetal gastrointestinal microbiota. *Critical Reviews in Microbiology*, 43(3), pp. 352–69.

27. Korpela, K., Costea, P., Coelho, L. P., et al., 2018. Selective maternal seeding and environment shape the human gut microbiome. *Genome Research*, 28(4), pp. 561–8.

28. Moore, R. E. and Townsend, S. D., 2019. Temporal development of the infant gut microbiome. *Open Biology*, 9(9), p. 190128.

29. Homann, C. M., Rossel, C. A. J., Dizzell, S., et al., 2021. Infants' first solid foods: impact on gut microbiota development in two intercontinental cohorts. *Nutrients*, 13(8), p. 2639.

30. Matsuyama, M., Morrison, M., Cao, K. A. L., et al., 2019. Dietary intake influences gut microbiota development of healthy Australian children from the age of one to two years. *Scientific Reports*, 9(1), p. 12476.

31. Koenig, J. E., Spor, A., Scalfone, N., et al., 2011. Succession of microbial consortia in the developing infant gut microbiome. *Proceedings of the National Academy of Sciences of the United States of America*, 108 (suppl. 1), pp. 4578–85.

32. Tannock, G. W., Lawley, B., Munro, K., et al., 2013. Comparison of the compositions of the stool microbiotas of infants fed goat milk formula, cow milk-based formula, or breast milk. *Applied and Environmental Microbiology*, 79(9), pp. 3040–8.

33. Bergström, A., Skov, T. H., Bahl, M. I., et al., 2014. Establishment of intestinal microbiota during early life: a longitudinal, explorative study of a large cohort of Danish infants. *Applied and Environmental Microbiology*, 80(9), pp. 2889–900.

34. Liu, R. T., Walsh, R. F. L. and Sheehan, A. E., 2019. Prebiotics and probiotics for depression and anxiety: a systematic review and meta-analysis of controlled clinical trials. *Neuroscience & Biobehavioral Reviews*, 102, pp. 13–23.

35. Eastwood, J., Walton, G., Van Hemert, S., Williams, C. and Lamport, D., 2021. The effect of probiotics on cognitive function across the human lifespan: a systematic review. *Neuroscience & Biobehavioral Reviews*, 128, pp. 311–27.

36. Basso, M., Johnstone, N., Knytl, P., et al., 2022. Systematic review of psychobiotic interventions in children and adolescents to enhance cognitive functioning and emotional behavior. *Nutrients*, 14(3), p. 614.

37. Baumann-Dudenhoeffer, A. M., D'Souza, A. W., Tarr, P. I., Warner, B. B. and Dantas, G., 2018. Infant diet and maternal gestational weight gain predict early metabolic maturation of gut microbiomes. *Nature Medicine*, 24(12), pp. 1822–9.

38. Matsuyama, M., Gomez-Arango, L. F., Fukuma, N. M., et al., 2019. Breastfeeding: a key modulator of gut microbiota characteristics in late infancy. *Journal of Developmental Origins of Health and Disease*, 10(2), pp. 206–13.

39. Moossavi, S., Sepehri, S., Robertson, B., et al., 2019. Composition and variation of the human milk microbiota are influenced by maternal and early-life factors. *Cell Host & Microbe*, 25(2), pp. 324–35.

40. Fehr, K., Moossavi, S., Sbihi, H., et al., 2020. Breastmilk feeding practices are associated with the co-occurrence of bacteria in mothers' milk and the infant gut: the CHILD cohort study. *Cell Host & Microbe*, 28(2), pp. 285–97.e4.

41. Butts, C. A., Paturi, G., Blatchford, P., et al., 2020. Microbiota composition of breast milk from women of different ethnicity from the Manawatu-Wanganui region of New Zealand. *Nutrients*, 12(6).

42. Borewicz, K., Suarez-Diez, M., Hechler, C., et al., 2019. The effect of prebiotic fortified infant formulas on microbiota composition and dynamics in early life. *Scientific Reports*, 9.

43. Donald, K., Petersen, C., Turvey, S. E., Finlay, B. B. and Azad, M. B., 2022. Secretory IgA: linking microbes, maternal

health, and infant health through human milk. *Cell Host & Microbe*, 30(5), pp. 650–9.

44. Kleist, S. A. and Knoop, K. A., 2020. Understanding the elements of maternal protection from systemic bacterial infections during early life. *Nutrients*, 12(4), p. 1045.

45. Zuurveld, M., van Witzenburg, N. P., Garssen, J., et al., 2020. Immunomodulation by human milk oligosaccharides: the potential role in prevention of allergic diseases. *Frontiers in Immunology*, 11.

46. Carr, L. E., Virmani, M. D., Rosa, F., et al., 2021. Role of human milk bioactives on infants' gut and immune health. *Frontiers in Immunology*, 12.

47. Laursen, M. F., Sakanaka, M., von Burg, N., et al., 2021. Bifidobacterium species associated with breastfeeding produce aromatic lactic acids in the infant gut. *Nature Microbiology*, 6(11), pp. 1367–82.

48. Milani, C., Duranti, S., Bottacini, F., et al., 2017. The first microbial colonizers of the human gut: composition, activities, and health implications of the infant gut microbiota. *Microbiology and Molecular Biology Reviews*, 81(4).

49. Borewicz, K., Gu, F. J., Saccenti, E., et al., 2020. The association between breastmilk oligosaccharides and faecal microbiota in healthy breastfed infants at two, six, and twelve weeks of age. *Scientific Reports*, 10(1).

50. Duranti, S., Lugli, G. A., Milani, C., et al., 2019. Bifidobacterium bifidum and the infant gut microbiota: an intriguing case of microbe-host co-evolution. *Environmental Microbiology*, 21(10), pp. 3683–95.

51. de Weerth, C., Aatsinki, A. K., Azad, M. B., et al., 2022. Human milk: from complex tailored nutrition to bioactive impact on child cognition and behavior. *Critical Reviews in Food Science and Nutrition*, 36, pp. 1–38.

52. Zhu, J., Dingess, K. A., Mank, M., Stahl, B. and Heck, A. J. R., 2021. Personalized profiling reveals donor- and lactation-specific trends in the human milk proteome and peptidome. *Journal of Nutrition*, 151(4), pp. 826–39.

53. Wells, J. C. K., 2018. Breast-feeding as 'personalized nutrition'. *European Journal of Clinical Nutrition*, 72(9), pp. 1234–8.

54. Morrow-Tlucak, M., Haude, R. H. and Ernhart, C. B., 1988. Breastfeeding and cognitive development in the first 2 years of life. *Social Science & Medicine*, 26(6), pp. 635–9.

55. Pereyra-Elías, R., Quigley, M. A. and Carson, C., 2022. To what extent does confounding explain the association between breastfeeding duration and cognitive development up to age 14? Findings from the UK Millennium Cohort Study. *Plos One*, 17(5), p. e0267326.

56. De Mola, C. L., Horta, B. L., Gonçalves, H., et al., 2016. Breastfeeding and mental health in adulthood: a birth cohort study in Brazil. *Journal of Affective Disorders*, 202, 115–19.

57. Oddy, W. H., Kendall, G. E., Li, J., et al., 2010. The long-term effects of breastfeeding on child and adolescent mental health: a pregnancy cohort study followed for 14 years. *The Journal of Pediatrics*, 156(4), pp. 568–74.

58. Girard, L. C., Doyle, O. and Tremblay, R. E., 2017. Breastfeeding, cognitive and noncognitive development in early childhood: a population study. *Pediatrics*, 139(4).

59. Heikkilä, K., Sacker, A., Kelly, Y., Renfrew, M. J. and Quigley, M. A., 2011. Breast feeding and child behaviour in the millennium cohort study. *Archives of Disease in Childhood*, 96(7), pp. 635–42.

60. Speyer, L. G., Hall, H. A., Ushakova, A., et al., 2021. Longitudinal effects of breast feeding on parent-reported child behaviour. *Archives of Disease in Childhood*, 106(4), pp. 355–60.

61. Lind, J. N., Li, R., Perrine, C. G. and Schieve, L. A., 2014. Breastfeeding and later psychosocial development of children at 6 years of age. *Pediatrics*, 134 (suppl. 1), pp. 36–41.

62. Carlson, A. L., Xia, K., Azcarate-Peril, M. A., et al., 2021. Infant gut microbiome composition is associated with non-social

fear behavior in a pilot study. *Nature Communications*, *12*(1), p. 3294.

63. Gao, W., Salzwedel, A. P., Carlson, A. L., et al., 2019. Gut microbiome and brain functional connectivity in infants: a preliminary study focusing on the amygdala. *Psychopharmacology (Berl.)*, *236* (5), pp. 1–11.

64. Vogel, S. C., Brito, N. H., and Callaghan, B. L., 2020. Early life stress and the development of the infant gut microbiota: implications for mental health and neurocognitive development. *Current Psychiatry Reports*, *22*(11), p. 61.

65. Fouhy, F., Watkins, C., Hill, C. J., et al., 2019. Perinatal factors affect the gut microbiota up to four years after birth. *Nature Communications*, *10*(1), p. 1517.

66. Beller, L., Deboutte, W., Falony, G., et al., 2021. Successional stages in infant gut microbiota maturation. *mBio*, *12*(6).

67. Stewart, C. J., Ajami, N. J., O'Brien, J. L., et al., 2018. Temporal development of the gut microbiome in early childhood from the TEDDY study. *Nature*, *562*, pp. 583–88.

68. Goyal, M. S., Venkatesh, S., Milbrandt, J., Gordon, J. I. and Raichle, M. E., 2015. Feeding the brain and nurturing the mind: linking nutrition and the gut microbiota to brain development. *Proceedings of the National Academy of Sciences of the United States of America*, *112*(46), pp. 14105–12.

69. Smith-Brown, P., Morrison, M., Krause, L. and Davies, P. S. W., 2016. Dairy and plant based food intakes are associated with altered faecal microbiota in 2 to 3 year old Australian children. *Scientific Reports*, *6*(1), p. 32385.

70. Berding, K., Holscher, H. D., Arthur, A. E. and Donovan, S. M., 2018. Fecal microbiome composition and stability in 4- to 8-year old children is associated with dietary patterns and nutrient intake. *Journal of Nutritional Biochemistry*, *56*, pp. 165–74.

71. Herman, D. R., Rhoades, N., Mercado, J., et al., 2020. Dietary habits of 2- to 9-year-old American children are associated with gut microbiome composition. *Journal of the Academy of Nutrition and Dietetics*, *120*(4), pp. 517–34.

72. Perrin, M. T., Fogleman, A. D., Newburg, D. S. and Allen, J. C., 2017. A longitudinal study of human milk composition in the second year postpartum: implications for human milk banking. *Maternal & Child Nutrition*, *13*(1).

73. Mandel, D., Lubetzky, R., Dollberg, S., Barak, S. and Mimouni, F. B., 2005. Fat and energy contents of expressed human breast milk in prolonged lactation. *Pediatrics*, *116* (3), pp. e432–5.

74. Dewey, K. G., 2001. Nutrition, growth, and complementary feeding of the breastfed infant. *Pediatric Clinics of North America*, *48*(1), pp. 87–104.

75. Onyango, A. W., Receveur, O. and Esrey, S. A., 2002. The contribution of breast milk to toddler diets in western Kenya. *Bulletin of the World Health Organization*, *80*(4), pp. 292–9.

76. Pietrzak-Fiećko, R. and Kamelska-Sadowska, A. M., 2020. The comparison of nutritional value of human milk with other mammals' milk. *Nutrients*, *12*(5), p. 1404.

77. Ballard, O. and Morrow, A. L., 2013. Human milk composition. *Pediatric Clinics of North America*, *60*(1), pp. 49–74.

78. Keshavan, M. S., Giedd, J., Lau, J. Y. F., Lewis, D. A. and Paus, T., 2014. Changes in the adolescent brain and the pathophysiology of psychotic disorders. *Lancet Psychiatry*, *1*(7), pp. 549–58.

79. Paus, T., Keshavan, M. and Giedd, J. N., 2008. Why do many psychiatric disorders emerge during adolescence? *Nature Reviews Neuroscience*, *9*(12), pp. 947–57.

80. Goddings, A. L., Mills, K. L., Clasen, L. S., et al., 2014. The influence of puberty on subcortical brain development. *NeuroImage*, *88*, pp. 242–51.

81. Mills, K. L, Goddings, A. L., Clasen, L. S., Giedd, J. N. and Blakemore, S. J., 2014. The developmental mismatch in structural brain maturation during adolescence. *Developmental Neuroscience*, *36*(3–4), pp. 147–60.

82. Mills, K. L., Goddings, A. L., Herting, M. M., et al., 2016. Structural brain development between childhood and adulthood: convergence across four longitudinal samples. *NeuroImage, 141*, pp. 273–81.

83. Chervonsky, E. and Hunt, C., 2019. Emotion regulation, mental health, and social wellbeing in a young adolescent sample: a concurrent and longitudinal investigation. *Emotion, 19*(2), pp. 270–82.

84. Dinan, T. G., Stanton, C. and Cryan, J. F., 2013. Psychobiotics: a novel class of psychotropic. *Biological Psychiatry, 74*(10), pp. 720–6.

85. Sarkar, A., Lehto, S. M., Harty, S., et al., 2016. Psychobiotics and the manipulation of bacteria-gut-brain signals. *Trends in Neurosciences, 39*(11), pp. 763–81.

86. Messaoudi, M., Violle, N., Bisson, J. F., et al., 2011. Beneficial psychological effects of a probiotic formulation (*Lactobacillus helveticus* R0052 and *Bifidobacterium longum* R0175) in healthy human volunteers. *Gut Microbes, 2*(4), pp. 256–61.

87. Tillisch, K., Mayer, E., Gupta, A., et al., 2017. Brain structure and response to emotional stimuli as related to gut microbial profiles in healthy women. *Psychosomatic Medicine, 79*(8), p. 905.

88. Chao, L., Liu, C., Sutthawongwadee, S., et al., 2020. Effects of probiotics on depressive or anxiety variables in healthy participants under stress conditions or with a depressive or anxiety diagnosis: a meta-analysis of randomized controlled trials. *Frontiers in Neurology, 11*, 421.

89. Bar-Haim, Y., Lamy, D., Pergamin, L., Bakermans-Kranenburg, M. J. and IJzendoorn, M. H. van, 2007. Threat-related attentional bias in anxious and nonanxious individuals: a meta-analytic study. *Psychological Bulletin, 133*(1), pp. 1–24.

90. Johnstone, N., Dart, S., Knytl, P., et al., 2021. Nutrient intake and gut microbial genera changes after a 4-week placebo controlled galacto-oligosaccharides intervention in young females. *Nutrients, 13*(12), p. 4384.

91. Jovanovic, T., Nylocks, K. M., Gamwell, K. L., et al., 2014. Development of fear acquisition and extinction in children: effects of age and anxiety. *Neurobiology of Learning and Memory, 113*, pp. 135–42.

92. Chu, C., Murdock, M. H., Jing, D., et al., 2019. The microbiota regulate neuronal function and fear extinction learning. *Nature, 574*(7779), pp. 543–8.

93. Kadosh, K. C., Haddad, A. D. M., Heathcote, L. C., et al., 2015. High trait anxiety during adolescence interferes with discriminatory context learning. *Neurobiology of Learning and Memory, 123*, pp. 50–7.

94. Sarkar, A., Harty, S., Johnson, K. V. A., et al., 2020. Microbial transmission in animal social networks and the social microbiome. *Nature Ecology and Evolution, 4*(8), pp. 1020–35.

Chapter

8

Old Age and Nutrition

Ivan Aprahamian, Andréia de Oliveira Pain and Sandra Maria Lima Ribeiro

Summary

Psychogeriatric patients commonly present nutritional disorders due to a higher burden of multimorbidity, polypharmacy or psychopathology. Different nutritional disorders are associated with geriatric syndromes and adverse health outcomes in these patients. Epidemiological and clinical evidence justify a basic nutritional assessment for malnutrition in older mental health patients, given that mental and physical components are rarely unrelated. However, several professionals that care for older mental health patients do not have a nutritional training background. Beyond nutritional evaluation, diet counselling and supplement recommendation may be even harder for non-specialists. In this chapter, we suggest a quick, simple and basic nutritional assessment, we evaluate the literature on the relationship between anthropometric and nutritional measurement and mental disorders in older adults, and we review the best evidence regarding nutritional management for these patients. Additionally, we review potential biological pathways of the association between nutrition and late-life mental illness.

Introduction

An older adult is defined by the United Nations as a person who is over 60 years of age, but this definition varies according to culture, geographic location, socioeconomic status and clinical conditions. Clinically, older age has particularities that go beyond the chronological age and is characterised by a more expressive burden of multimorbidity, polypharmacy, common age-related syndromes (i.e. geriatric syndromes, such as delirium, cognitive impairment and falls) and situations or diseases that pose a greater risk of loss of autonomy or independence. Nutritional disorders are prevalent at this stage of life and are associated with several mental disorders, such as dementia and depression. Deviations from nutritional status, namely malnutrition, encompass undernutrition and overweight, which are particularly important in the geriatric clinic. For example, overweight mainly includes obesity and a series of chronic diseases associated with metabolic syndrome (high blood pressure, insulin resistance or diabetes and dyslipidaemia). On the other hand, undernutrition refers to a reduced intake or assimilation of nutrients (both macro and micronutrients) and has been shown to be at the beginning of processes such as sarcopenia and frailty (Figure 8.1). It is also important to differentiate nutritional risk from malnutrition, which is quickly identified using screening tools. Based on the identification of nutritional risk, a more objective assessment of the nutritional condition is recommended.

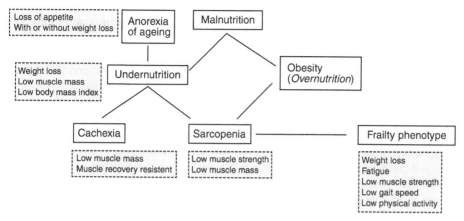

Figure 8.1 The relation between malnutrition and geriatric syndromes.

Frailty is a syndrome highly associated with late-life psychiatric disorders and is an important predictor variable of adverse health outcomes (1, 2). The relationship between frailty and psychogeriatric conditions such as cognitive and mood disorders appears to be bidirectional, which demands continuous clinical attention during the care plan. This relation leads to a practical implication which consists of a paradigm shift in the treatment of mental disorders, from a highly centred use of psychotropics and psychotherapies to multi-disciplinary multimorbidity management, prescription of physical activity reduction of polypharmacy and nutritional evaluation (1–3). In this sense, the clinics and basic understanding of nutrition are fundamental to the good practice of geriatric medicine. The complexity of the aged organism requires a great integration in the care of the body and mind, such components being inseparable in older patients. According to our experience, a cohesive mental health-care plan must adopt items such as diet and physical activity counselling. In this way, we believe it is essential for health providers who care for older people with mental disorders to have a minimum of knowledge about nutritional care.

In this chapter, we will approach the nutritional diagnosis in older adults with mental disorders in a practical way and summarise the most relevant evidence of the association between clinical nutrition and the most common late-life mental disorders, such as mood disorders and cognitive impairment, deriving recommendations for clinical practice.

Basic Nutritional Assessment of the Older Person with Mental Health Disorders

With the exception of nutritionists, the practice of nutritional assessment is generally not included in the curriculum of health-care professionals such as psychiatrists, psychogeriatricians, psychologists and other team members who care for older adults with mental health disorders. At the same time, these professionals are not expected to have much time for a nutritional assessment that is not essential to ensure basic and relevant aspects of diagnosis and treatment. In this way, we selected anthropometric measurements and assessment instruments that are simple, easy and quick to use.

Ageing is characterised by numerous body changes which have repercussions on physical and mental capacities. Most of these changes have important associations, direct or indirect, with nutritional status. By definition, nutritional status is an indicator of health status in terms of the concentration and availability of nutrients from the diet and present in the body (4, 5). For a comprehensive assessment of nutritional status, different methods are often used as described in Table 8.1.

Appetite changes usually precede weight loss. Appetite is usually assessed subjectively by the patient. The loss of appetite is especially relevant in anorexia of ageing, a geriatric syndrome, which can occur primarily to ageing or secondarily to depression or dementia, among other causes. Anorexia of ageing is a worrying condition as it can lead to reduced energy and nutrient intake, and is consequently one of the main causes of protein-energy malnutrition, sarcopenia and frailty, leading to an increased risk of mortality (6, 7). Different data suggests that the prevalence of anorexia of ageing is somewhere between 15% and 30% in independent older people, and more than 30% at hospital and 42% in residents of long-stay institutions (6). Social, environmental and lifestyle factors also affect food intake (7). For example, cephalic responses to the environment are often associated with a 'thinking about food' stimulation. In this context, it is expected that a person who eats alone (considering the limited social contact and restriction of social participation of many older people) has less appetite and eats less than someone who eats with a partner (6, 8). Identifying and treating anorexia can prevent weight loss, which requires a long recovery time and is associated with malnutrition, frailty and sarcopenia. Anorexia can also be measured using the Simplified Nutritional Assessment Questionnaire (SNAQ), which takes approximately 1 minute (Figure 8.2). A score equal to or less than 14 points indicates anorexia and predicts a weight loss of 5% in 6 months, being a warning sign for the need for intervention by a multi-disciplinary team for further evaluation. The SNAQ can also be used as an objective measure of appetite improvement in patients with depressive disorders or dementia. In late-life depressive disorders, anorexia plays an important role in nutrition. In a previous study in a geriatric outpatient clinic, we found about one-fifth of our sample to have appetite loss (9). Most of our patients did not present nutritional risk according to standardised instruments and anthropometric measurements. In this study, depressive symptoms were significantly more associated with loss of appetite (9). In another study by our group with older outpatients, we observed that high scores on psychometric depression instruments (even without somatic complaints), such as the Geriatric Depression Scale and the PHQ-9, and major depressive disorder were associated with anorexia of ageing (10). Anorexia was more common in patients with major depressive disorder compared to non-depressed patients (30.7% vs. 7.7%) and was associated with weight loss. The SNAQ continuous score and its 14-point cut-off were significantly associated with the diagnosis of major depression and the instruments used to assess symptomatology (GDS and PHQ-9) (10). Finally, anorexia can be a predictor of geriatric syndromes, such as frailty, with a worse prognosis in mood and cognition disorders (11).

Weight loss is a major indicator of nutritional risk and a later stage of anorexia. According to the European Society for Clinical Nutrition and Metabolism (ESPEN), estimated losses of 5% in 6 months or 10% over 6 months, or significant decreases in body mass index (BMI = weight (kg)/height squared; e.g. BMI <20 kg/h2) or muscle mass, are characteristics of malnutrition (12, 13). However, for the diagnosis of malnutrition, the recent consensus recommendation from the Global Leadership Initiative on Malnutrition (GLIM) establishes the combination of at least one phenotypic criterion (non-volitional

Table 8.1 Principles of the assessment of nutritional status (ABCD) with emphasis on those related to the presence of cognitive and depressive disorders

Method	Description	Clinical importance to mental health disorders
Anthropometry	Assessment of quantity, quality and distribution of body dimensions and components (fat, muscle mass, mineral mass and body water), which is more related to macronutrients. The use of anthropometric measurements is the simplest and most inexpensive way to carry out a nutritional assessment; however, today more advanced and sensitive techniques can be considered, such as electrical bioimpedance, dual-energy X-rays (DXA or DEXA), imaging methods (such as nuclear magnetic resonance) and computed tomography scan.	Overweight, as well as underweight, have been linked to mental disorders. Body fat distribution is strongly associated with chronic adverse outcomes.
Biochemistry	Measurements of nutrients' concentrations and chemical compounds in body fluids and tissues are able to identify the state of the organism in a more sensitive way than anthropometry, as they identify steps prior to incorporation into body mass. In clinical practice, these measurements are performed on whole blood, plasma or serum. Biochemical measurements can identify molecules related to macronutrients (e.g. blood glucose, lipids, proteins and amino acids) but are of great importance in identifying micronutrients (vitamins, minerals and other non-nutrient compounds with nutritional relevance).	Omega-3 polyunsaturated fatty acids have a range of neurobiological activities such as modulation of neurotransmitters, anti-inflammation, antioxidation and neuroplasticity. Vitamins B6 and B12 and folic acid are essential in the one-carbon metabolism, responsible among other things for the synthesis of neurotransmitters.
Clinical evaluation	Clinical assessment of nutritional status is understood as the identification of signs and symptoms indicative of nutritional deviations, e.g. pallor and reduced energy due to iron deficiency or	It is a cheap and logical first step to identify nutritional disorders.

Table 8.1 (cont.)

Method	Description	Clinical importance to mental health disorders
	skin dryness due to deficiencies of essential fatty acids, among others.	
Diet evaluation	Diet assessment is essential in the nutritional assessment process, since most important interventions result from this evaluation. Diet assessment can be performed by direct observation, but in practice tools such as 24-hour food consumption assessment, food diaries or food frequency lists are used. The analysis of these tools can be done by identifying nutrients and food compounds and then comparing them with reference studies and/or by identifying dietary patterns, which can be determined a priori or later. A priori identification is the most used technique in clinical practice, e.g. adherence to predetermined standards such as the Mediterranean diet or the MIND diet.	Identification of specific nutrient intake and/or eating patterns related to mental disorders.

weight loss, low BMI or reduced muscle mass) and an etiological criterion (reduced food intake/malabsorption or disease with inflammation) (14). Malnutrition has a wide epidemiological variation, with a prevalence of less than 10% in community-dwelling older people and up to 30% in those residing in a long-stay institution (15, 16). It has a high association with unfavourable outcomes such as increased rates of infections and pressure injuries, longer hospital stays, prolonged convalescence after acute illness and increased mortality (17). In this sense, the calculation of BMI and calf circumference is important.

Although BMI cannot determine the exact proportion of body fat, it is a screening evaluation widely used in clinical practice for the detection of nutritional disorders and has been recommended by the World Health Organization (WHO) since 1995. It is important to note that although the cut-off points for this index are well established for the adult population, there is still much discussion about the best values for older adults, leading to different values according to different regions of the world. The BMI is able to identify from underweight to obesity in different degrees/severity. Several studies carried out in different age groups have generally indicated a positive association between being obese and having symptoms or a diagnosis of depression. However, studies that include or are exclusive to older people show great disparities.

Noh and colleagues, using data from the Korean Longitudinal Study of Aging (KLoSA), investigated the association between BMI and depressive symptoms in 7,672 people between

SNAQ

Administration Instructions: Ask the subject to complete the questionnaire by circling the correct answers and then tally the results based upon the following numerical scale: a 1, b 2, c 3, d 4, e 5. The sum of the scores for the individual items constitutes the SNAQ score. SNAQ score = 14 indicates significant risk of at least 5% weight loss within six months.

1. My appetite is:
a. very poor
b. poor
c. average
d. good
e. very good
2. When I eat
a. I feel full after eating only a few mouthfuls
b. I feel full after eating about a third of meal
c. I feel full after eating over half a meal
d. I feel full after eating most of the meal
e. I hardly ever feel full
3. Food tastes
a. very bad
b. bad
c. average
d. good
e. very good
4. Normally I eat
a. less than one meal a day
b. one meal a day
c. two meals a day
d. three meals a day
e. more than three meals a day
SNAQ score:

Component

SARC-F

Component	Question	Scoring
Strength	How much difficulty do you have in lifting and carrying 10 1b?	None = 0 Some = 1 A lot or unable = 2
Assistance in walking	How much difficulty do you have walking across a room?	None = 0 Some = 1 A lot or unable = 2
Rise from a chair	How much difficulty do you have transferring from a chair or bed?	None = 0 Some = 1 A lot or unable = 2
Climb stairs	How much difficulty do you have climbing a flight of 10 stairs?	None = 0 Some = 1 A lot or unable = 2
Falls	How much difficulty do you have the past year?	None = 0 Some = 1 A lot or unable = 2

Figure 8.2 Common instruments to evaluate direct or indirect nutritional risk in older adults: the FRAIL questionnaire, SARC-F, the Simplified Nutritional Assessment Questionnaire (SNQ) and the Mini Nutritional Assessment (MNA).

Last name:			First name:		
Sex:	Age:	Weight, kg:	Height, cm:	Date:	

Complete the screen by filling in the boxes with the appropriate numbers. Total the numbers for the final screening score.

Screening

A Has food intake declined over the past 3 months due to loss of appetite, digestive problems, chewing or swallowing difficulties?
0 = severe decrease in food intake
1 = moderate decrease in food intake
2 = no decrease in food intake ☐

B Weight loss during the last 3 months
0 = weight loss greater than 3 kg (6.6 lbs)
1 = does not know
2 = weight loss between 1 and 3 kg (2.2 and 6.6 lbs)
3 = no weight loss ☐

C Mobility
0 = bed or chair bound
1 = able to get out of bed / chair but does not go out
2 = goes out ☐

D Has suffered psychological stress or acute disease in the past 3 months?
0 = yes   2 = no ☐

E Neuropsychological problems
0 = severe dementia or depression
1 = mild dementia
2 = no psychological problems ☐

F1 Body Mass Index (BMI) (weight in kg) / (height in m)^2 ☐
0 = BMI less than 19
1 = BMI 19 to less than 21
2 = BMI 21 to less than 23
3 = BMI 23 or greater ☐

IF BMI IS NOT AVAILABLE, REPLACE QUESTION F1 WITH QUESTION F2.
DO NOT ANSWER QUESTION F2 IF QUESTION F1 IS ALREADY COMPLETED.

F2 Calf circumference (CC) in cm
0 = CC less than 31
3 = CC 31 or greater ☐

Screening score ☐☐
(max. 14 points)

			Save
12–14 points:	☐	Normal nutritional status	Print
8–11 points:	☐	At risk of malnutrition	Reset
0–7 points:	☐	Malnourished	

Ref. Vellas B, Villars H, Abellan G, et al. *Overview of the MNA® – Its History and Challenges.* J Nutr Health Aging 2006; 10:456–456.
Rubenstein LZ, Harker JO. Salva A. Guigoz Y. Vellas B. *Screening for Undernutrition in Geriatric Practice: Developing the Short-Form Mini Nutritional Assessment (MNA-SF).* J. Geront 2001;56A: M366–377.
Guigoz Y. *The Mini Nutritional Assessment (MNA®) Review of the Literature – What does it tell us?* J Nutr Health Aging 2006; 10:466–487.
Kaiser MJ, Bauer JM, Ramsch C, et al. *Validation of the Mini Nutritional Assessment Short-Form (MNA®-SF): A practical tool for identification of nutritional status.* J Nutr Health Aging 2009; 13:782–788.
® Societe des Produits Nestle SA, Trademark Owners.

FRAIL SCALE

F_atigue – "Are you fatigued?"

R_esistance – "Can you walk up 1 flight of stairs?"

A_mbulation – "Can you walk 1 block?"

I_llness (greather than 5)* - "Do you have more than 5 illnesses?"
*Hypertension, diabetes, cancer (other than a minor skin cancer), chronic lung disease, heart attack, congestive heart failure, angina, asthma, arthritis, stroke, and kidney disease

L_oss of Weight (>5% over 1 year) – "Have you lost more than 5% of your weight in the past 6 months?"

3 - 5 = frail/ 1 - 2 = prefrail/ 0 = robust

Figure 8.2 (cont.)

50 and 102 years old (56.9% women) (18). BMI values were classified according to the WHO revised Asia-Pacific criteria as underweight (less than 18.5 kg/m^2), normal weight (between 18.5 kg/m^2 and 23 kg/m^2), overweight (between 23 kg/m^2 and 25 kg/m^2), obese (between 25 kg/m^2 and 30 kg/m^2) or severely obese (more than 30 kg/m^2). Depressive symptoms were identified by the Korean version of the Center for Epidemiological Studies Depression (CES-D) tool with 10 items. After adjusting for sociodemographic variables, the authors identified a U-shaped curve, indicating that both undernutrition (from the underweight classification) and overnutrition (specifically from severe obesity) were significantly associated with a higher prevalence of depressive symptoms. However, some characteristics related to BMI were observed when analysing men and women separately; the group of men with the lowest prevalence of depressive symptoms was predominantly classified as overweight, and among women, the lowest prevalence of depressive symptoms was in the normal weight range.

More recently, another publication related to KLoSA explored these different relationships in sex (19). The authors used more complex statistical methods to identify 'if' and 'how' the relationships between depressive symptoms and cognitive function, mediated by BMI, differed between the sexes. In addition to assessing depressive symptoms using the Korean version of the CES-D, they also assessed cognitive function using the Korean version of the Mini-Mental State Examination (K-MMSE). The authors identified that depressive symptoms were significantly associated with cognitive impairment, which was directly and indirectly associated with reduced BMI. However, the indirect relationship between depressive symptoms and BMI-mediated cognitive function was significant only in men over 70 years of age. This Korean data points to the complex role of BMI in late-life neuropsychiatric disorders. It is worth noting the potential limitations of these studies, such as the involvement of only Korean older adults and its cross-sectional designs.

Therefore, to expand the scope of the discussions in this chapter, we have included a systematic review conducted in 2010 by Luppino and colleagues (20). This meta-analysis with only longitudinal studies investigated relationships between depression, overweight and obesity, considering the possible bidirectional relationship between overweight (BMI between 25 and 29.99 kg/m^2) or obesity (BMI >30 kg/m^2) and depression. For the 15 selected studies (58,745 people), odds ratios (OR) with or without adjustments were calculated and sub-groups were also analysed in order to identify possible mediators (between sex, age and severity of depression). Being obese at baseline increased the risk of developing depression at follow-up (unadjusted OR=1.55; 95% CI=1.22–1.98; $p<0.001$). The associations were more relevant in studies from the American continent than in Europe and more pronounced for depressive disorders than for depressive symptoms. Being overweight increased the risk of depression at follow-up (unadjusted OR=1.27; 95% CI=1.07–1.51; $p<0.01$), and these associations were significant only in adults, not in younger people. The opposite direction indicated that depression was a predictor of obesity at follow-up (OR=1.58; 95% CI=1.33–1.87; $p<0.001$), but not overweight.

The association between BMI, particularly overweight and obesity, and depressive symptoms and disorders presents several confounding variables in old age, such as the presence of comorbidities associated with metabolic syndrome, in addition to the side effects of antidepressant medications and several other drugs commonly used by older people, which can also induce obesity. More recently, a robust meta-analysis investigated the evidence and association between obesity and depression exclusively in older adults (aged over 60 years) (21). The authors performed the search in six electronic databases from inception to November 2019. Cross-sectional, longitudinal and case-control studies were included, with depression or depressive symptoms identified by different scales or clinical interviews, and obesity was also identified by different techniques (BMI, waist circumference, waist to hip ratio and body fat percentage, among others). Nineteen studies were evaluated in this systematic review and 14 were analysed by meta-analysis. Surprisingly, the results indicated that older people who were overweight or obese by BMI had a lower chance of depression than those classified as normal weight (pooled OR=0.847; 95% CI=0.789–0.908; $p<0.001$ and pooled OR=0.795; 95% CI=0.658–0.960; $p=0.017$, respectively). Obesity identified by waist circumference was not significantly associated with depression (pooled OR=0.722; 95% CI=0.465–1,119; $p=0.145$). The other methods for determining obesity were not meta-analysed.

It can be assumed that the different results can be attributed to the presence or absence of comorbidities. There are certain factors in addition to BMI in the nutritional assessment of older people with depressive or cognitive symptoms that warrant consideration. The association between BMI, particularly overweight and obesity, and depressive symptoms and disorders presents the presence of comorbidities as a confounding variable, particularly those associated with the metabolic syndrome. In addition, the side effects of antidepressant medications can induce obesity.

Calf circumference can be used as a surrogate technique to estimate muscle mass if it is less than 31 cm (22, 23). Calf circumference may be limited because of obesity, ethnicity or lower-limb oedema. The loss of muscle mass is a fundamental component for the diagnosis of sarcopenia, together with the loss of muscle strength. Another way to assess the potential loss of muscle mass and sarcopenia is through the use of the SARC-F instrument alone or together with calf circumference (23). The SARC-F is an easy-to-use instrument and serves to screen for the presence of sarcopenia when its score is equal to or more than 4 points (Figure 8.2). The greatest limitation of the instrument is its low sensitivity, despite its high specificity (24). Sarcopenia is associated with both depressive (25) and cognitive (26) disorders in older adults and can predict negative health outcomes similar to those associated with malnutrition in patients with mental disorders. We conducted a prospective observational study with 105 older inpatients hospitalised because of severe depression (27). Anthropometric measures were most predictive of worse outcomes such as falls and readmission.

Finally, a useful instrument for the assessment of nutritional risk in the geriatric clinic is the Mini Nutritional Assessment (MNA) (28). The MNA already includes anthropometric measurements such as BMI and arm and calf circumferences (Figure 8.2). This instrument is divided into two stages. The first is a screening that investigates changes in food intake, weight, mobility and psychological status (stress and neuropsychological problems), in addition to BMI. The screening criteria were scored according to greater or lesser alteration (12–14 points: normal nutritional status; 8–11 points: at risk of malnutrition; 0–7 points: malnourished) and added to the second stage of the instrument, which is made up of the global assessment. A total result more than 23.5 points indicates that the patient is in a normal nutritional status; a score between 17 and 23.5 indicates they are at risk of malnutrition; and a score less than 17 indicates they are malnourished. Either the screening alone or the complete instrument can be used, depending on the time available for evaluation.

Nutrition Counselling and Late-Life Mental Illness: What Recommendations Are Evidence-Based?

The emerging field of nutritional psychiatry focusses on the consequences of and associations between eating habits, diet and supplement use, and behaviour. After the nutritional assessment process in older people who present behavioural symptoms, nutritional strategies that can attenuate the inflammatory and antioxidant effects can be considered. In fact, any diet, when properly combined in terms of pro- and anti-inflammatory compounds and nutrients, is capable of providing benefits. Several nutrients, non-nutrient compounds such as phytochemicals or even supplements aimed at intestinal modulation can be useful. Lately, nutrition has been studied comprehensively, leaving the paradigm of evaluating an isolated nutrient to better understand the impact of nutritional habits and dietary profiles. Recent trends have been to use food combinations in the form of dietary patterns (patterns determined a priori). Next, we will present some studies that demonstrate how research in this regard has been conducted.

Nutritional counselling in geriatric psychiatry can be divided into two parts: diets and supplements. In 2014, Lay and colleagues conducted a systematic review with meta-analysis where 21 studies were included (29). These studies found that higher consumption of fruits, vegetables, fish and grains was associated with a reduced risk of depression. Some evidence has indicated that there is a bidirectional correlation between depression and diet quality in older adults. Depression can lead to poorer diet quality and diversity; individuals with current depression are more likely to have poorer eating habits, which is likely due to the short-term calming effects of antidepressant medications and their long-term ill effects (30). Using this perspective, in 2017, our group published a study with the aim of investigating fruit and vegetable intake (FVI) and physical activity (PA) as predictors of clinically relevant levels of depressive symptoms (CRLDS) in African Americans (31). Baseline data was extracted from wave 1 (2000/1) of the African American Health (AAH) study, a population-based longitudinal study of African Americans in St Louis. At wave 8, participants self-reported FVI and completed the Yale Physical Activity Scale. At both waves 8 and 10, the CES-D 11-item scale was used to identify those who met the criteria for CRLDS. Sequential logistic regression modelling was used to examine the associations of components of FVI/PA with CRLDS, both cross-sectionally (n=680) and longitudinally (n=582). Modelling employed gender, age, perceived income adequacy and education as potential confounders. Cross-sectionally, vigorous PA and leisure walking PA were independently associated with lower odds of CRLDS in all but the fifth model and green vegetables in all models. Longitudinally, green vegetables and the interaction between total FVI score, total PA score and other factors at wave 8 were most consistently associated with CRLDS at wave 10. In both cross-sectional and longitudinal models, the socioeconomic variables showed an association as risk factors for CRLDS. Therefore, green vegetables, total FVI and various aspects of PA showed protective effects regarding CRLDS. Therefore, the promotion of such lifestyles is likely to help prevent CRLDS in this population.

A Mediterranean diet may have protective effects against cognitive decline in older adults because of the combination of foods and nutrients potentially protective against cognitive dysfunction or dementia, such as monounsaturated fatty acids, fish, vitamin B12, folate and antioxidants (vitamin E, carotenoids, flavonoids). Additionally, the anti-inflammatory effects of antioxidant ingredients, vitamins and flavonoids present in vegetables and other foods may explain their protective role against depression. Furthermore, the benefit of a Mediterranean diet for depression in old age may also be due to its effects on vascular health and has been shown to maintain a high level of vascular health and prevent many of the usual problems of ageing.

The Mediterranean diet is the dietary recommendation that has been most tested in depression and cognition. In this book, the Mediterranean diet has been covered in more detail in Chapter 3. In general, it consists of the abundant use of olive oil; high consumption of fruits, vegetables, legumes, cereals and nuts; regular and moderate intake of red wine with meals; and moderate consumption of fish, seafood, poultry and fermented dairy products. The consumption of red meat, processed products and sweets is limited. Three observational studies, totalling 3,539 people, reported lower depressive symptoms and diagnosis of depression among people more adherent to the Mediterranean diet (32–34). It is worth emphasising that in one of these studies, the Mediterranean diet was combined with principles of the Dietary Approaches to Stop Hypertension (DASH) diet. Similar to the Mediterranean diet, the DASH diet specifies a high consumption of plant-based foods but also limits the intake of saturated and total fat, cholesterol and sodium (<2400 mg/daily). The beneficial effects of the Mediterranean diet are most consistent for depression. In a meta-analysis involving more than 41,000 people in 15 cohort studies and 2 clinical trials, global cognitive improvement was observed, especially in episodic memory (35). The DASH and MIND (Mediterranean–DASH Diet Intervention for Neurodegenerative Delay) diets also improved cognition and reduced the risk of neurodegeneration (36, 37). The MIND diet emphasises the consumption of natural plant-based foods as well as red fruits and leafy greens, limiting animal foods and saturated fats, with restrictions of cheese, butter/margarine and fried foods. Finally, a recent clinical trial observed a strong relationship between the Mediterranean diet and the promotion of overall healthier ageing through several biomarkers expressing less frailty and better cognitive function, in addition to being negatively associated with inflammatory markers and changes in the gut microbiota (38). Our group conducted a cross-sectional study to evaluate the association between adherence to the Mediterranean diet with the presence of common mental health disorders (CMD) in Brazilian older adults, adopting two different concepts of the diet (39). The sample included 545 older people from the 2015 Health Survey of São Paulo City (cross-sectional population-based study). CMD were identified through the Self-Reporting Questionnaire-20. Data from two 24-hour dietary recalls was used to construct two diet patterns according to the Mediterranean diet score: traditional diet (including only foods with characteristics of the original diet) and Brazilian-Mediterranean (including foods with non-Mediterranean characteristics). Moderate and high adherence to the traditional diet were associated with a lower prevalence of CMD (OR=0.59; 95% CI=0.35–0.98 and OR=0.42; 95% CI=0.18–0.96, respectively) after adjustment for sociodemographic, lifestyle and health status variables. In turn, the presence of CMD was not significantly associated with any level of adherence to the Brazilian-Mediterranean diet. Therefore, moderate and high adherence to the traditional diet were found to reduce the risk of mental disorders in Brazilian older adults. Nevertheless, an increased intake of non-Mediterranean food components can limit this effect.

Nutritional supplements are popular among seniors. Several vitamins have been linked to a better ageing process, especially for the brain. Some of the most popular supplements marketed to improve memory are fish oils (omega-3 fatty acids), B vitamins (most commonly folate, B6 and B12) and vitamin D (40). Vitamins A, C, E and D and B vitamins were not associated with cognitive improvement or reduced neurodegeneration. Controversial evidence comes from the B vitamins, where meta-analyses have reported associations between B-vitamin compound supplementation and less brain atrophy in mild cognitive impairment, but without observing any cognitive improvement (41). In mood disorders, evidence is also insufficient or negative with B-complex or vitamin D supplementation (42, 43), although the use of folic acid/methylfolate as an adjunct to selective-serotonin reuptake inhibitors and serotonin-norepinephrine reuptake inhibitor treatment in major depressive disorder has been associated with reduced symptomatology (44).

Omega-3 fatty acids, including eicosapentaenoic (EPA), docosahexaenoic (DHA) and alpha-linolenic (ALA) acids, have been evaluated for cognitive and depressive disorders for their anti-inflammatory properties and potential influence on neurogenesis and neuronal function (45). Despite this, evidence of its use for cognitive improvement, prevention of dementia or depression and improvement of depressive symptoms is still insufficient. S-adenosylmethionine (SAMe), an endogenous intracellular metabolite of amino acids and enzymatic co-substrate involved in the biosynthesis of hormones and neurotransmitters, has been implicated in depression and cognition. It is a safe compound with minimal interactions and has shown good results in monotherapy and adjunctive therapy in unipolar depression. However, the effects are small and more clinical trials are needed, including especially an exclusive older adult population (46, 47). There are a number of literature reviews with meta-analyses of the possible effects of pre-, pro- and symbiotic substances on the modulation of late and cognitive conditions, but the results are still modest. It should be noted that the specific studies involve older adults. Our group carried out a clinical study with a small number of older people with the aim of investigating the effect of a symbiotic substance on symptoms of brain disorders and inflammation (48). Forty-nine older adults were studied, receiving a symbiotic or placebo. At the end of the experiment, both groups reduced their percentage of body fat, tumour necrosis factor and serum diamine oxidase; interleukin-10 was significantly increased only in the symbiotic group. Depressive symptomatology at the end of the study was explained negatively by the percentage of body fat, tumour necrosis factor, serum diamine oxidase, interleukin-10, female sex and placebo group. Therefore, we found weaker effects of the symbiotic on depressive symptoms.

Inflammaging, Gut Microbiome and Mental Illness: Potential Pathophysiological Associations

Most probably, the association between depression and obesity permeates the concept of low-grade systemic inflammation, particularly that linked to ageing. Over the course of life, damage accumulates, culminating in the loss of resilience. Lifelong antigenic stimulation can lead to an imbalance in the immune system and consequent low-grade systemic inflammation (inflammaging), which has been linked to many age-related conditions and diseases (49). Currently, some contributor mechanisms associated with ageing have been proposed to explain inflammaging. Here, considering the nutritional status of old adults, we will briefly address the adipose tissue and the gut.

The ageing-related increase and redistribution of body fat stand out in visceral white adipose tissue (50). The high-fat content in this tissue allows the infiltration of M1 macrophages and T lymphocytes. These immune cells, and the adipocytes themselves, release cytokines and chemokines, which settles an inflammatory profile (51). In addition to these processes, the existing adipose tissue vasculature does not support the tissue's expansion, reducing the entry of oxygen and activating the hypoxia-inducible factor-1 that targets inflammatory genes. Systemically, the increase in body fat entails higher cellular exposure to saturated fatty acids, indirectly activating the toll-like receptor signalling and possibly altering macrophage lipid metabolism (52).

However, adipose tissue and dietary fat are not the only contributors to ageing-related systemic inflammation. In fact, the contribution of the gut, adipose tissue and diet raises the concept of metaflammation, a metabolic disorder featured by cellular oxidative stress and increased plasma proinflammatory cytokine levels, principally triggered by nutrients and metabolic surplus. The role of metabolic inflammation is well established in the pathogenesis of insulin resistance, mainly through stimulation of the proinflammatory cell signalling pathway, with activation of the transcription factors, namely nuclear factor-kappa B and activator protein-1 mediated by toll-like receptor-4 (53). Therefore, inflammaging and metaflammation share similar molecular mechanisms.

Regarding the gut, its microbiota can release inflammatory products (54). Many ageing-related factors can modify the gut microbiota, favouring the growth of pathogenic bacteria (i.e. *Fusobacteria, Clostridia, Eubacteria*) and the reduction of some beneficial bacteria (i.e. *Firmicutes, Bacteroides, Bifidobacterium*). These beneficial bacteria are able to ferment polysaccharides and originate short-chain fatty acids (SCFAs). The SCFAs, besides several metabolic functions, have fundamental immunological roles. Therefore, bacterial unbalance and the reduced production of SCFAs are associated with abnormal activation of the gut-associated lymphoid tissue, modifying the tolerance pattern of the immune cells (55). Changes in the gut environment harm its barrier function, allowing the passage of bacterial fragments (i.e. lipopolysaccharides) to the blood flow. These fragments bind to specific pattern-recognising receptors, mainly the toll-like receptor-4; these bindings trigger inflammatory signalling cascades that ultimately stimulate innate immune responses with the generation of proinflammatory cytokines, chemokines, eicosanoids and reactive oxygen species. It is essential to highlight that the production of inflammatory cytokines constitutes a feedback cycle since these molecules stimulate the activity of toll-like receptors. This inflammatory picture is named metabolic endotoxemia and has local and systemic consequences. For instance, it impairs endothelial cell function and contributes to atherosclerosis; it leads to hepatic steatosis and insulin resistance; in the pancreas, it favours β-cell dysfunction; in skeletal muscle, it increases the risk of sarcopenia (56); and in the brain, it increases neuroinflammation (57).

Therefore, all processes related to inflammaging cause an imbalance between circulating inflammatory cytokines. Many of these molecules are able to cross the blood–brain barrier, increasing neuroinflammation and consequently altering the synthesis of neurotransmitters, decreasing the production of serotonin and increasing the production of neurotoxic molecules (58).

Conclusions

Nutritional disorders are common among older people with mental illness. They are a biological cornerstone of the burden for several important geriatric syndromes, such as frailty, anorexia and sarcopenia, which present a bidirectional relationship with neuropsychiatric disorders. In this sense, there are no thresholds between mental and physical health in older adults, and basic nutritional evaluation and counselling must be part of the routine of allied professionals who care for psychogeriatric patients. Only a few anthropometric measures and simple instruments for the assessment of appetite, muscle and nutrition are sufficient to improve the health of these patients. We suggest an objective geriatric evaluation concerning general nutritional health to any allied professional (Figure 8.3). In this flow diagram, we suggest the evaluation of frailty using the FRAIL questionnaire, an accessible and quick instrument to screen for this condition (59, 60). Anorexia, undernutrition, low muscle mass and weight loss are all associated with frailty at some level. The identification of frailty leads to indirect nutritional screening and vice versa. The evidence for nutritional intervention in older adults is mostly centred on diet patterns.

The Mediterranean diet and its derivatives show the best reliable data for late-life depressive and neurocognitive disorders. We support the prescription of this diet to psychogeriatric patients and also a high level of vigilance against a low level of B-complex vitamins (Figure 8.4). The Mediterranean diet appears to reduce symptoms of depression,

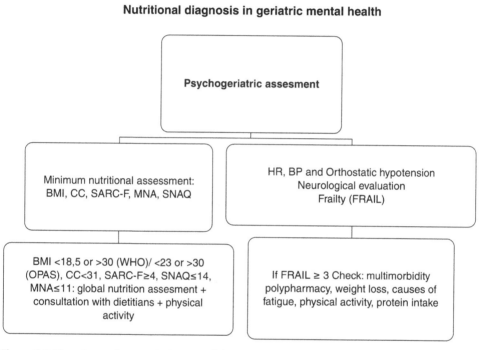

Nutritional diagnosis in geriatric mental health

Psychogeriatric assesment

Minimum nutritional assessment:
BMI, CC, SARC-F, MNA, SNAQ

HR, BP and Orthostatic hypotension
Neurological evaluation
Frailty (FRAIL)

BMI <18,5 or >30 (WHO)/ <23 or >30 (OPAS), CC<31, SARC-F≥4, SNAQ≤14, MNA≤11: global nutrition assesment + consultation with dietitians + physical activity

If FRAIL ≥ 3 Check: multimorbidity polypharmacy, weight loss, causes of fatigue, physical activity, protein intake

Figure 8.3 Flow diagram for a practical nutritional diagnosis in geriatric medicine.

RECOMMENDATIONS	
Mediterranean diet	High amounts of: Olive oil, non-refined grains, fruits, vegetables, legumes, potatoes, seeds, nuts, beans
	Limited/restricted: Red meat, processed meat, sweets
MIND	High amounts of: Whole grains, green leafy vegetables, berries, other vegetables, nuts, beans
	Limited/restricted: Cheese, butter/margarine, fast/fried food
DASH	High amounts of: Grains, fruits, vegetables, legumes, nuts, seeds, low-fat dairy
	Limited/restricted: Sodium < 2400 mg/d
Complex B vitamins	Controversial, but some studies show benefits.

Figure 8.4 Nutritional recommendations to the psychogeriatric patient.

reduce the incidence of depression and improve general cognitive performance and recent memory. No single vitamin or nutritional supplement showed a significant result in mental illness compared with anti-inflammatory and antioxidative diet patterns. Changing diet habits is difficult, especially among psychogeriatric patients, but in this field there is no magic pill that substitutes for a healthy diet. Future studies are needed to shed more light on dietary habits, the use of multiple nutritional supplements, integrated care plans including nutritional counselling, metabolomic-guided or microbiome-guided nutritional plans, and many other beneficial potential interventions for late-life mental health patients.

References

1. Aprahamian, I., Borges, M. K., Hanssen, D. J. C., Jeuring, H. W. and Oude Voshaar, R. C., 2022. The frail depressed patient: a narrative review on treatment challenges. *Clinical Interventions in Aging*, *17*, pp. 979–90.

2. Borges, M. K., Canevelli, M., Cesari, M. and Aprahamian, I., 2019. Frailty as a predictor of cognitive disorders: a systematic review and meta-analysis. *Frontiers in Medicine (Lausanne)*, 6, p. 26.

3. Borges, M. K., Jeuring, H. W., Marijnissen, R. M., et al., 2022. Frailty and affective disorders throughout adult life: a 5-year follow-up of the Lifelines Cohort Study. *Journal of the American Geriatrics Society*, *12*, pp. 3424–35.

4. Ribeiro, S. M. L., Melo, C. M. and Tirapegui, J., 2018. *Avaliação Nutricional: teoria e prática*. 2nd ed. Guanabara Koogan.

5. Gibson, R., 2005. *Principles of nutritional assessment*. 2nd ed. Oxford University Press.

6. Cox, N. J., Morrison, L., Ibrahim, K., et al., 2020. New horizons in appetite and the anorexia of ageing. *Age Ageing*, *49*(4), pp. 526–34.

7. Hara, L. M., Freiria, C. N., Silva, G. M., Fattori, A. and Corona, L. P., 2019. Anorexia of aging associated with nutrients intake in Brazilian elderly. *The Journal of Nutrition, Health and Aging*, 23 (7), pp. 606–13.

8. Cox, N. J., Ibrahim, K., Sayer, A. A., Robinson, S. M. and Roberts, H. C., 2019. Assessment and treatment of the anorexia of aging: a systematic review. *Nutrients*; *11* (1), p. 144.

9. Zukeran, M. S., Valentini Neto, J., Romanini, C. V., et al., 2022. The association between appetite loss, frailty, and psychosocial factors in community-dwelling older adults. *Clinical Nutrition ESPEN*, *47*, pp. 194–8.

10. Aprahamian, I., Romanini, C. V., Lima, N. A., et al., 2021. The concept of anorexia of aging in late life depression: a cross-sectional analysis of a cohort study. *Archives of Gerontology and Geriatrics*, *95*, pp. 345–55.

11. de Lima, E. S., Zukeran, M. S., Valentini Neto, J., et al., 2022. Factors related to malnutrition and their association with frailty in community-dwelling older adults registered at a geriatric clinic. *Experimental Gerontology*; *165*, p. 111865.

12. Cederholm, T., Bosaeus, I., Barazzoni, R., et al., 2015. Diagnostic criteria for malnutrition: an ESPEN consensus statement. *Clinical Nutrition*, *34*(3), pp. 335–40.

13. Cederholm, T., Barazzoni, R., Austin, P., et al., 2017. ESPEN guidelines on definitions and terminology of clinical nutrition. *Clinical Nutrition*, *36*(1), pp. 49–64.

14. Jensen, G. L. and Cederholm, T., 2018. Global leadership initiative on malnutrition: progress report from ASPEN clinical nutrition week 2017. *Journal of Parenteral and Enteral Nutrition*, *42*(2), pp. 266–7.

15. Kaiser, M. J., Bauer, J. M., Rämsch, C., et al., 2010. Frequency of malnutrition in older adults: a multinational perspective using the mini nutritional assessment.

Journal of the American Geriatrics Society, 58(9), pp. 1734–8.

16. Cereda, E., Pedrolli, C., Klersy, C., et al., 2016. Nutritional status in older persons according to healthcare setting: a systematic review and meta-analysis of prevalence data using MNA®. *Clinical Nutrition,* 35(6), pp. 1282–90.

17. Agarwal, E., Miller, M., Yaxley, A. and Isenring, E., 2013. Malnutrition in the elderly: a narrative review. *Maturitas, 76* (4), pp. 296–302.

18. Noh, J. W., Kwon, Y. D., Park, J., et al., 2015. Body mass index and depressive symptoms in middle aged and older adults. *BMC Public Health, 15,* p. 310.

19. Yeom, H. E. and Kim, Y.-J., 2022. Age and sex-specific associations between depressive symptoms, body mass index and cognitive functioning among Korean middle-aged and older adults: a cross-sectional analysis. *BMC Geriatrics, 22,* p. 412.

20. Luppino, F. S., de Wit, L. M., Bouvy, P. F., et al., 2010. Overweight, obesity, and depression: a systematic review and meta-analysis of longitudinal studies. *Archives of General Psychiatry, 67*(3), pp. 220–9.

21. Mingming, Y., Yuexian, S., Libin, G. and Wenru, W., 2022. 'Jolly fat' or 'sad fat': a systematic review and meta-analysis of the association between obesity and depression among community-dwelling older adults. *Aging and Mental Health, 26* (1), pp. 13–25.

22. Sousa-Santos, A. R., Barros, D., Montanha, T. L., Carvalho, J. and Amaral, T. F., 2021. Which is the best alternative to estimate muscle mass for sarcopenia diagnosis when DXA is unavailable? *Archives of Gerontology and Geriatrics, 97,* p. 104517.

23. Santos, L. P., Gonzalez, M. C., Orlandi, S. P., et al., 2019. New prediction equations to estimate appendicular skeletal muscle mass using calf circumference: results from NHANES 1999–2006. *Journal of Parenteral and Enteral Nutrition, 43*(8), pp. 998–1007.

24. Voelker, S. N., Michalopoulos, N., Maier, A. B. and Reijnierse, E. M., 2021.

Reliability and concurrent validity of the SARC-F and its modified versions: a systematic review and meta-analysis. *Journal of the American Medical Directors Association, 22*(9), pp. 1864–76.

25. Chang, K. V., Hsu, T. H., Wu, W. T., Huang, K. C. and Han, D. S., 2017. Is sarcopenia associated with depression? A systematic review and meta-analysis of observational studies. *Age and Ageing, 46* (5), pp. 738–46.

26. Cabett Cipolli, G., Sanches Yassuda, M. and Aprahamian, I., 2019. Sarcopenia is associated with cognitive impairment in older adults: a systematic review and meta-analysis. *The Journal of Nutrition, Health and Aging, 23*(6), pp. 525–31.

27. Lobato, Z. M., Almeida da Silva, A. C., Lima Ribeiro, S. M., et al., 2021. Nutritional status and adverse outcomes in older depressed inpatients: a prospective study. *The Journal of Nutrition, Health and Aging, 25*(7), pp. 889–94.

28. Cereda, E., 2012. Mini nutritional assessment. *Current Opinion in Clinical Nutrition & Metabolic Care, 15*(1), pp. 29–41.

29. Lay, J. S., Hiles, S., Bisquera, A., et al., 2014. A systematic review and meta-analysis of dietary patterns and depression in community-dwelling adults. *The American Journal of Clinical Nutrition, 99,* pp. 181–97.

30. Jacka, F. N., 2017. Nutritional psychiatry: where to next? *EBioMedicine, 17,* pp. 24–9.

31. Ribeiro, S. M. L., Malmstrom, T. K., Morley, J. E. and Miller, D. K., 2017. Fruit and vegetable intake, physical activity, and depressive symptoms in the African American Health (A AH) study. *Journal of Affective Disorders, 220,* pp. 31–7.

32. Masana, M. F., Haro, J. M., Mariolis, A., et al., 2018. Mediterranean diet and depression among older individuals: the multinational MEDIS study. *Experimental Gerontology, 110,* pp. 67–72.

33. Vicinanza, R., Bersani, F. S., D'Ottavio, E., et al., 2020. Adherence to the Mediterranean diet moderates the association between multimorbidity and

depressive symptoms in older adults. *Archives of Gerontology and Geriatrics, 13* (88), p. 104022.

34. Cherian, L., Wang, Y., Holland, T., et al., 2021. DASH and Mediterranean-DASH Intervention for Neurodegenerative Delay (MIND) diets are associated with fewer depressive symptoms over time. *The Journals of Gerontology Series A*, 76(1), pp. 151–6.

35. Loughrey, D. G., Lavecchia, S., Brennan, S., Lawlor, B. A. and Kelly, M. E., 2017. The impact of the Mediterranean diet on the cognitive functioning of healthy older adults: a systematic review and meta-analysis. *Advances in Nutrition*, 8, pp. 571–86.

36. Morris, M. C., Tangney, C. C., Wang, Y., et al., 2015. MIND diet associated with reduced incidence of Alzheimer's disease. *Alzheimer's & Dementia Journal, 11*, pp. 1007–14.

37. van den Brink, A., Brouwer-Brolsma, E. M., Berendsen, A. A. M. and van de Rest, O., 2019. The Mediterranean, Dietary Approaches to Stop Hypertension (DASH), and Mediterranean-DASH intervention for neurodegenerative delay (MIND) diets are associated with less cognitive decline and a lower risk of Alzheimer's disease: a review. *Advances in Nutrition*, 10, pp. 1040–65.

38. Ghosh, T. S., Rampelli, S., Jeffery, I. B., et al., 2020. Mediterranean diet intervention alters the gut microbiome in older people reducing frailty and improving health status: the NU-AGE 1-year dietary intervention across five European countries. *Gut*, 69, pp. 1–11.

39. Bastos, A. A., Nogueira, L. R., Neto, J. V., et al., 2020. Association between the adherence to the Mediterranean dietary pattern and common mental disorders among community-dwelling elders: 2015 Health Survey of São Paulo, SP, Brazil. *Journal of Affective Disorders, 265*, pp. 389–94.

40. Solfrizzi, V., Agosti, P., Lozupone, M., et al., 2018. Nutritional interventions and cognitive-related outcomes in patients with late-life cognitive disorders: a systematic review. *Neuroscience & Biobehavioral Reviews*, 95, pp. 480–98.

41. McGrattan, A. M., McEvoy, C. T., McGuinness, B., McKinley, M. C. and Woodside, J. V., 2019. Effect of dietary interventions in mild cognitive impairment: a systematic review. *British Journal of Nutrition, 120*(12), pp. 1388–405.

42. de Koning, E. J., Lips, P., Penninx, B. W. J. H., et al., 2019. Vitamin D supplementation for the prevention of depression and poor physical function in older persons: the D-Vitaal study, a randomized clinical trial. *The American Journal of Clinical Nutrition, 110*(5), pp. 1119–30.

43. Young, L. M., Pipingas, A., White, D. J., Gauci, S. and Scholey, A., 2019. A systematic review and meta-analysis of B vitamin supplementation on depressive symptoms, anxiety, and stress: effects on healthy and 'at-risk' individuals. *Nutrients, 11*(9), p. E2232.

44. Altaf, R., Gonzalez, I., Rubino, K. and Nemec, E. C., 2nd,2021. Folate as adjunct therapy to SSRI/SNRI for major depressive disorder: systematic review and meta-analysis. *Complementary Therapies in Medicine, 61*, p. 102770.

45. Burckhardt, M., Herke, M., Wustmann, T., et al., 2016. Omega-3 fatty acids for the treatment of dementia. *Cochrane Database of Systematic Reviews*, 4, p. CD009002.

46. Galizia, I., Oldani, L., Macritchie, K., et al., 2016. S-adenosyl methionine (SAMe) for depression in adults. *Cochrane Database of Systematic Reviews*, 10, p. CD011286.

47. Sharma, A., Gerbarg, P., Bottiglieri, T., et al., 2017. S-Adenosylmethionine (SAMe) for neuropsychiatric disorders: a clinician-oriented review of research. *The Journal of Clinical Psychiatry*, 78(6), pp. 656–67.

48. Louzada, E. R. and Ribeiro, S. M. L., 2020. Synbiotic supplementation, systemic inflammation, and symptoms of brain disorders in elders: a secondary study from a randomized clinical trial. *Nutritional Neuroscience*, 23(2), pp. 93–100.

49. Franceschi, C., Bonafè, M., Valensin, S., et al., 2000. Inflammaging: an evolutionary perspective on immunosenescence. *Annals of the New York Academy of Sciences, 908*, pp. 244–54.

50. Zorena, K., Jachimowicz-Duda, O., Ślęzak, D., Robakowska, M. and Mrugacz, M., 2020. Adipokines and obesity: potential link to metabolic disorders and chronic complications. *International Journal of Molecular Sciences*, *21*(10), p. 3570.

51. Lee, Y. S., Wollam, J. and Olefsky, J. M., 2018. An integrated view of immunometabolism. *Cell*, *172*, pp. 22–40.

52. Nguyen, M. T., Favelyukis, S., Nguyen, A. K., et al., 2007. A subpopulation of macrophages infiltrates hypertrophic adipose tissue and is activated by free fatty acids via toll-like receptors 2 and 4 and JNK-dependent pathways. *Journal of Biological Chemistry*, *282*, pp. 35279–92.

53. Lee, J. Y., Sohn, K. H., Rhee, S. H. and Hwang, D., 2001. Saturated fatty acids, but not unsaturated fatty acids, induce the expression of cyclooxygenase-2 mediated through toll-like receptor 4. *Journal of Biological Chemistry*, *276*, pp. 16683–9.

54. Franceschi, C., Garagnani, P., Parini, P., Giuliani, C. and Santoro, A., 2018. Inflammaging: a new immune-metabolic viewpoint for age-related diseases. *Nature Reviews Endocrinology*, *14*, 576–90.

55. André, P., Laugerette, F. and Féart, C., 2019. Metabolic endotoxemia: a potential underlying mechanism of the relationship between dietary fat intake and risk for cognitive impairments in humans? *Nutrients*, *11*(8), p. 1887.

56. Livshits, G. and Kalinkovich, A., 2019. Inflammaging as a common ground for the development and maintenance of sarcopenia, obesity, cardiomyopathy and dysbiosis. *Ageing Research Reviews, 56*, p. 100980.

57. Di Benedetto, S., Müller, L., Wenger, E., Düzel, S. and Pawelec, G., 2017. Contribution of neuroinflammation and immunity to brain aging and the mitigating effects of physical and cognitive interventions. *Neuroscience & Biobehavioral Reviews, 75*, pp. 114–28.

58. Castanon, N., Luheshi, G. and Layé, S., 2015. Role of neuroinflammation in the emotional and cognitive alterations displayed by animal models of obesity. *Frontiers in Neuroscience, 9*, p. 229.

59. Dent, E., Morley, J. E., Cruz-Jentoft, A. J., et al., 2019. Physical frailty: ICFSR international clinical practice guidelines for identification and management. *The Journal of Nutrition, Health and Aging, 23* (9), pp. 771–87.

60. Aprahamian, I., Lin, S. M., Suemoto, C. K., et al., 2017. Feasibility and factor structure of the FRAIL Scale in older adults. *Journal of the American Medical Directors Association, 18*(4), pp. 367.e11–e18.

Broad-Spectrum Micronutrients and Mental Health[*]

Julia J. Rucklidge, Jeanette M. Johnstone, Amelia Villagomez, Noshene Ranjbar and Bonnie J. Kaplan

Summary

This chapter summarises evidence relating to the importance of nutrient intake from diet and supplementation to brain health. Circumstances that may contribute to an individual requiring additional nutrients beyond what are available in diet, such as consumption of nutritionally depleted food, individual differences in biological need, long-term medication use and gut–brain health needs, are detailed. These factors support the use of a broad spectrum of nutrients to address personal metabolic needs or environmentally induced nutrient depletions. The evidence for treating psychological symptoms with supplementary nutrients is reviewed, summarising research using broad-spectrum micronutrients in the treatment of mental health issues including aggression, autism, attention deficit hyperactivity disorder, anxiety and stress, mood disorders, and psychosis. The breadth and consistency of the findings highlight the importance of receiving a complete foundation of nutrients to optimise brain health. Documented safety and lack of toxicity provide reassurance that this treatment approach does not result in serious or long-term adverse events. The question of pre-treatment nutrient level testing is discussed. Finally, we offer practical suggestions to clinicians interested in incorporating this information into their clinical practice, discussing these suggestions within the context of informed consent.

Other chapters in this book describe the research that supports the importance of eating nutrient-dense food for optimising mental health. In this chapter, we focus on the circumstances that may predispose an individual to require additional nutrients beyond the levels they can get from their diet. In addition, the evidence base for treating psychiatric problems with supplementary broad-spectrum micronutrients will be reviewed. By 'broad-spectrum', we mean the full array of about 30 essential minerals and vitamins necessary for optimising brain health, not just a select few. Finally, we offer practical suggestions for health professionals who want to incorporate this information into their clinical practice.

---

[*] Parts of this chapter have been adapted from Rucklidge, J. J., Johnstone, J. M. and Kaplan, B. J. 2021. Nutrition provides the essential foundation for optimizing mental health. *Evidence-Based Practice in Child and Adolescent Mental Health*, 6(1), pp. 131–54.

Nutrition Is Essential for Maintaining a Healthy Brain

Minerals and vitamins (micronutrients) contribute to healthy brain functioning in several ways: supporting brain metabolism, enabling mitochondria to function, modifying genetic expression, fighting excess inflammation and protecting from environmental toxins. A wealth of research demonstrates an *association* between eating a nutrient-dense diet and better mental health, with the strength of the association confirmed through meta-analyses (1–4). However, over and above these observational studies, prospective longitudinal studies and randomised controlled trials (RCTs) show that the relationship is causal (5–12): consuming a whole-foods diet rich in micronutrients (vitamins and minerals) can improve resilience, lower the risk of developing a mental health problem, reduce the risk of suicide and treat mental health symptoms. In addition, a number of these studies show that an ultra-processed diet, characterised by packaged foods containing manufactured chemicals and typically high in poor-quality fats, salt and sugar, generally *precedes* poor mental health.

When Might Individuals Need More Nutrients Than They Can Obtain from Their Diet?

Both environmental and individual factors may result in an individual requiring an increased intake of nutrients above the usual dietary reference ranges.

Nutritionally Depleted Food

Neither plants nor humans can synthesise minerals. Plants absorb minerals from the soil and then use them to synthesise vitamins. Over the last 70 years, the nutrient density of our food supply has been decreasing (13). This nutrient depletion may result from several factors including an emphasis on crop yield over nutritional value, high carbon dioxide levels, climate change and the use of herbicides. Modern agricultural practices tend to emphasise crop yield to increase financial margins, creating a 'dilution effect' of lower nutrient levels relative to carbohydrates (14). Many years of tilling the soil, even with rotating crops, can deplete minerals. Food producers use fertiliser, the primary components of which are nitrogen, phosphorous and potassium (NPK). While these three minerals are important, plants require 15–16 essential minerals for defence against insects, best growth and the ability to synthesise vitamins (15). The good news is that modern regenerative agricultural practices, such as no-till farming, can improve soil minerals (16).

High levels of atmospheric carbon dioxide are concerning to nutrient density because even though carbon helps plants grow, it also leads to plants with more sugars and fewer micronutrients. The result is larger plants and greater sweetness in the yield, but the produce may provide fewer nutrients needed for brain health. One study of eight strains of rice exposed to increased carbon dioxide under controlled conditions found lower levels of vitamins, minerals and protein (17). Another study looked at nutrient balance in spring wheat grown naturally over three consecutive seasons (18). Higher carbon dioxide levels led to larger plants and a higher yield, resulting in an increase in carbohydrates, but protein declined by more than 7%, and iron and manganese both decreased. Similar results have been found in studies of other crops. As the planet gets hotter, many crops will likely become even higher in carbohydrates and lower in protein and micronutrients.

Another possible contributor to nutrient depletion of crops is the heavy use of glyphosate in places such as North America. Glyphosate, a herbicide and principal ingredient of

Roundup®, was initially patented in the USA in 1961 as a descaling agent to remove mineral deposits in pipes and boilers, and it has been applied to crops to kill weeds since 1974. A 2019 study showed that glyphosate disturbs the human blood–brain barrier, making it more permeable (19). Permeability means that some molecules intended to be excluded by the blood–brain barrier might be able to pass through, potentially causing adverse effects in the brain. It is also relevant that while there is still debate on the topic, some research suggests that glyphosate makes dietary minerals such as iron, manganese and nickel *less* available for the body to absorb (20) and decreases soil health (21), factors that may also affect plant nutrient density.

Although methodological criticisms regarding the comparison of nutrient content across time have been raised (14) (e.g. crops having multiple varieties requiring different sampling or storage), significant changes reported in several countries suggest there is cause for concern. Modern agricultural practices focussed on plant yield rather than nutrient density may explain why some people do not obtain adequate doses of nutrients from food. Because plant nutrient levels play a vital role in human brain health, these issues that affect crop nutrient levels warrant more research.

Individual Differences

Aside from metabolic pathways' requirements for an abundance of nutrients for efficient enzymatic activity, personal differences may contribute to an individual's need for higher intake. In 2002, Ames summarised 50 genetic mutations associated with slowed metabolic pathways that may be remedied with high-dose vitamin cofactors, suggesting that some individuals may have an inherited need for higher amounts of nutrient cofactors, a phenomenon known for decades in relation to physical health (22).

In summary, research has identified that some people inherit the need for an above-average supply of nutrients for metabolic pathways to work efficiently for optimal physical health. It is possible that some psychiatric symptoms may also result from metabolic dysfunction caused by insufficient mineral and vitamin cofactors in the brain, an idea first proposed in the 1960s by Nobel Laureate Linus Pauling (23). As many mental disorders run in families, Pauling hypothesised that the genes for mental illness may be the ones involved in the regulation of essential nutrients for brain metabolism. If so, nutrient supplementation to raise nutrients to a sufficient level, based on individual needs, may remedy mental health issues. As the Ames paper showed, restoring near-normal physical functioning is possible when enzymes with drastically reduced binding activity become supersaturated with the necessary cofactors through nutrient supplementation (22).

Long-Term Medication Use

Another factor that may increase the need for supplemental nutrients is the use of certain medications. For example, mood stabilisers deplete folic acid, vitamin D, vitamin B_6 and vitamin B_{12}, as well as minerals such as copper, selenium and zinc (24). Metformin reduces B_{12}; contraceptives decrease B_6, folate, magnesium and vitamins C and E; and aspirin negatively affects vitamin C levels (25). Clinicians need to be aware that these medications may reduce nutrient stores and impact brain health. Increasing an individual's nutrient supply through micronutrient supplementation may alleviate the depletion caused by medication (26, 27).

Gut–Brain Health

The association between digestive and mood problems has been known for centuries (28). Recent studies examining the human gut microbiome have identified that digestive problems may be caused by gut dysbiosis, or an imbalance in the gut-microbial communities that are associated with disease. Previous chapters in this book (see Chapters 2, 3 and 4) have discussed the crucial communication between the gut and the brain, identifying a number of communication channels through which the microbiome can influence neural pathways in the brain. These channels include the nervous system (via the vagus nerve), the immune system (via cytokines) and the endocrine system (via the hypothalamic–pituitary–adrenal (HPA) axis) (29–31). Many studies highlight how the gut microbiota might affect the expression of behavioural symptoms (32, 33).

Some research has suggested an association between certain bacterial strains and disorders such as attention deficit hyperactivity disorder (ADHD), schizophrenia and depression, although the results of these studies have been inconsistent (34, 35). Unfortunately, the science cannot yet define what constitutes a healthy gut microbiome for optimal brain function. Based on the cited studies, microbiome/microbial diversity appears to be important (36), and the less optimal the microbiome, the more likely there could be mental health problems. Several factors may negatively impact gut-microbial diversity including antibiotics, stress, infection and environmental toxins, while a diet rich in plant-based foods supports microbial diversity (34, 37). As such, one of the first recommendations for improving gut health is to improve the quality of the foods eaten and reduce the consumption of ultra-processed industrialised products. However, for some individuals, supplemental micronutrients may be necessary as well to improve gut health and brain functioning. One study showed that micronutrient supplementation increases bacterial diversity, which is associated with symptom improvement in children with ADHD (38). These results, though preliminary, highlight the possibility that nutrient supplementation may positively alter bacterial composition and underscore that nutrient insufficiencies may be a causal factor in both dysbiosis and mental health symptoms.

How Supplementary Nutrients Might Improve Mental Health

We have reviewed several reasons why eating a healthy diet may not be sufficient to ensure optimal mental health for everyone. Environmental factors such as depleted soil minerals and climate change can influence the nutrient density of the food we consume. In addition, individual differences, medication use and gut health all provide plausible reasons why nutrient requirements may vary, resulting in a greater need for nutrients in some individuals than what can be obtained from diet alone.

The question of whether nutrient supplementation may have positive effects on mental health is not new. Scientists first investigated this possibility by studying one nutrient at a time (e.g. thiamine, selenium or calcium). Some studies revealed small positive effects (39–41), but most of the research was largely negative. A number of systematic reviews and meta-analyses have highlighted the concentrated effort to find a single nutrient that would alleviate symptoms associated with an array of psychiatric issues such as mood (42, 43), psychosis (44), ADHD (45) or antisocial behaviours (46). These studies report modest to low benefit from single nutrient supplementation (47). The complex interplay of nutrients, working together for optimal brain metabolism, underscores why the search for a single nutrient to resolve complex psychiatric symptoms is unrealistic. Therefore, in reviewing the evidence base for micronutrient supplementation for mental health, we will focus on the studies of micronu-trients given *in combination* as the treatment; in particular, studies that used the full array of approximately 30 vitamins and minerals that are viewed as essential for health. We will refer to this combination as broad-spectrum micronutrient supplementation (BSMS).

ADHD

The historical evidence for the use of micronutrients in the treatment of ADHD has been obscured by early studies that tended to use either very small doses, showing no benefit, or mega-doses, resulting in toxicity (48). In the past two decades, several studies have employed BSMS to treat core ADHD symptoms at doses between recommended dietary allowance and below upper tolerable intake level for most ingredients. Although the open-label trials varied in length and micronutrient composition, all of them resulted in signifi-cant improvements in behavioural functioning, including core ADHD symptoms and/or emotion regulation (49–51). These were then followed by three RCTs.

The first RCT (52) randomised 80 medication-free adults diagnosed with ADHD to receive either BSMS or placebo for 8 weeks. Greater improvement on ADHD rating scales compared with placebo was found for self-report (ES=0.61) and observer ratings (ES=0.59), but not clinician ratings (ES=0.23). Clinicians rated 48% of those taking the nutrients as 'much' or 'very much' improved compared with 21% of the placebo group (X^2=6.189, p=0.013, OR=3.4; Figure 9.1). Those randomised to BSMS, who entered the trial with a moderately to severely low mood, reported a greater improvement in mood compared with the placebo group (between-group ES=0.64).

A replication followed in 93 medication-free children aged 7–12, randomly assigned to either BSMS or placebo capsules for 10 weeks (53). Clinician-rated inattention (ES=0.41) and overall functioning (ES=0.48) improved significantly more in children who took the micro-nutrients than those who took placebo. There were no group differences in parent- and teacher-rated ADHD symptoms as well as clinician-rated hyperactivity/impulsivity. Across all raters (parents, teachers and clinicians), there was significantly greater improvement in

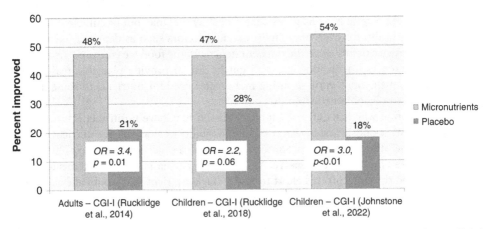

Figure 9.1 Percentage identified as 'much' to 'very much' improved across groups based on the Clinician Global Impression (CGI-I).
OR=odds ratio.

aggression (ES=0.52) and emotion regulation (ES=0.66) for those children who took the micronutrients compared to placebo. A meta-analysis confirms the consistency of findings across these two RCTs, noting significant effects on clinician-rated inattention, global functioning, Clinician Global Impression (CGI-I) and CGI-I-ADHD (54).

The participants in both of these RCTs were followed for 1 year, with about 80% of those still taking the micronutrients being identified as in remission from their ADHD symptoms (about one-fifth of the original number of participants) versus about 40% of those on medications and about 20% of those who stopped all treatments (55, 56). The two main reasons cited for stopping the nutrients in both studies were cost and the number of capsules required. Continued symptom improvement over time was reported for participants who stayed on the nutrients, suggesting that the benefit of micronutrient treatment takes time to reach its full potential. Further, those who switched from micronutrients to stimulant medications were more likely to have problems with mood or anxiety compared to those who stayed on nutrients at the 1-year follow-up assessment (56).

A third RCT conducted across three sites in the USA and Canada (57) reported remarkably similar results to the New Zealand trial (53). Of 135 randomised, 126 children (93%) aged 6–12 completed the trial. Fifty-four per cent of the micronutrient and 18% of the placebo group were identified as responders based on a measure of global impression of improvement (OR=2.97; $p<0.001$; Figure 9.1). ADHD measures improved significantly for both groups ($p<0.01$), with no significant group differences (ES=0.07). The micronutrient group grew 6 mm more than the placebo group (ES=1.15).

In summary, open-label pilot studies and three RCTs provide promising data for the clinical benefits of BSMS in ADHD populations.

Aggression

A broad spectrum of minerals and vitamins (sometimes combined with omega-3s) can reduce aggression and violent incidents based on case studies, open-label studies and multiple RCTs. The results have been reported across a range of populations, from aggressive children to incarcerated adults (50, 53, 58–65). The earliest randomised trial was more than 20 years ago, when researchers conducted a fully blinded 3-month RCT in 62 incarcerated youth aged 13–17. Those randomised to receive BSMS exhibited a 28% greater decrease in rule violations compared with those receiving the placebo, for both non-violent (ES=0.70) and violent (ES=0.52) offences (59).

Another RCT conducted by the same researchers found schoolchildren aged 6–12 who received BSMS for 1 school year also improved (63). The 40 children in the experimental group who were randomised to receive BSMS exhibited 47% fewer antisocial behaviours requiring discipline than the 40 children who received a placebo. The antisocial behaviours monitored in the study included threats, fighting, vandalism, defiance, endangering others and disorderly conduct.

Other studies in incarcerated adults have reported similar findings (58, 61). Evidence for the benefit of BSMS has continued to emerge from studies of children with explosive rage, conduct disorder and ADHD with mood dysregulation (50, 53, 62, 66). These human studies complement the long-standing literature on lab animals, which supports the relationship between poor nutrition and aggression (67). In summary, there is ample evidence that BSMS can reduce aggression.

Anxiety and Stress

Stress, although an inevitable part of life, may contribute to nutrient insufficiency. Wired to survive, our bodies preferentially prioritise micronutrient-dependent functions required for short-term survival (e.g. the fight/flight response) at the expense of longer-term functions, like concentration (68). The Triage Theory (68) refers to the preferential sequence in which the fight/flight response takes priority over other functions. In situations of both acute and chronic stress, supplementing with micronutrients has been shown to be an effective way to replenish micronutrients and reduce stress in adults. Studies on stressors ranging from natural and humanmade disasters to workplace stress (69–71) have all documented the benefit of BSMS. Stress levels reduced to the non-clinical range in these studies, and in one the rate of probable PTSD reduced from 65% to 19% over a 4-week period.

Autism Spectrum Disorders (ASD)

A pilot RCT involving 20 children with ASD found that those taking micronutrients showed improvements in sleep and gastrointestinal problems, along with some suggestive trends for improved behaviour, eye contact and receptive language (72). These same researchers followed up with a larger RCT in 141 children and adults with autism and reported positive effects from a modified version of the formula compared to placebo in reducing tantrums (ES=0.51) and hyperactivity (ES=0.37), as well as improving receptive language (ES=0.40) and overall functioning (ES=0.46), with no significant effects on play, sociability, expressive language, sleep, cognition and eye contact (73). The formulas in both studies contained 29 nutrients and participants were monitored for 3 months. Next, the researchers conducted an effectiveness trial comparing micronutrients combined with a variety of other therapies (including essential fatty acids, Epsom salts, digestive enzymes, carnitine and a gluten-free/dairy-free diet) versus no treatment over 1 year. There was significant benefit in those who received the comprehensive treatment approach, including improvements in non-verbal IQ, symptoms of ASD, social responsiveness, sensory profile and aberrant behaviour (74).

A case-control study (75) systematically followed 44 children and adults with ASD (age range 2–28 years) taking BSMS, some for up to 2 years. These individuals were later matched by age, gender and symptom severity to 44 children and adults from the same clinic whose families had chosen conventional medications to treat ASD symptoms. The clinician was blinded to the treatment the participant received. Measures of parent- and teacher-rated irritability and hyperactivity showed significant benefit for the micronutrient group over the medication group, with medium between-group effect sizes. In addition, clinician ratings of self-injurious behaviour intensity were lower post-treatment, with no change in the medication group. The decreased intensity of self-injurious behaviour in the micronutrient group was unexpected and warrants further clinical studies, as these behaviours are among the most disturbing for families.

Mood Disorders

Numerous studies, including clinical observations and open-label trials of BSMS (64, 76–78), as well as case studies (79) and database analyses in adults (80) and children (26) with bipolar disorder, show significant improvement in mental health symptoms along with a reduction in the amount of medication required to maintain symptom control for most of the participants.

Two challenges exist in understanding the possible benefit of supplements for symptoms of depression. The first is that in many studies, participants did not exhibit significant depression at baseline. Not surprisingly, those participants showed little benefit from supplementation, which could be a floor effect because there was little room for improvement (81).

The second challenge is that most of the studies conducted on depression have used only a few selected nutrients rather than the broad spectrum of vitamins and minerals needed for optimal brain functioning. The findings on selected nutrients are mixed: some show benefit but most studies show the nutrients to be no better than placebo (82–84).

Premenstrual Syndrome (PMS)

PMS regularly affects 20–30% of all women, and 1.2–6.4% will experience an even more severe form known as premenstrual dysphoric disorder (PMDD). PMDD includes symptoms of severe depression, mood swings and anxiety. Studies as far back as the 1980s demonstrate the benefit of giving additional nutrients to treat PMS symptoms, with trials reporting a 50% reduction of PMS complaints in the first 1–3 months of taking the micronutrients (85, 86).

A more recent study confirmed the benefit of both B_6 alone and BSMS. B_6 was chosen given its documented benefits for treating PMS (87). A blinded RCT demonstrated efficacy for both approaches: 72% of the BSMS group and 60% of the vitamin B_6 group were in remission for PMS symptoms after three cycles (88). In addition, the women who took BSMS during this study showed a greater improvement than the B_6 group in health-related quality of life.

Psychosis

Other than two case studies, one in a child and one in an adult successfully treated with BSMS (89, 90), the only research that has been conducted specifically on micronutrients and psychosis involved 19 patients who gradually reduced their medications as they added BSMS (27). The study started as an RCT with a 1-month open-label lead-in when everyone received the nutrients. At the end of the month, when the participants were due to be randomised with a 50% chance of receiving a placebo, none were willing to risk being in the placebo group. All stated they were feeling better taking nutrients. The researchers were forced to change their study design and monitor these participants over 2 years instead, comparing their progress to 31 patients who had chosen not to be in the trial.

At 15 months, the group taking micronutrients and gradually reducing their doses of medication showed significantly fewer psychosis symptoms than the medication-only group. This difference was even stronger at the 2-year mark (27). When participants took the micronutrients, and required smaller doses of their medication to be effective, they experienced fewer medication side effects.

Substance Use and Addiction

The link between smoking and nutrition was first observed in 1956 by Roger Williams. He reported a 50% success rate in reversing alcohol substance abuse by improving participants' nutrient intake, and from this work he speculated that much of the dependence on addictive substances was due to nutrient insufficiency. Preliminary studies in the 1980s also showed the potential of micronutrients to enable people to overcome various forms of addiction, including to alcohol and cocaine (91). In 2018, the first known RCT was published investigating the impact of BSMS to reduce or stop using cigarettes altogether (92). One hundred and seven smokers were randomised to take either the nutrients or a placebo, and all participants received assistance from Quit New Zealand, also known as Quitline, which offers online support and ideas on how to distract, delay and decrease cigarette consumption. Based on the participants who received the full intervention (pills + Quitline), regardless of whether they completed the study, 42% of the micronutrient group achieved full abstinence for 12 weeks versus 23% of the placebo group. The micronutrients were comparable to or better than other smoking cessation treatments, but with far fewer side effects. This quit rate was higher than that observed with smoking cessation medication such as Varenicline (12-week quit rate: 22%), as well as Nicotine Replacement Therapy + Quitline (12-week quit rate: 26%). Further, participants taking the active nutrient formula smoked fewer cigarettes during the quit-attempt phase and up to 4 weeks post-quitting. Because of the high dropout rate (58%), generalisability is limited.

Supplementation during Pregnancy

A few studies have focussed on the prevention of postnatal depression using nutritional supplements. One study showed that a broad-spectrum multivitamin and mineral supplement taken during the preconception period decreased symptoms of depression for women with evidence of prenatal mood problems (93).

However, very few studies have investigated micronutrients for the treatment of anxiety and depression *during* pregnancy. Research that followed the infants of mothers who used multivitamins of any type during pregnancy found that nutrient use was associated with a reduced risk of autism at 3 years and ADHD at 7 years (94, 95), highlighting that additional nutrients during pregnancy may reduce the risk of the development of psychiatric disorder in those infants. Further studies are underway (96).

Safety and Lack of Toxicity of Broad-Spectrum Micronutrients

To date, no serious adverse effects have been attributed to BSMS. Several of the studies have collected safety data from blood tests, heart rate monitoring and blood pressure before and after exposure to the nutrients, typically over 2 or 3 months, some over several years. In all of these studies, amounting to several hundred blood tests before and after micronutrient use, no evidence of clinically meaningful short- or long-term harm has emerged (52, 53, 74, 97, 98).

The most commonly reported side effects have been mild and transitory (headaches, stomach aches) and can be avoided by taking capsules on a full stomach and with plenty of water. A minority of study participants reported feeling more agitated; lowering the dose tended to reduce the agitation for many. In all of the RCTs, these minor side effects have occurred equally in both the micronutrient and placebo groups (52, 53).

It is important to note these safety results are based mostly on studies conducted with participants who are *not concurrently taking psychiatric medications*. Taking the nutrients with medication needs to be monitored carefully by the prescriber and doses often need to be adjusted – see the next section for details.

Another safety consideration is that study participants report fewer adverse effects from micronutrients relative to medications. For instance, in the study comparing nutrients to medications for the treatment of autism-related symptoms, the 44 people with autism who were taking prescription medications experienced 6.5 times as many adverse events as the 44 people with autism taking micronutrients alone (75).

Alongside safety issues, clinicians often wonder about whether the nutrient interventions are only useful to people who have an identified deficiency in a particular nutrient, such as vitamin D or zinc. A number of studies have revealed that a baseline deficiency, as indicated by blood nutrient levels, was not useful for predicting who would benefit clinically from supplementation. Two of the ADHD RCTs reported that a few nutrients modestly predicted outcome (100, 101), but the three main findings were: (1) the vast majority of the baseline nutrient levels fell in the normal range across both studies (72% of the samples had nutrient levels in the 'normal' range) and pre-treatment nutrient levels were not associated with ADHD symptom severity; (2) nutrient levels before treatment did not reliably predict who would respond to the treatment, meaning that people who had 'normal'-range nutrient levels had a similar response rate to those who had 'abnormal' nutrient levels; and (3) change in a nutrient biomarker did not correlate with symptom improvement (102). Other researchers have also found that serum levels of specific micronutrients (e.g. vitamin D, folate and B12) are poor predictors of response to nutrient interventions for people with mood and psychotic disorders (103). The term 'nutrient deficiency' may be misleading as it suggests that individuals are deficient relative to the average population. If an individual's nutritional needs are higher than the average population, then nutrient levels will not assist in identifying who is deficient relative to their own individual metabolic needs. Therefore, based on the current published evidence, nutrient testing is not a prerequisite in considering the possible benefit of nutrient supplementation.

Clinical Application

The majority of the evidence in children and adults described in this chapter comes from two formulas developed in Canada (EMPowerplus™ and Daily Essential Nutrients™); the research for these two formulas has been conducted by independent researchers who did not receive any funding from the manufacturers. The manufacturers do provide the active and placebo capsules for scientific research. Cited in the references are most of the 40 peer-reviewed publications on these two formulas. In addition, there are combinations of nutrients that have been studied for aggression in Europe (various brands) and for autism in the USA (ANRC Essentials Plus™), which have also been tested in controlled trials.

It is noteworthy that the typical over-the-counter vitamin/mineral formulas for children, of which 22 were examined in a New Zealand study, contain only small doses of the micronutrients compared to the amounts in the formulas for which research has shown mental health benefit (104). A systematic review and meta-analysis of micronutrients for psychiatric conditions also highlighted the limited ingredient range and low dosage of many studied formulas (54). Typically, the cost of micronutrients is paid by the family, and if prescribed by a physician, a health-care savings account can be used to purchase them. Funding for micronutrient supplements is currently an issue that could be resolved if insurance companies and the public health-care system covered the cost. Research from two case studies demonstrated that BSMS treatment cost less than 10% of conventional inpatient care (89, 90).

For psychiatrists, general physicians or other prescribing clinicians, the growing research on the use of BSMS for mental health provides a foundation for educating patients and families about the importance of nutrition in brain and behavioural health. Historically, information about nutritional approaches to mental health and studies on nutrient supplementation have not been included in medical or other clinician education or training curricula; hence, the expanding research in the field provides significant challenges (in addition to opportunities) in clinical practice. The following general clinical considerations are offered as an introduction, with recommendations for further training and education for practising clinicians.

For patients with ADHD who are not already on psychotropic medications, who prefer to begin with a nutritional (non-medication) approach to their treatment, and for whom the cost is not prohibitive ($50–100 per month currently, depending on dose and formulation), it is reasonable to explore the option of a BSMS trial. As part of the informed consent process, it is important to provide education about the pros and cons of a nutritional approach and the use of BSMS. It must be acknowledged that large long-term studies do not yet exist on BSMS, and that nutritional supplements, unlike medications, are not subject to the Federal Drug Administration (FDA) approval processes. The clinician can inform the patient or family that the current data on BSMS shows a good safety profile and studies have demonstrated improvements with ADHD symptoms, particularly irritability, explosive rage and emotion dysregulation. Patients need to be made aware that although broad-spectrum micronutrients are not medications, they can have profound effects on the body (and mind) and require close monitoring and communication with the patient's physician or other prescribing clinician. BSMS can have positive (or rarely, negative) effects on sleep, energy, mood and bowel movements; for example, if taken late in the evening, the B vitamins in the BSMS can contribute to insomnia, or those with pre-existing gastrointestinal issues can see a worsening, likely secondary to difficulty with absorbing and metabolising the micronutrients.

Although BSMS has a good safety profile in clinical trials with medication-free participants, there have been repeated clinical observations that BSMS potentiates (or amplifies) the effect of psychotropic medications. Therefore, once BSMS is added at therapeutic levels, the patient may begin to experience medication side effects that were not present on the same dose of medication prior to initiation of BSMS. The mechanism of action for potentiation is not fully known; however, with increased availability of vitamins and minerals which serve as cofactors, there may be more efficient synthesis of neurotransmitters. Secondly, some vitamins and minerals act as inhibitors of the cytochrome enzymes involved in drug metabolism, thereby effectively increasing their level in the body. To address potentiation, it is recommended that medication dosage be decreased in small increments while the BSMS is titrated up to full dose. This is a delicate balance, as too large a decrease of psychotropic medications can cause withdrawal symptoms. It is strongly recommended that clinicians wishing to use BSMS for patients taking psychotropic medication (including non-psychiatric medication that has psychotropic effects such as thyroid medication and glucocorticoids) seek additional training on how to cross-titrate BSMS and medications. During the cross-titration process, ongoing communication between patient and clinician about improvements and/or side effects is essential for optimal treatment outcomes. Given the risk for potentiation and the need for a medical review prior to initiation of BSMS, it is strongly recommended that non-prescribing clinicians who believe that BSMS may be appropriate for a patient ask their patient to discuss their interest with their physician/prescribing clinician prior to initiation.

BSMS can also be used for patients who are seeking to lower their dose of medications and for those who have experienced an inadequate response to psychopharmacological treatment and want augmentation or alternative approaches to address residual symptoms. In these cases, peer supervision and additional training of the prescribing clinician is paramount. From clinical experience, with training and mindful titration of BSMS, many patients can experience symptom improvements, reduced side effects and an overall sense of enhanced health on lower doses of medications such as stimulants, antidepressants, anti-anxiety agents, antipsychotics and mood stabilisers (75). Additionally, those experiencing inadequate response to BSMS alone can receive augmentation with psychotropic medications, introduced at low doses and titrated slowly. Additional clinical scientists, research investment and clinical studies are needed to address the nuances of indications, optimal dosing, titration and potentiation.

Time to response may be within days to weeks, depending on the unique patient. From clinical experience, for those not on medications who need to be cross-tapered, mood regulation improvement is often seen within 2 weeks of initiating BSMS. Given most of the clinical trials were around 8–10 weeks in duration, it is reasonable for clinicians to conduct a 3-month trial before concluding that a patient is unresponsive to BSMS intervention. Research indicates that best outcomes emerge in those who stay on the BSMS for at least 1 year (55, 56).

For strict and relative contraindications, see Table 9.1. Prostate cancer is considered a strict contraindication as a prospective study found that using above the recommended doses of three commercial multivitamins was associated with an increased rate of prostate cancer spread (105), though not in the incidence of *de novo* cancer. The implications of this finding for other cancers are not known.

Both EMPowerplus™ and Daily Essential Nutrients™ have recommended dosages and titration schedules created by the manufacturers, which can be obtained by contacting them directly. Dosage is 4–12 capsules per day depending on the selected formula, the patient's age and the symptoms being targeted. For example, the dosage of Daily Essential Nutrients™ used in the Micronutrients for ADHD in Youth (MADDY) trial (57) of paediatric ADHD was the following: for ages 6–8, participants were titrated up to three

Table 9.1 Contraindications for using broad-spectrum micronutrients

Strict contraindications for the use of BSMS	Relative contraindications for the use of BSMS
Wilson disease (risk for copper overload)	Inability to reduce recreational drug use, including high caffeine or nicotine intake, alcohol use (concern for potentiation)
Hemochromatosis and hemosiderosis (risk for iron overload)	Legally or medically required treatment with central nervous system active agents at fixed dosages (concern for potentiation)
Phenylketonuria (EMPowerplus™ contains phenylalanine, but Daily Essential Nutrients™ does not)	Severe hyperlipidaemia or severe protein malnutrition (concern for increased susceptibility to vitamin A toxicity)
Trimethylaminuria (risk for choline overload)	Liver or renal disease, especially alcohol-related (theoretical)
Prostate cancer (theoretical)	Confirmed malignant cancer of any type (theoretical)
	Epilepsy (concern for potentiation of anti-seizure medications)

capsules three times a day by day 5. Participants were able to decrease to six capsules per day if there were side effects. Participants aged 9 and above had the same titration schedule, but at week 4 they had the option to increase to four capsules three times a day if they did not have any side effects and there was insufficient improvement. Of note, the participants were not on any psychotropic medications during the MADDY trial. In the adult trials using Daily Essential Nutrients™, participants were titrated up to 12 capsules per day in three divided doses over the course of 1 week (106). For the stress studies, four to eight pills of EMPowerplus™ were used. For individuals who are unable to tolerate capsules, a powdered formulation is also available that can be made into a smoothie. Additionally, capsules can be opened and poured into apple sauce/yogurt; however, some children do not tolerate the taste.

There are no official treatment guidelines for baseline blood work to be done prior to initiation and/or later as follow-up testing. Out of caution, some clinicians may choose to do baseline screening, which may include a complete blood count, comprehensive metabolic profile, and calcium, phosphate, magnesium, copper and ceruloplasmin, vitamin B12, 25-OH vitamin D, folate, and iron studies. In the absence of large studies of long-term use, it may be prudent to do occasional follow-up laboratory testing. There is no current evidence to suggest these two formulas cause any significant adverse events (see previous section on safety). Since BSMS does not contain omega-3s or significant amounts of iron and vitamin D, these may need to be added separately in cases of individual deficiencies. For an expanded review of BSMS in clinical practice, please see chapter 6 of *Complementary and Integrative Treatments in Psychiatric Practice* (99).

Conclusions

Research evidence underscores the importance of eating a healthy diet for achieving and maintaining optimal mental health, and given the robust evidence across multiple different research methodologies, including observational, prospective and randomised controlled trials and meta-analyses, clinicians have a responsibility to talk to their clients about this connection. For some clients, eating a whole-foods diet may not be sufficient to optimise their brain health. This chapter provided the rationale for why it may be necessary for some individuals struggling with mental health issues to consider supplementary nutrients. Considerations include both individual and environmental factors, such as chronic stress, medication use, gut health, individual biochemistry and consuming nutrient-depleted food. All of these factors argue for a broad spectrum of nutrients to be consumed in order to address personal deficiencies and metabolic needs or environmentally induced nutrient depletions.

The evidence base for treating psychological problems with supplementary nutrients highlighted the potential effectiveness of a broad spectrum of micronutrients for ADHD, autism, aggression, stress, anxiety, mood disorders and psychosis. The breadth and consistency of the research show the importance of receiving a good foundation of nutrients for supporting psychiatric problems. Documented safety and lack of toxicity provide reassurance that this treatment approach does not result in serious adverse events or substantial or continuing side effects.

In any discussion of nutrient supplementation, it is essential that supplements are not viewed as a substitute for a healthy diet. Given this field is rapidly expanding, with studies underway to further investigate mechanisms of action, others replicating and adding greater methodological rigour to the published studies, and further RCTs exploring the efficacy of micronutrients in the treatment of a variety of disorders, clinicians will have a wealth of data available to inform their work. This review provides foundational knowledge, as well as resources for further exploration for clinicians motivated to educate themselves about the field of nutrition and mental health.

References

1. O'Neil, A., Quirk, S. E., Housden. S., et al., 2014. Relationship between diet and mental health in children and adolescents: a systematic review. *American Journal of Public Health, 104*(10), pp. e31–42.

2. Firth, J., Marx, W., Dash, S., et al., 2019. The effects of dietary improvement on symptoms of depression and anxiety: a meta-analysis of randomized controlled trials. *Psychosomatic Medicine, 81*(3), pp. 265–80.

3. Rios-Hernandez, A., Alda, J. A., Farran-Codina, A., Ferreira-Garcia, E. and Izquierdo-Pulido, M., 2017. The Mediterranean diet and ADHD in children and adolescents. *Pediatrics, 139*(2).

4. Sanchez-Villegas, A., Delgado-Rodriguez, M., Alonso, A., et al., 2009. Association of the Mediterranean dietary pattern with the incidence of depression: the Seguimiento Universidad de Navarra/University of Navarra follow-up (SUN) cohort. *Archives of General Psychiatry, 66*(10), pp. 1090–8.

5. Francis, H. M., Stevenson, R. J., Chambers, J. R., et al., 2019. A brief diet intervention can reduce symptoms of depression in young adults: a randomised controlled trial. *PLoS One, 14*(10), p. e0222768.

6. Jacka, F. N., Kremer, P. J., Berk, M., et al., 2011. A prospective study of diet quality and mental health in adolescents. *PLoS One, 6*(9), p. e24805.

7. Jacka, F. N., O'Neil, A., Opie, R., et al., 2017. A randomised controlled trial of dietary improvement for adults with major depression (the 'SMILES' trial). *BMC Medicine, 15*(1), p. 23.

8. Li, Y., Lv, M. R., Wei, Y. J., et al., 2017. Dietary patterns and depression risk: a meta-analysis. *Psychiatry Research, 253*, pp. 373–82.

9. Parletta, N., Zarnowiecki, D., Cho, J., et al., 2019. A Mediterranean-style dietary intervention supplemented with fish oil improves diet quality and mental health in people with depression: a randomized controlled trial (HELFIMED). *Nutritional Neuroscience, 22*(7), pp. 474–87.

10. Nanri, A., Mizoue, T., Poudel-Tandukar, K., et al., 2013. Dietary patterns and suicide in Japanese adults: the Japan Public Health Center-based Prospective Study. *British Journal of Psychiatry, 203*(6), pp. 422–7.

11. Opie, R. S., O'Neil, A., Itsiopoulos, C. and Jacka, F. N., 2015. The impact of whole-of-diet interventions on depression and anxiety: a systematic review of randomised controlled trials. *Public Health Nutrition, 18*(11), pp. 2074–93.

12. Bayes, J., Schloss, J. and Sibbritt, D., 2022. The effect of a Mediterranean diet on the symptoms of depression in young males (the 'AMMEND' study): a randomized control trial. *The American Journal of Clinical Nutrition, 116*(2), pp. 572–80.

13. Davis, D. R., Epp, M. D. and Riordan, H. D., 2004. Changes in USDA food composition data for 43 garden crops, 1950 to 1999. *Journal of the American Nutrition Association, 23*(6), pp. 669–82.

14. Marles, R. J., 2017. Mineral nutrient composition of vegetables, fruits and grains: the context of reports of apparent historical declines. *Journal of Food Composition and Analysis, 56*, pp. 93–103.

15. Datnoff, L. E., Elmer, W. H. and Huber, D. M. (eds.), 2007. *Mineral nutrition and plant disease*. American Phytopathological Society.

16. Montgomery, D. R., Biklé, A., Archuleta, R., Brown, P. and Jordan, J., 2022. Soil health and nutrient density: preliminary comparison of regenerative

and conventional farming. *PeerJ, 10,* p. e12848.

17. Zhu, C., Kobayashi, K., Loladze, I., et al., 2018. Carbon dioxide (CO2) levels this century will alter the protein, micronutrients, and vitamin content of rice grains with potential health consequences for the poorest rice-dependent countries. *Science Advances, 4*(5), p. eaaq1012.

18. Hogy, P., Wieser, H., Kohler, P., et al., 2009. Effects of elevated CO2 on grain yield and quality of wheat: results from a 3-year free-air CO2 enrichment experiment. *Plant Biology (Stuttgart), 11*(suppl. 1), pp. 60–9.

19. Martinez, A. and Al-Ahmad, A. J., 2019. Effects of glyphosate and aminomethylphosphonic acid on an isogeneic model of the human blood-brain barrier. *Toxicology Letters, 304,* pp. 39–49.

20. Zobiole, L. H., Oliveira, R. S., Visentainer, J. V., et al., 2010. Glyphosate affects seed composition in glyphosate-resistant soybean. *Journal of Agricultural and Food Chemistry, 58*(7), pp. 4517–22.

21. Kanissery, R., Gairhe, B., Kadyampakeni, D., Batuman, O. and Alferez, F., 2019. Glyphosate: its environmental persistence and impact on crop health and nutrition. *Plants (Basel, Switzerland), 8*(11), p. 499.

22. Ames, B. N., Elson-Schwab, I. and Silver, E. A., 2002. High-dose vitamin therapy stimulates variant enzymes with decreased coenzyme binding affinity (increased K(m)): relevance to genetic disease and polymorphisms. *The American Journal of Clinical Nutrition, 75*(4), pp. 616–58.

23. Pauling, L., 1968. Orthomolecular psychiatry. *Science, 160,* pp. 265–71.

24. Kaplan, B. J. and Shannon, S., 2007. Nutritional aspects of child and adolescent psychopharmacology. *Pediatric Annals, 36* (9), pp. 600–9.

25. Mohn, E. S., Kern, H. J., Saltzman, E., Mitmesser, S. H. and McKay, D. L., 2018. Evidence of drug-nutrient interactions with chronic use of commonly prescribed medications: an update. *Pharmaceutics, 10*(1).

26. Rucklidge, J. J., Gately, D. and Kaplan, B. J., 2010. Database analysis of children and adolescents with bipolar disorder consuming a micronutrient formula. *BMC Psychiatry, 10*(1), p. 74.

27. Mehl-Madrona, L. and Mainguy, B., 2017. Adjunctive treatment of psychotic disorders with micronutrients. *Journal of Alternative and Complementary Medicine, 23*(7), pp. 526–33.

28. Phillips, J. G. P., 1910. The treatment of melancholia by the lactic acid bacillus. *British Journal of Psychiatry, 56*(234).

29. Cenit, M. C., Sanz, Y. and Codoner-Franch, P., 2017. Influence of gut microbiota on neuropsychiatric disorders. *World Journal of Gastroenterology, 23*(30), pp. 5486–98.

30. Mathee, K., Cickovski, T., Deoraj, A., Stollstorff, M. and Narasimhan, G., 2020. The gut microbiome and neuropsychiatric disorders: implications for attention deficit hyperactivity disorder (ADHD). *Journal of Medical Microbiology, 69*(1), pp. 14–24.

31. Mitrea, L., Nemeş, S.-A., Szabo, K., Teleky, B.-E. and Vodnar, D.-C., 2022. Guts imbalance imbalances the brain: a review of gut microbiota association with neurological and psychiatric disorders. *Frontiers in Medicine, 9,* p. 813204.

32. Szopinska-Tokov, J., Dam, S., Naaijen, J., et al., 2020. Investigating the gut microbiota composition of individuals with attention-deficit/hyperactivity disorder and association with symptoms. *Microorganisms, 8*(3).

33. Berding, K. and Cryan, J. F., 2022. Microbiota-targeted interventions for mental health. *Current Opinion in Psychiatry, 35*(1), pp. 3–9.

34. Cryan, J. F., O'Riordan, K. J., Cowan, C. S. M., et al., 2019. The microbiota-gut-brain axis. *Physiological Reviews, 99*(4), pp. 1877–2013.

35. Borkent, J., Ioannou, M., Laman, J. D., Haarman, B. C. M. and Sommer, I. E. C., 2022. Role of the gut microbiome in three

major psychiatric disorders. *Psychological Medicine*, 52(7), pp. 1–21.

36. Bastiaanssen, T. F. S., Cowan, C. S. M., Claesson, M. J., Dinan, T. G. and Cryan, J. F., 2019. Making sense of . . . the microbiome in psychiatry. *The International Journal of Neuropsychopharmacology*, 22(1), pp. 37–52.

37. Robertson, R. C., Seira Oriach, C., Murphy, K., et al., 2017. Omega-3 polyunsaturated fatty acids critically regulate behaviour and gut microbiota development in adolescence and adulthood. *Brain, Behavior, and Immunity*, 59, pp. 21–37.

38. Stevens, A. J., Purcell, R. V., Darling, K. A., et al., 2019. Human gut microbiome changes during a 10 week randomised control trial for micronutrient supplementation in children with attention deficit hyperactivity disorder. *Scientific Reports*, 9(1), p. 10128.

39. Benton, D., Griffiths, R. and Haller, J., 1997. Thiamine supplementation mood and cognitive functioning. *Psychopharmacology (Berlin)*, 129(1), pp. 66–71.

40. Benton, D. and Cook, R., 1991. The impact of selenium supplementation on mood. *Biological Psychiatry*, 29(11), pp. 1092–8.

41. Thys-Jacobs, S., Starkey, P., Bernstein, D. and Tian, J., 1998. Calcium carbonate and the premenstrual syndrome: effects on premenstrual and menstrual symptoms. Premenstrual Syndrome Study Group. *American Journal of Obstetrics and Gynecology*, 179(2), pp. 444–52.

42. Kaplan, B. J., Crawford, S. G., Field, C. J. and Simpson, J. S., 2007. Vitamins, minerals, and mood. *Psychological Bulletin*, 133(5), pp. 747–60.

43. Sarris, J., Mischoulon, D. and Schweitzer, I., 2011. Adjunctive nutraceuticals with standard pharmacotherapies in bipolar disorder: a systematic review of clinical trials. *Bipolar Disorders*, 13(5–6), pp. 454–65.

44. Firth, J., Stubbs, B., Sarris, J., et al., 2017. The effects of vitamin and mineral supplementation on symptoms of schizophrenia: a systematic review and meta-analysis. *Psychological Medicine*, 47(9), pp. 1515–27.

45. Rucklidge, J. J., Johnstone, J. and Kaplan, B. J., 2009. Nutrient supplementation approaches in the treatment of ADHD. *Expert Review of Neurotherapeutics*, 9(4), pp. 461–76.

46. Benton, D., 2007. The impact of diet on anti-social, violent and criminal behaviour. *Neuroscience & Biobehavioral Reviews, 31* (5), pp. 752–74.

47. Firth, J., Teasdale, S. B., Allott, K., et al., 2019. The efficacy and safety of nutrient supplements in the treatment of mental disorders: a meta-review of meta-analyses of randomized controlled trials. *World Psychiatry*, 18(3), pp. 308–24.

48. Heilskov Rytter, M. J., Andersen, L. B., Houmann, T., et al., 2015. Diet in the treatment of ADHD in children: a systematic review of the literature. *Nordic Journal of Psychiatry*, 69(1), pp. 1–18.

49. Gordon, H. A., Rucklidge, J. J., Blampied, N. M. and Johnstone, J. M., 2015.Clinically significant symptom reduction in children with attention-deficit/hyperactivity disorder treated with micronutrients: an open-label reversal design study. *Journal of Child and Adolescent Psychopharmacology*, 25(10), pp. 783–98.

50. Kaplan, B. J., Fisher, J. E., Crawford, S. G., Field, C. J. and Kolb B., 2004. Improved mood and behavior during treatment with a mineral-vitamin supplement: an open-label case series of children. *Journal of Child and Adolescent Psychopharmacology*, 14(1), pp. 115–22.

51. Rucklidge, J. J., Taylor, M. and Whitehead, K., 2011. Effect of micronutrients on behavior and mood in adults with ADHD: evidence from an 8-week open label trial with natural extension. *Journal of Attention Disorders*, 15(1), pp. 79–91.

52. Rucklidge, J. J., Frampton, C. M., Gorman, B. and Boggis, A., 2014. Vitamin-mineral treatment of attention-deficit hyperactivity disorder in adults: double-blind randomised

placebo-controlled trial. *British Journal of Psychiatry*, 204(4), pp. 306–15.

53. Rucklidge, J. J., Eggleston, M. J. F., Johnstone, J. M., Darling, K. and Frampton, C. M., 2018. Vitamin-mineral treatment improves aggression and emotional regulation in children with ADHD: a fully blinded, randomized, placebo-controlled trial. *Journal of Child Psychology and Psychiatry*, 59(3), pp. 232–46.

54. Johnstone, J., Hughes, A., Goldenberg, J. Z., Romijn, A. R. and Rucklidge, J. J., 2020. Multinutrients for the treatment of psychiatric symptoms in clinical samples: a systematic review and meta-analysis of randomized controlled trials. *Nutrients*, 12(11).

55. Rucklidge, J. J., Frampton, C. M., Gorman, B. and Boggis, A., 2017. Vitamin-mineral treatment of ADHD in adults: a 1-year naturalistic follow-up of a randomized controlled trial. *Journal of Attention Disorders*, 21(6), pp. 522–32.

56. Darling, K. A., Eggleston, M. J. F., Retallick-Brown, H. and Rucklidge, J. J., 2019 Mineral-vitamin treatment associated with remission in attention-deficit/ hyperactivity disorder symptoms and related problems: 1-year naturalistic outcomes of a 10-week randomized placebo-controlled trial. *Journal of Child and Adolescent Psychopharmacology*, 29(9), pp. 688–704.

57. Johnstone, J. M., Hatsu, I., Tost, G., et al., 2022. Micronutrients for attention-deficit/ hyperactivity disorder in youths: a placebo-controlled randomized clinical trial. *Journal of the American Academy of Child and Adolescent Psychiatry*, 61(5), pp. 647–61.

58. Gesch, C. B., Hammond, S. M., Hampson, S. E., Eves, A. and Crowder, M. J., 2002. Influence of supplementary vitamins, minerals and essential fatty acids on the antisocial behaviour of young adult prisoners: randomised, placebo-controlled trial. *British Journal of Psychiatry*, 181, pp. 22–8.

59. Schoenthaler, S., Amos, S., Doraz, W., et al., 1997. The effect of randomized vitamin-mineral supplementation on violent and non-violent antisocial behavior among incarcerated juveniles. *Journal of Nutritional and Environmental Medicine*, 7, pp. 343–52.

60. Tammam, J. D., Steinsaltz, D., Bester, D. W., Semb-Andenaes, T. and Stein, J. F., 2016. A randomised double-blind placebo-controlled trial investigating the behavioural effects of vitamin, mineral and n-3 fatty acid supplementation in typically developing adolescent schoolchildren. *British Journal of Nutrition*, 115(2), pp. 361–73.

61. Zaalberg, A., Nijman, H., Bulten, E., Stroosma, L. and van der Staak, C., 2010. Effects of nutritional supplements on aggression, rule-breaking, and psychopathology among young adult prisoners. *Aggressive Behavior*, 36(2), pp. 117–26.

62. Hambly, J. L., Francis, K., Khan, S., et al., 2017. Micronutrient therapy for violent and aggressive male youth: an open-label trial. *Journal of Child and Adolescent Psychopharmacology*, 27(9), pp. 823–32.

63. Schoenthaler, S. and Bier, I., 2000. The effect of vitamin-mineral supplementation on juvenile delinquency among American schoolchildren: a randomized, double-blind placebo-controlled trial. *Journal of Alternative and Complementary Medicine*, 6(1), pp. 7–17.

64. Kaplan, B. J., Hilbert, P. and Tsatsko, E., 2015. Micronutrient treatment for children with emotional and behavioral dysregulation: a case series. *Journal of Medical Case Reports*, 9, p. 240.

65. Schoenthaler, S., Gast, D., Giltay, E. J. and Amos, S., 2021. The effects of vitamin-mineral supplements on serious rule violations in correctional facilities for young adult male inmates: a randomized controlled trial. *Crime & Delinquency*, 69(4), pp. 822–40.

66. Kaplan, B. J. and Leung, B., 2011. Multi-micronutrient supplementation for the treatment of psychiatric symptoms. *Integrative Medicine: A Clinician's Journal*, 10(3).

67. Valzelli, L., 1984. Reflections on experimental and human pathology of

aggression. *Progress in Neuro-Psychopharmacology & Biological Psychiatry*, 8(3), pp. 311–25.

68. McCann, J. C. and Ames, B. N., 2009. Vitamin K, an example of triage theory: is micronutrient inadequacy linked to diseases of aging? *The American Journal of Clinical Nutrition*, 90(4), pp. 889–907.

69. Rucklidge, J. J., Andridge, R., Gorman, B., et al., 2012. Shaken but unstirred? Effects of micronutrients on stress and trauma after an earthquake: RCT evidence comparing formulas and doses. *Human Psychopharmacology*, 27(5), pp. 440–54.

70. Kaplan, B. J., Rucklidge, J., Romijn, A. and Dolph, M., 2015. A randomized trial of nutrient supplements to minimize psychological stress after a natural disaster. *Psychiatry Research*, 228, pp. 373–9.

71. Young, L., Pipingas, A., White, D., Gauci, S. and Scholey, A., 2019. A systematic review and meta-analysis of B vitamin supplementation on depressive symptoms, anxiety, and stress: effects on healthy and 'at-risk' individuals. *Nutrients*, 11(9), p. 2232.

72. Adams, J. B. and Holloway, C., 2004. Pilot study of a moderate dose multivitamin/mineral supplement for children with autism spectrum disorder. *Journal of Alternative and Complementary Medicine*, 10(6), pp. 1033–9.

73. Adams, J. B., Audhya, T., McDonough-Means, S., et al., 2011. Effect of a vitamin/mineral supplement on children and adults with autism. *BMC Pediatrics*, 11, p. 111.

74. Adams, J. B., Audhya, T., Geis, E., et al., 2018. Comprehensive nutritional and dietary intervention for autism spectrum disorder: a randomized, controlled 12-month trial. *Nutrients*, 10(3), p. 369.

75. Mehl-Madrona, L., Leung, B., Kennedy, C., Paul, S. and Kaplan, B. J., 2010. Micronutrients versus standard medication management in autism: a naturalistic case-control study. *Journal of Child and Adolescent Psychopharmacology*, 20(2), pp. 95–103.

76. Kaplan, B. J., Simpson, J. S., Ferre, R. C., et al., 2001. Effective mood stabilization with a chelated mineral supplement: an open-label trial in bipolar disorder. *The Journal of Clinical Psychiatry*, 62(12), pp. 936–44.

77. Popper, C., 2001. Do vitamins or minerals (apart from lithium) have mood-stabilising effects? *The Journal of Clinical Psychiatry*, 62(12), pp. 933–5.

78. Frazier, E. A., Gracious, B., Arnold, L. E., et al., 2013. Nutritional and safety outcomes from an open-label micronutrient intervention for pediatric bipolar spectrum disorders. *Journal of Child and Adolescent Psychopharmacology*, 23(8), pp. 558–67.

79. Kaplan, B. J., Crawford, S. G., Gardner, B. and Farrelly, G., 2002. Treatment of mood lability and explosive rage with minerals and vitamins: two case studies in children. *Journal of Child and Adolescent Psychopharmacology*, 12(3), pp. 205–19.

80. Gately, D. and Kaplan, B., 2009. Database analysis of adults with bipolar disorder consuming a multinutrient formula. *Clinical Medicine: Psychiatry*, 4, pp. 3–16.

81. Blampied, M., Bell, C., Gilbert, C. and Rucklidge, J. J., 2020. Broad spectrum micronutrient formulas for the treatment of symptoms of depression, stress, and/or anxiety: a systematic review. *Expert Review of Neurotherapeutics*, 20(4), pp. 351–71.

82. Bot, M., Brouwer, I., Roca, M., et al., 2019. Effect of multinutrient supplementation and food-related behavioral activation therapy on prevention of major depressive disorder among overweight or obese adults with subsyndromal depressive symptoms: the MooDFOOD randomized clinical trial. *JAMA*, 321(9), pp. 858–68.

83. Sarris, J., Byrne, G., Stough, C., et al., 2019. Nutraceuticals for major depressive disorder – more is not merrier: an 8-week double-blind, randomised, controlled trial. *Journal of Affective Disorders*, 245, pp. 1007–15.

84. Berk, M., Turner, A., Malhi, G., et al., 2019. A randomised controlled trial of a mitochondrial therapeutic target for bipolar depression: mitochondrial agents,

N-acetylcysteine, and placebo. *BMC Medicine*, 17(1), p. 18.

85. London, R., Bradley, L. and Chiamori, N., 1991. Effect of a nutritional supplement on premenstrual symptomatology in women with premenstrual syndrome: a double-blind longitudinal study. *Journal of the American Nutrition Association*, 10(5), pp. 494–9.

86. Chakmakjian, Z., Higgins, C. E. and Abraham, G. E., 1985. The effect of a nutritional supplement, Optivite for women, on premenstrual tension syndromes. II. Effect on symptomatology, using a double blind cross-over design. *The Journal of Applied Nutrition*, 37(1), pp. 12–7.

87. Wyatt, K., Dimmock, P., Jones, P. and O'Brien, S., 1999. Efficacy of vitamin B-6 in the treatment of premenstrual syndrome: systematic review. *The BMJ*, 318(7195), pp. 1375–81.

88. Retallick-Brown, H., Blampied, N. and Rucklidge, J., 2020. A pilot randomized treatment-controlled trial comparing vitamin B6 with broad-spectrum micronutrients for premenstrual syndrome. *Journal of Alternative and Complementary Medicine*, 26(2), pp. 88–97.

89. Rodway, M., Vance, A., Watters, A., et al., 2012. Efficacy and cost of micronutrient treatment of childhood psychosis. *BMJ Case Reports*, 10, pp. 1–7.

90. Kaplan, B. J., Isaranuwatchai, W. and Hoch, J. S., 2017. Hospitalization cost of conventional psychiatric care compared to broad-spectrum micronutrient treatment: literature review and case study of adult psychosis. *International Journal of Mental Health Systems*, 11, p. 14.

91. Blum, K., Allison, D., Trachtenberg, M. C., Williams, R. W. and Loeblich, L. A., 1988. Reduction of both drug hunger and withdrawal against advice rate of cocaine abusers in a 30-day inpatient treatment program by the neuronutrient Tropamine. *Current Therapeutic Research*, 43(6), pp. 1204–14.

92. Reihana, P., Blampied, N. and Rucklidge, J., 2018. Novel mineral–vitamin treatment for reduction in cigarette smoking: a fully blinded randomized placebo-controlled trial. *Nicotine & Tobacco Research*, 21(11), pp. 1496–505.

93. Nguyen, P., DiGirolamo, A., Gonzalez-Casanova, I., et al., 2017. Impact of preconceptional micronutrient supplementation on maternal mental health during pregnancy and postpartum: results from a randomized controlled trial in Vietnam. *BMC Women's Health*, 17(1), p. 44.

94. Schmidt, R., Iosif, A.-M., Guerrero Angel, E. and Ozonoff, S., 2019. Association of maternal prenatal vitamin use with risk for autism spectrum disorder recurrence in young siblings. *JAMA Psychiatry*, 76(4), pp. 391–8.

95. Virk, J., Liew, Z., Olsen, J., et al., 2017. Pre-conceptual and prenatal supplementary folic acid and multivitamin intake, behavioral problems, and hyperkinetic disorders: a study based on the Danish National Birth Cohort (DNBC). *Nutritional Neuroscience*, 21(5), pp. 1–9.

96. Bradley, H. A., Campbell, S. A., Mulder, R. T., et al., 2020. Can broad-spectrum multinutrients treat symptoms of antenatal depression and anxiety and improve infant development? Study protocol of a double blind, randomized, controlled trial (the 'NUTRIMUM' trial). *BMC Pregnancy and Childbirth*, 20(1), pp. 1–19.

97. Rucklidge, J. J., Eggleston, M. J. F., Ealam, B., Beaglehole, B. and Mulder, R. T., 2019. An observational preliminary study on the safety of long-term consumption of micronutrients for the treatment of psychiatric symptoms. *Journal of Alternative and Complementary Medicine*, 25(6), pp. 613–22.

98. Simpson, S., Crawford, S., Goldstein, E., et al., 2011. Systematic review of safety and tolerability of a complex micronutrient formula used in mental health. *BMC Psychiatry*, 11, p. 62.

99. Popper, C., Kaplan, B. J. and Rucklidge, J. J., 2017. Single and broad-spectrum micronutrient treatments in psychiatry practice. In P. L. Gerbarg, P. R. Muskin and R. P. Brown (eds.), *Complementary and integrative treatments in psychiatric practice* (pp. 75–104). American Psychiatric Association Publishing.

100. Rucklidge, J. J., Johnstone, J., Gorman, B., Boggis, A. and Frampton, C. M., 2014. Moderators of treatment response in adults with ADHD treated with a vitamin-mineral supplement. *Progress in Neuro-Psychopharmacology & Biological Psychiatry, 50*, pp. 163–71.

101. Rucklidge, J. J., Eggleston, M. J. F., Darling, K. A., et al., 2019. Can we predict treatment response in children with ADHD to a vitamin-mineral supplement? An investigation into pre-treatment nutrient serum levels, MTHFR status, clinical correlates and demographic variables. *Progress in Neuro-Psychopharmacology & Biological Psychiatry, 89*, pp. 181–92.

102. Rucklidge, J. J., Eggleston, M. J. F., Boggis, A., et al., 2019. Do changes in blood nutrient levels mediate treatment response in children and adults with ADHD consuming a vitamin-mineral supplement? *Journal of Attention Disorders, 25*(8), pp. 1107–19.

103. van der Burg, K., Cribb, L., Firth, J., Karmacoska, D. and Sarris, J., 2019. Nutrient and genetic biomarkers of nutraceutical treatment response in mood and psychotic disorders: a systematic review. *Nutritional Neuroscience, 24*(4), pp. 1–17.

104. Rucklidge, J. J., Harris, A. and Shaw, I., 2014. Are the amounts of vitamins in commercially available dietary supplement formulations relevant for the management of psychiatric disorders in children? *The New Zealand Medical Journal, 127* (1392), pp. 73–85.

105. Roswall, N., Larsen, S., Friis, S., et al., 2013. Micronutrient intake and risk of prostate cancer in a cohort of middle-aged, Danish men. *Cancer Causes & Control, 24*, pp. 1129–35.

106. Blampied, M., Bell, C., Gilbert, C., et al., 2018. Study protocol for a randomized double blind, placebo controlled trial exploring the effectiveness of a micronutrient formula in improving symptoms of anxiety and depression. *Medicines, 5*(2), p. 56.

Epigenetics

Lynda Sedley

Summary

Like microorganisms, the human subspecies can be characterised by subtle differences at the genomic and epigenomic levels. The divergence is due to epigenetic adaptations to variations in environmental conditions and dietary staples. It is evident that environments or food choices which may be essential to sustain life in one population may be toxic to another. However, the recognition of evolutionary biodiversity has been largely ignored with universal nutritional standards and fortification of dietary staples with epigenetic modulators. Because of environmental concerns, global consumption of plants as a primary food is rising; epigenetic adaptation of biological pathways and microbiomes is required to adjust for the loss of bioactive molecules previously obtained from animal-based diets. The resulting epigenetic inflexibility may lead to over- or under-compensation of biological pathways and disease.

This chapter discusses the modern interpretation of epigenetics as the complex plasticity of the epigenome and its DNA sequence, demonstrating the potential for modulation of epigenetic pathways through nutritional, microbiome and environmental modifications.

Introduction

In 1942, embryologist Conrad Waddington proposed the name 'epigenotype' to describe the complex developmental processes between genotype and phenotype (1). There have been many perspectives; today, epigenetics refers to the regulation of gene expression without an alteration in the DNA sequence (2). However, this description may also require revision, as the more we learn about the epigenetic modulation of chromatin, the more we discover about the diversity and plasticity of its sequence.

The Epigenome

The epigenome is a highly dynamic histone chromatin complex composed of salt bridges, hydrogen bonds, and hydrophobic and hydrophilic electrostatic interactions between DNA, ribonucleic acid (RNA) and histone proteins (3).

For a long time, we have considered the basic structure of the genome to be composed of four primary nucleotides – guanine (G), thymine (T), adenine (A) and cytosine (C) – which are supported by a phosphate backbone forming a double-helical structure through hydrogen bonding of base pairs (4). Any deviation from this structure was speculated to be mutagenic. We now understand that the genome is far more structurally versatile than previously thought (5). The Watson-Crick model of base pairing describes only one of the many ways nucleotides can pair through hydrogen bonding (6).

Alongside epigenetic modifications, nucleotides contribute to chemical versatility through adopting isomeric forms, known as tautomers (keto $\leftrightharpoons$ enol) (7). Tautomers differ in the position of hydrogen (8). Computerised molecular dynamic (MD) simulations of Grotthuss' mechanism of water (H_2O) molecules have helped to describe how proton (H^+) hopping influences the tautomerisation of nucleic acids (9) and amino acids (10). Rare tautomeric nucleotides are proposed to enhance the structural and functional diversity of RNA (5).

Chromatin

Chromatin is dynamic. The chemical composition of chromatin determines the structural organisation, protein interactions, gene accessibility and expression (11).

Histones

Four positively charged core histones, rich in lysine and arginine, comprise the histone octamer, a heterotetramer of histone H3 and H4 and two dimers of H2A-H2B (12). Histone tails maintain chromatin stability through charge-specific electrostatic inter- actions with each other and DNA (3). All histones except H4 have several variants which are cell- and phase-specific and can be exchanged by histone chaperones or chromatin remodelling complexes (CRC) when required. There are 11 human variations of linker histone (H1), most of which are found within a major cluster on chromosome 6 (13). Histone proteins contain amino acid domains of serine, proline, lysine and lysine (SPKK), which prefer to bind to AT-rich segments of DNA (14). The N terminal tails of all core histones (15) plus an additional C terminal tail for H2A extend out of the surface of the nucleosome, comprising 28% of the core histone mass (16). The majority of histone modifications occur at the N terminal tails; core modifications have also been demonstrated (17) (Figure 10.1).

Nucleosome

A 145–7-bp segment of DNA wraps the cylindrical octamer 1.66 times, forming a nucleosome. Nucleosomes are connected by a segment of linker DNA (18) (Figure 10.1).

H1 contribute to structural support and condensation of nucleosomes by bridging linker DNA (19). H1 are associated with nucleosome repeat length (NRL), which is the average spacing between nucleosomes (13). Half to all nucleosomes contain a H1 (20). Studies in chicken embryos suggest it may be possible for a nucleosome to bind two H1 (21). The nucleosome is composed of 6% more protein than DNA and is responsible for the first level of DNA compaction known as the 10-nm fibre (3) (Figure 10.1).

Studying Nucleosomes

To study nucleosome arrays, Widlund and colleagues extracted murine nucleosome DNA and found TATA elements containing adenosine extensions TATAAA/C form the most stable nucleosomes (22).

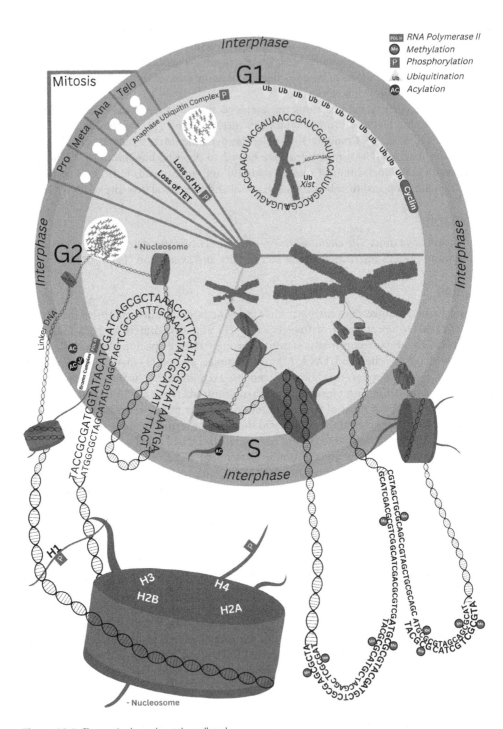

Figure 10.1 Chromatin throughout the cell cycle.
Epigenetic modulation, X chromosome inactivation, expansion and compaction of chromatin throughout the cell cycle. Adapted from 306.

Shortly thereafter, Widom and Lowary (1998) created the AT-rich sequence known as the Widom 601 sequence to study nucleosome positioning arrays. Widom's sequences had slightly fewer TATA elements and more CTA elements. Interestingly, the CTA trinucleotides did not have typical complementary bases (23). This may be due to the sequence being derived from mature chicken erythrocytes which, unlike mammalian erythrocytes, retain their nuclei and the chromosomes remain completely heterochromatic and inactive (24).

The Histone Code

It has been over 30 years since Strahl and Allis proposed the controversial histone code hypothesis, where specific modifications to one or more histones, either sequentially or in combination, provide instruction for other proteins to orchestrate downstream genomic events (25).

Histone Post-Translational Modification

After the histone code proposal there was an explosion of interest in and the discovery of post-translational histone (PTM) modifying elements, including but not limited to methylation, acetylation, phosphorylation, o-glycosylation, ADP ribosylation, ubiquitination, sumoylation, citrullination, succinylation, dopaminylation, serotonylation, nitrosylation, glutathionylation, crotonylation, hydroxylation, propoinylation, butyrylation and carbonylation (26).

A histone-modifying element is a functional group with a unique atomic charge distribution that can attach to a specific amino acid residue of the histone tail (27). Electromagnetic energy transfer via modifications disrupts the established electrostatic interactions, contributing to dynamic structural changes which enable or disable interactions with proteins (27).

Modifications are unique to each cell and cell-phase and are often the product of an enzymatic reaction (28). Communication between histone modifications can occur at the same amino acid residue, on the same tail or between different tails (29). Amino acid residues within histone tails are encoded for simplicity. For example, the addition of a methyl group at histone 3, lysine 9 can be described as H3K9me (30). The proteins responsible for these modifications belong to the epigenetic hierarchy of readers, writers and erasers which are categorised by their binding domains, and often work together, forming large protein complexes (31).

Methylation

Methylation is the enzymatic or non-enzymatic attachment of a single carbon alkyl methyl group to an amino acid, nucleotide or protein (32).

One-Carbon Metabolism

One-carbon metabolism (1 CM) is the primary biological process responsible for the supply and storage of endogenous alkyl (CH_3) units for epigenetic and non-epigenetic purposes (32). CH_3 is transferred to homocysteine in a cobalamin-dependent enzymatic reaction by the enzyme 5-methyltetrahydrofolate-homocysteine methyltransferase (MTR) in the final step of methionine re-synthesis (33). Methionine is then adenylated by ATP forming s-adenosyl-methionine (SAM or AdoMet), the primary adenosyl and CH3 and donor for protein methylation. Methionine adenosyl-transferase genes *MAT1a*, *MAT2a* and *MAT2b* transcribe the subunits of the protein responsible for SAM synthesis and have regulatory and catalytic roles in ATP-dependent adenylation and methylation (34) (Figure 10.2b). MAT enzymes are regulated by a large group of highly specific promoter binding transcription factors (35) and epigenetic marks (36).

CH_3 molecules are added to medicines to provide a steric hindrance and inhibit interactions with neighbouring molecules (37). Fruit, vegetables, antioxidants (38) and cytochrome P450 metabolism of pharmaceuticals (39) contribute to the carbon pool via the production of formaldehyde (40). Our environment contributes to the pool of endogenous CH_3 through ultraviolet oxidation of the atmospheric greenhouse gas methane ($CH_4 = CH_3 + H$) (41). The microbiome plays an essential role in regulating CH_3 availability through the production of CH_3 carriers such as folate (42). Methanogenic archaea play an important role in maintaining homeostasis through the synthesis of methane (43).

Radical SAM

Radical SAM is a SAM-dependent superfamily of proteins found in over 126 species (44). There are currently eight known human radical SAM proteins (45). Radical SAM proteins bind an auxiliary iron-sulphur (4fe-4S) cluster with three sulphur-containing cysteine residues CXXXCXXC (46). The remaining unbound iron from the cluster binds an alpha-amino and alpha-carboxylate group of SAM (46). This structure facilitates the cleavage of a 5'deoxyadenosyl radical via electron transfer from the 4fe-4S cluster to the sulphur atom of SAM and cleavage of the CH_3 radical (47). The 5'deoxyadensyl radical is an extremely powerful single-electron oxidant that can translocate hydrogen from a molecule (48). CH_3 cleavage is reversible and may self-regulate the redox reaction through the atomic spin at the iron centre (49).

DNA polymerase and DNA repair proteins contain 4fe-4S clusters (50). 4fe-4S clusters can replace zinc in proteins containing zinc finger domains (ZFD) or work in conjunction with zinc, suggesting radical methylation may play a much larger role in epigenetic modifications than previously thought (51).

Histone Methylation

Histone methylation is regulated by a specific set of writer enzymes referred to as methyltransferases. Histone methylation can repress (H3K9me) or promote gene expression (H3K4me) depending on which histone amino acid residue is modified (52).

Histone Demethylation

Histone demethylation can occur by three known biological processes. A specific set of eraser enzymes referred to as demethylases enzymatically remove histone methylation marks (52). The jumonji C domain-containing demethylases are regulated by the tricarboxylic acid cycle (TCA) and produce succinate as a by-product from the metabolism of the ketone alpha-ketoglutarate (αKG) (53).

The lysyl oxidase family of enzymes (LOX) deaminate methylated histone lysine residues. The ability to produce multiple transcript isoforms gives LOX a diverse specificity for histone lysine residues (54).

Cathepsin is a protease enzyme that shares sequence homology with the plant enzyme papain. Cathepsin is found in the nucleus and is shown to modify histones through cleavage of the tail. Histone modifications are said to play a role in tail cleavage specificity, but conflicting results suggest more research is needed to determine how histone modifications influence the site of cleavage (55).

Cyclic Biological Processes

The human body is designed to work in perfect harmony with its environment. Epigenetic mechanisms rely on our environment for cues and cyclic biological processes rely on the infinite fluctuation of epigenetic mechanisms to adapt to changing conditions.

Circadian Rhythm

The central circadian rhythm (CR) is driven by fluctuating epigenetic mechanisms, resulting in oscillations of biochemical, physiological and behavioural functions that occur every 24 hours (56). Dysregulation of the CR has been implicated in most psychiatric and metabolic pathologies (57).

Photoreceptors that receive environmental cues for the central sleep/wake circadian pacemaker are found abundantly in the eye. Light-induced cues are absorbed by pigmented photoactive chromophores and converted to intracellular signals in the central pacemaker located in the suprachiasmatic nucleus (56).

Cryptochromes (*CRY*) are a family of mammalian photoreceptors containing a flavin adenine dinucleotide (FAD) and pterin chromophore (56). CRY regulate CR through negative feedback inhibition of *CLOCK* genes (58). *CRY* genes have been associated with depression (59) and sleep regulation (60).

When exposed to light, FAD drives electron transfer from an excited state to its reduced form, resulting in a rearrangement of chemical bonds. The pterin chromophore acts as a light harvester, transferring energy to the catalytic centre of the photoreceptor (61).

Photoreceptors and *CLOCK* genes are found in peripheral tissues and demonstrate cell-specific clocks independent of the central pacemaker. For example, feeding rhythms are synchronised by the CR of the liver (62). CR drives cell division, where key genes responsible for cell division are driven by circadian genes and disruptions to the CR have been implicated in various cancers (63).

Cell Cycle

During the cell cycle, chromatin displays many levels of compaction to allow for the changing conditions of transcription, replication and mitosis (18).

Cells with high turnover rates such as gastrointestinal epithelial cells may go through all phases of the cell cycle within a 24-hour period, whereas other cells may remain in G0–G1 until senescence (64) (Figure 10.1).

Cell Cycle: G2 Phase

10-nm Fibre

G2 is considered the metabolically active phase of the cell cycle. In low-salt in vitro conditions, the 10-nm fibre is euchromatic and resembles beads on a string (65). Longer NRLs are associated with active transcription and allow for greater protein interactions (66).

Promoter regions of euchromatin are generally nucleosome depleted regions (NDR). However, even during G2, approximately one-third of the genome remains heavily condensed (67). AT-rich segments of DNA are associated with transcription (68). TATA box elements are found in high frequency at gene promotors and are a key recognition site for transcription factor (TF) binding (69). In euchromatin, a nucleosome can be found approximately 100–200 bp upstream of a transcription start site (TSS) (–nucleosome) and a second nucleosome can be found immediately downstream (+nucleosome) (66) (Figure 10.1).

Acylation: G2 Phase

The earliest-discovered protein acylation (Ac) was histone lysine acetylation (70). Acetyltransferase enzymes (FAT) have many roles in regulating gene expression and are commonly associated with euchromatin and active gene expression (52). Sometimes histone acetyltransferases are referred to as HATs and lysine acetyltransferases are referred to as KATs (71). Acetylation of H4K16 is one of the most-studied histone modifications which is shown to be essential for maintaining the 10-nm fibre (72).

Acetylation is regulated by compartmental acetyl CoA availability through oxidation of fatty acids and pyruvate (73). Acetyl CoA (4^-) is a high-energy acetylated tetra-anion and pantothenic acid containing adenosine triphosphate ribonucleoside (74). Histone acetyltransferase (HAT) enzymes write the electro-negative acetyl (CH_3CO) moiety from acetyl CoA to a specific positively charged amino group (NH^+1) of lysine at the N terminal, reducing the electro-positivity and contributing to specific structural change (73).

Each additional acylation contributes to greater relaxation of the electromagnetic interactions between the negatively charged DNA backbone and the positively charged histones. Cleavage of the acetyl moiety from acetyl CoA contributes to the pool of high-energy ATP for ATP-dependent CRC or phosphorylation, further contributing to an open state of chromatin (75).

The repertoire of histone acylation has recently expanded with the identification of fatty acids and other acyl-containing metabolic by-products showing histone and non-histone acylation properties (76). Several classes of histone acetyltransferase enzymes, KAT2A, Tip60 and MOF, can utilise the alternative acyl substrates, and their activity depends on the size and electromagnetic charge of the substrate. Histone lysine acetyltransferase KAT23B seems to be highly versatile, whereas KAT2A has a higher affinity for the penta-anion succinyl-CoA (5^-) than for acetyl CoA (4^-) because of its greater electro-negativity (73).

Deacetylation

Histone deacetylase enzymes (HDACs) erase the applied acylations. Humans have 18 known HDACs which have been divided into four classes. Classes I, II and IV require zinc ($Zn2^+$) for catalytic mechanisms (77).

Nicotinamide adenosine dinucleotide (NAD^+) is a redox photocatalyst and cofactor for class III sirtuin HDAC reactions (78). NAD^+ contains two chromophores (79) and its role is to initiate an electron transport chain in a reduction reaction, forming NADH (78). NAD^+ is reduced via the transfer of hydrogen from the cleavage site of acetyl-lysine, ultimately producing free nicotinamide and a 2'-o-acetylated-adenine dinucleotide phosphate ribose (77). However, like acylation, the reaction mechanisms differ depending on the length and electrochemical properties of each acyl substrate (80). Nicotinamide is a known inhibitor of sirtuin (77); however, its inhibition also depends on the rate of deacylation and the substrate chain length (80).

Two classes of sirtuin inhibitors (HDACi) have been defined: those that interact with NAD^+ binding sites and those that interact with acetyl binding sites (77). The microbiome contributes to epigenetic mechanisms through the production of short-chain fatty acid

(SCFA) metabolites (81) such as lactate and butyrate. SCFAs regulate epigenetic mechanisms such as HDAC and acylation (77) through interception at acetyl binding sites (82).

Transcription

Transcriptional activation occurs in three stages: the opening of chromatin structure, the assembly of a preinitiation complex (PIC) and the transition to productive transcription by RNA polymerase II (POL II) (83). Ultimately, Pol II produces a complementary strand of pre-messenger RNA (pre-mRNA) (18). Transcription start sites (TSS) begin at the 5' prime untranslated region (5'UTR) of a gene, usually preceding a methionine start codon (AUG). However, we are beginning to see a growing number of genes using alternative or multiple start codons (84). Dihydrofolate reductase enzyme (DHFR) uses AUG and the alternative ACG, AAG start codons (85).

It was long thought that nucleosomes were inaccessible to protein and rendered inactive. We now understand that pioneer transcription factors (TF) can bind nucleosome DNA and recruit transcription machinery for the activation of transcription. Pioneer TF OCT4 regulates embryonic differentiation by competing with H1 at the linker DNA entrance to the nucleosome (86). However, for transcription to occur, POL II must overcome the tight nucleosomal barrier (87).

Mechanism of Intranucleosome Transcription

When POL II approaches an encountered nucleosome, it partially uncoils the nucleosome from behind, slowly forming a small intranucleosomal loop and pausing to allow for uncoiling (88). This pause and partially uncoiled DNA is said to initiate TF recruitment and mark the position of histone acetylation for greater relaxation of chromatin (89) (Figure 10.1).

Acetylation and Transcription

HATs with co-activating functions are recruited to TSS but are insufficient to promote histone acetylation on their own (89).

Chromatin Remodelling Complexes

CRCs are multi-protein complexes that use energy from ATP hydrolysis to change the position of a nucleosome by sliding, altering or displacing histones. Four primary CRC families have been characterised: SWI/SNF, INO80, ISWI/NURD and CHD (18). Brahma (BRM) and Brahma Related Gene 1 (BRD1) are the human homologous subunits of the yeast SWI/SNF CRC (90). SWI/SNF can remodel nucleosomes without losing a histone or displace an entire histone octamer which can be inserted into a new segment of DNA (18). SWI/SNF subunit variations can be switched during different stages of development to enhance AT binding specificity (91).

Bromodomain Readers

Bromodomain proteins contain an acetyl-lysine binding pocket that can bind acetylated chromatin and other acetylated proteins (18). Both SWI/SNF subunits contain bromodomains and read lysine-acetylated proteins to promote transcription (92). SWI/SNF can recruit many TFs, forming very large complexes that can interact directly with DNA, protein and other modifications, like methylation (93) (Figure 10.1).

Transcription Factors

TFs recruited to the PIC can promote the enhancement, insulation and/or activation of transcription (93). TFs were traditionally classified by their mechanism of action; however, this conception has been questioned because of TFs' ability to recruit multiple cofactors with opposing effects (94). Approximately 1,639 TFs have been catalogued which are regulated by PTM to assist in recruitment, duration of binding and structural diversity (94).

TSS-associated TF and HATs can also contain bromodomains; therefore, while promoting acetylation, they can bind acetylated proteins and be bound by other proteins with bromodomains, ultimately forming large multi-protein acetylated complexes (95) (Figure 10.1).

Compartmentalisation

Liquid–liquid phase separation distinguishes the nucleoplasm from the cytoplasm (96). Multi-bromodomain proteins can induce droplet-like phase separation of acetylated chromatin distinctly different to unmodified chromatin. Chromatin may adopt different phase-separated states to influence the dynamic properties and cell epigenetic requirements (97).

Cell Cycle: Interphase

30-nm Fibre

The second level of DNA compaction is observed in vitro where the coiling of the 10-nm fibre results in a 40-fold reduction in DNA length and a fibre diameter of approximately 30 nm (18). Three early models exist:

- Single-start solenoid (Klug, 1979) (98).
- Two-start helical ribbon (Worcel, 1981) (99) and reproduced by Woodcock in 1984 (100).
- Two-start cross-linked fibre (2SCLF) (Williams, 1986) (101).

In 2014, a replica was produced of the widely accepted 30-nm 2SCLF model using cryo-electron microscopy (EM) which defined the nucleosomes as stacked in a dyad head to head through their octamer surfaces and zig-zagging back and forth, twisting against each other. Three tetranucleosomal units are attached by straight linker DNA (102).

Because of the many variables in laboratory procedures, the structure of the 30-nm fibre has been the subject of much debate (103). Despite the controversy, the 30-nm fibre is said to exist through interphase and has been associated with both active and restricted transcription (98).

In physiological conditions, DNA and chromatin spontaneously flow like a wave, fluctuating in conformations as though breathing. DNA breathing is modulated in vitro with modification of salt concentrations or temperature (104). Observing chromatin's true form has been difficult experimentally. Scientists are turning to MD computational simulations to provide greater insight into the physical properties and dynamic interactions of biological structures (105).

The hydration of DNA plays an important role in the dynamics and function of the epigenome (106). The coupling of DNA to H_2O molecules allows for ultra-fast vibrational energy exchange and molecular communication (107). The most recent model describes a fluid/liquid-like chromatin which condenses into an irregular polymorphic ensemble, where nucleotides engage in a steady flow of interactions with a wide range of molecules (103).

A recent MD simulation explains why we see model variations in vitro. Constraining the nucleosome DNA to remain unnaturally and permanently attached to the histone core in physiological salt concentrations of 0.15% NaCl directs chromatin into the two-start 30-nm zig-zag structure equivalent to the cryo-EM model. However, when constraints are relaxed comparable to the natural flow of molecular exchange through compartments, the chromatin transforms into the fluid-like structure (103).

Chromosome Territories

Hi-C technology, a method that probes the three-dimensional structures of whole genomes, showed chromosomes are defined to territories within the nucleus during interphase. Chromosomes are shown to segregate spatially to form two genome-wide compartments which can be differentiated by the level of density and the quantification of active genes. The dense DNA regions resemble a globule segregated into fractions that enable easy unfolding of any genomic locus (108). Segments from the territories of the same chromosome or from different chromosomes can form hubs around interchromatin granules, like nuclear speckles which contain nuclear equipment and interact for a common cause, such as splicing or gene repression (109).

Topological Associated Domains

Hi-C technology has allowed us to visualise the early descriptions of looped extrusions from highly condensed chromosomes which we now refer to as topological associated domains (TADs) (110). The spatial organisation of the genome is linked to its biological function through TADs (111). For example, *Lox* gene overlaps with genes associated with tissue repair members of the extracellular matrix (112).

The human genome contains approximately 10,000 TADs which contain sub-domains within these boundaries (113). TADs are defined by distinct histone marks and the loops are anchored to the chromosome axis at the TAD boundary by a CCCTC binding factor insulator protein encompassing cell-specific promoters and enhancers (110).

Cell Cycle: DNA Replication (S Phase)

During replication, chromatin doubles in mass as DNA is replicated for cell division (mitosis). The nucleosome structure is disrupted at the replication fork and the strands of DNA are separated. Replication occurs in three stages: initiation, elongation and termination. Each stage requires a highly organised set of proteins. Once DNA is replicated, nucleosomes are rapidly generated on both the parent and daughter chromosomes (18) (Figure 10.1).

Acetylation

Maintenance of the genome throughout the cell cycle relies on newly synthesised histones and the assembly of new nucleosomes (114). Histones are transcribed during replication and inserted into new nucleosomes as they are synthesised. The H1 transcriptome increases only during replication and falls back to basal levels thereafter (115). Histones are acetylated and the acetyl is removed upon insertion into the nucleosome (18) (Figure 10.1).

Phosphorylation

H1 phosphorylation progresses incrementally during the cell cycle, becomes maximal during the late G2 phase and decreases sharply by the end of the telophase (13) (Figure 10.1). During replication, both phosphorylated and unphosphorylated H1 forms exist. H1 phosphorylation remains maximal on the original chromosome until the citrullination of the H1 arginine residue displaces the phosphorylated histone and decompacts the chromatin for replication (116).

DNA Methylation

Cells deficient in DNA methylation struggle to complete replication (117). DNA methylation is the most widely studied epigenetic modification and may also be one of the least understood. It is the prevailing assumption that DNA methylation occurs only at consecutive C and G dinucleotides joined by a phosphate bond, known as CpG (18).

In 1987, Woodcock and colleagues showed most of the DNA methylation in the human was not CpG and 54.5% DNA methylation in splenic tissue was applied to minor dinucleotides CpA, CpT and CpC (118). In 1970, Hayatsu demonstrated the modification of cytosine carbon 6 with the addition of a sulphur salt (119). Today this method is known as sodium bisulphite sequencing and is used to better understand DNA methylation. Bisulphite sequencing has allowed us to identify functional non-CpG methylation (120) such as CpA, which comprises 25% of all modified C in embryonic stem cells (121), an epigenetic mark which is lost upon differentiation (122).

Clusters of CpG known as islands (CpGi) are found in 60% of gene promoters and are usually found unmethylated but may be methylated in a tissue- or cell-phase-specific manner (123). Unmethylated CpGi provide ideal conditions for binding of Zn-containing proteins for modification by methylation or crosstalk between histone methylation through the binding of TFs which can recruit and establish activating histone methylation modifications such as H3K4 (124). Tissue-specific modifications associated with gene inactivation can occur at CpG island shores and are found approximately 2,000 bases from CpGi (125).

DNA methylation in the body of genes has been compared in the inactive and active X chromosomes. Gene-body methylation promotes gene expression in the active X chromosome and has a direct inverse relationship with the CpGi of the inactive X chromosome (126). Most DNA methylation occurs during embryogenesis and is maintained during replication and differentiation (127).

DNA Methyltransferase

DNA methyltransferases (DNMT) is responsible for the covalent nucleophilic enzymatic transfer of a CH_3 to cytosine from SAM produced by 1 CM. Five human DNMTs have been identified (127). DNMT methylates the carbon 5 of cytosine by flipping the DNA (128), resulting in 5'methylcytosine (5'mC), known as the fifth nucleotide base. DNMT3a, DNMT3b and DNMT1 were first recognised for their roles in establishing and maintaining methylation during replication. DNMT3a and DNMT3b initiate methylation and are known as de novo methyltransferases (129). DNMT1 acts only on hemi-methylated sites during replication to complete the double-stranded DNA methylation for daughter cells and is known as the maintenance methyltransferase (18) (Figure 10.1).

We are only beginning to understand the complex network of interactions responsible for establishing and maintaining DNA methylation. Both forms of DNMT can form large complexes and are recruited to DNA in a wide variety of situations and cell phases and have distinct roles (127).

The CH_3 of 5'mC provides a steric hindrance to proteins and prevents the cysteine–cytosine interactions of zinc-finger-domain-containing ZF proteins (130).

Zinc Finger Domains

The cysteine XX cysteine (CXXC) motif within DNMT and other ZF proteins plays an important role in epigenetic regulation because of its ability to recognise unmodified CpG dinucleotides. Epigenetic ZFD-CXXC proteins can be divided into four classes: those associated with activating H3K4 methylation, DNA methylation, histone demethylation and DNA hydroxymethylation (131).

DNMTs recognise unmethylated cytosine through binding of their conserved sulphur-containing CXXC domains, forming an adduct with the sixth carbon of cytosine (132). The tandem bromodomain within DNMT1 is autoinhibitory and can be positioned on DNA to block de novo methylation and therefore only methylate hemi-methylated CpG (133). Experimental mutation of the CXXC domain in DNMT1 is shown to prevent binding to DNA in the replication fork (134).

Passive and Active Demethylation

To date, no direct enzymatic or radical removal of CH_3 from DNA has been described. DNA demethylation can occur passively during replication in the absence of maintenance DNMT or actively by TET oxidation and base excision repair (BER) (30).

Ten-Eleven Translocase

Ten-eleven translocase (TET) proteins take part in active demethylation and belong to a family of oxygen (O_2), iron and αKG-dependent dioxygenase enzymes (135). TET1 is enriched at gene promoters and its CpG targeting potential is due to its conserved CXXC ZFD which contains 8 cysteine residues and expands over 126 nucleotides with 8 potential interactions with unmethylated cytosines. The ZFD interacts with a euchromatic region in the minor groove of the DNA but, unlike other ZF proteins, TET demonstrates a flexible binding capacity that is unbiased to unmethylated cytosines. TET can shift binding to the next available non-methylated cytosine using a base-flipping mechanism to target the methylated base (136).

TET oxidation takes part in active DNA demethylation through the oxidation of 5'mC and thymine (135), forming 5'hydroxymethylcystosine (5'hmC) (132) and 5'hydroxymethyluluracil (5'hmU), respectively (137). If required, TET can continue to oxidise 5'hmC to 5'formycytosine (5'fC) and 5'formylcarboxycytosine (5'caC) by remaining bound to the DNA and blocking any further interaction with DNMT (138).

It was once thought that 5'hmC, 5'fC and 5'caC were transient and subsequently converted back to an unmodified cytosine by the BER pathway; however, we now understand that this may occur only when required (139).

5'hydroxymethylcytosine

5'hmC is considered the sixth base and is the most abundant of the oxidised bases (136). TET is frequently found at gene promoters, yet these regions tend to be largely depleted of 5'hmC (138). 5'hmC is found in much greater proportions in gene bodies (136).

5'formylcytosine

5'fC may be considered the seventh base. Although rare in mammalian genomes, it is shown to interact with more proteins than 5'mC and 5'hmC (140). Using a more stable isotope than previous studies, 5'fC was described as a stable nucleotide (141). 5'fC binds several key genes in the epigenomic hierarchy, including those associated with embryonic development, CRC and DNA repair (139). Interestingly, the formylated bases tend to cluster in CpG repeats, particularly of CRCs and TFs, and are shown to be directly associated with a unique structure of the DNA double helix through interactions with intramolecular H_2O (140).

5'hydroymethyluracil

5'hmU may be considered the eighth base. The newly discovered base increases genomic flexibility (137) and hydrophobicity and is shown to be essential for structural integrity and nucleotide–protein interactions (142).

Cell Cycle: Mitosis

Human chromatin can further compact 10,000-fold and is essential for advancing the cell cycle through mitosis (18).

TET and Differentiation

Most genes show a decrease of 5'hmC upon induction of differentiation. TET interacts with cell-cycle-dependent CDK1/cyclin B complex in embryonic stem cells, maintaining its stability and preventing differentiation (143). Cells lacking TET and 5'hmC are prone to differentiation (143). SWI/SNF associates with TET (144) to induce changes in CpGi DNA methylation to promote transcription (90). The electro-negative reactive hydroxyl motif produced by oxidation of 5'mC and thymine can be further modified, directly changing the electromagnetic interactions because of a loss of the methylated steric hindrance (143). 5'hmC enrichment is associated with greater RNA expression and therefore TET and 5'hmC are associated with euchromatin (117).

The repeated CH_3 of highly methylated CpGi is like a beacon to repressive TF which are recruited to restrict access by TET proteins and prevent further oxidation of cytosine or thymine. This is required to establish a heterochromatin state and advance the cell to the mitotic phase (138) (Figure 10.1).

Histone Methylation and Heterochromatin

Heterochromatin protein 1 (HP1) is a chromodomain protein that interacts with specific methylated histone residues such as H3K9me3 to promote heterochromatin. Through the recruitment of histone methyltransferase SUV39H1, HP1 can induce the propagation of H3k9me3 across the genome, establishing large heterochromatin domains (145). The binding of HP1 is influenced by alternative histone marks such as phosphorylation of H3Y41 (146). Recently, it was discovered that unphosphorylated HP1 is soluble, but when phosphorylated or bound to DNA, HP1 forms liquid-like droplets and phase separates (147). In line with the modern dynamical descriptions of the genome (106), the HP1 solvent may control molecular entry via sequestration and repulsion of specific molecules, while enabling ultra-fast propagation of heterochromatin across the genome (147).

Cell Cycle: Metaphase

Highly dense metaphase chromosomes are examined and karyotyped by cytogenetic staining or the more recent fluorescent in situ hybridisation (FISH). Lighter bands are gene-rich and contain mostly facultative heterochromatin (148). Dark bands (G) or bright bands (Q) contain AT-rich sequences, <50% CG, are gene-poor, consist mostly of constitutive heterochromatin and non-coding DNA, and are associated with inactivity (149). However, we now understand that even the most constitutively inactive heterochromatin is capable of gene expression (150). Repetitive non-coding DNA which was once considered junk plays a critical regulatory role of coding and non-coding genes (151).

Endogenous Retroviruses and Retrotransposons

Endogenous retroviruses (ERVs) are responsible for the mammalian evolution of the centromere through retro-transposition in the placenta (152). Retrotransposons comprise approximately half of the genome (153). Long interspersed nuclear elements (LINE) L1, L2 and L3 are non-coding RNA (ncRNA) mobile elements which are transcribed using a self-coded reverse transcriptase and preferentially transpose to alternative AT-rich sequences within the genome (154). L1 is responsible for the deposition of alu short interspersed nuclear elements (SINE) (155) and over 8,000 processed pseudogenes (156). Repetitive elements comprise 50% of the genome (153), making at least 40% of the mammalian genome the product of reverse transcription (154). L1 is epigenetically regulated with high complexity. Immobile L1 is 90% methylated and the loss of methylation through modification of 5'mC results in transposition and redeposition into the genome elsewhere. The CpG residues of a site upstream of the L1 promoter bind the TF Yin Yang 1 (YY1), which prevents the loss of 5'mC. Loss of YY1 or DNMT increases transposition (157).

Activation of L1 is essential for differentiation, embryogenesis, neurogenesis and development (158). Increased copy numbers of L1 due to hypomethylation are implicated in metabolic disease, cancer, major depression (159), neurological disease, schizophrenia and bipolar disorder (160).

Non-Coding RNA

Protein-coding genes comprise less than 5% of the genome (153). Pseudogenes influence epigenetic mechanisms and can operate on a coding and non-coding basis (161).

Introns which were once considered excised genomic debris are now known to have highly specific functionality (162). NcRNA broadly defines all RNA which lacks evidence of protein translation capabilities (163). It is estimated that 98% of human transcripts come from ncRNA which are divided into classes based on their size: short (22–3), medium (50–200) and long (>200) (52). NcRNA recognise their target sequences and transfer information in a highly compact, energy-efficient manner, which may have been a crucial step in evolution to address accelerating regulatory requirements (162) (see Table 10.1).

X Chromosome Inactivation

XIST is a lncRNA pseudogene transcribed from the X chromosome to establish X chromosome inactivation (Xi) (171). Commencing with a loss of H3K27 acetylation and a gain of H2AK119 ubiquitination (172), XIST recruits several histone-modifying complexes during the interphase and spreads its RNA from the site of transcription, progressively coating the chromosome and forming a phase-separated Barr body which is isolated and mostly inactive (150) (Figure 10.1).

Many lncRNA are transcribed cis-antisense to other genes (170). XIST and TSIX is an example of a cis-antisense pair (173) where the transcription of TSIX on the antisense strand blocks XIST transcription on the active X chromosome by recruiting DNMT3a for methylation and repression (174). It is estimated that >1,600 genes are capable of antisense transcription (175).

Table 10.1 Non-coding RNA

Transfer RNA (tRNA)	• Adaptors for triplet nucleotide code (AUG) for amino acid translation. • The human genome contains approximately 497 tRNAs (153).
Ribosomal RNA (rRNA)	• Catalyse peptide bonds during translation (153).
Micro RNA (miRNA)	• 22 nucleotide length. • The human genome contains approximately 2,300 miRNAs (163). • 60% of protein-coding genes are targeted by miRNA for post-transcriptional repression (164). • Epi-miRNA is the term used to describe miRNAs that regulate epigenetic mechanisms (165).
Small non-coding RNA (sncRNA)	• Many subclasses. • Range between 20 and 29 nucleotides (166).
Small interfering RNA (siRNA)	• Derived from retrotransposons (167). • Bind miRNA like a primer for removal. • Generate a unique double-stranded siRNA which is transposed back into the genome (168).
Piwi interfering RNA (piRNA)	• 25–33 nucleotides in length. • Largest class of small ncRNA (52). • Found in clusters in retro-transposon remnants (169). • Can be translated in antisense and sense from their promoter (52). • The complex piRNA pathway is a conserved defence RNA silencing system that directs epigenetic mechanisms to protect the genome, particularly germ cells, from transposable elements (169).
Long non-coding RNA (lncRNA)	• Involved in genomic imprinting and gene dose compensation (170).

After the initial X inactivation, all subsequent daughter cells inherit the same inactive X (176). Understanding the patterns of Xi in humans has been difficult because of inbreeding in animal models (177). Approximately 15–20% of genes within the Xi of women escape inactivation. Escape regions lack repressive H3K27me3 and are enriched in active acetylating marks (150).

Ubiquitination

Three key classes of genes control the cell cycle: cyclin, cyclin-dependent kinases and cyclin-dependent kinase inhibitors. Scheduled proteolytic degradation of these proteins by ubiquitin-proteasome system (UPS) is essential in the regulation of the cell cycle. Ubiquitin is a 76-amino acid protein which attaches to a target protein with the involvement of three critical enzymes: ubiquitin-activating enzyme E1, ubiquitin-conjugating enzyme E2 and ubiquitin-ligase E3. UPS anaphase-promoting complex is activated by phosphorylation during mid-mitosis and mediates proteolytic degradation of mitotic cyclins throughout the G1 phase (178) (Figure 10.1).

Genomic Imprinting

Small nucleolar RNA (snoRNA) is transcribed from introns of protein-coding genes and lncRNA. A cluster of snoRNA is contained within an imprinted region of chromosome 15. This imprinted control region (ICR) is responsible for Prader-Willi and Angelman syndromes. The ICR is also responsible for controlling the expression of an essential component of the UPS, E3 ubiquitin-ligase. The ICR is heavily DNA methylated on the maternal chromosome retaining a repressive H3K9me3 mark, whereas the paternal ICR remains unmethylated and the promoters are actively marked with H3K4me. A sense-transcribed E3 ubiquitin-ligase (UBE3a) is transcribed from both chromosomes but is also transcribed as a lncRNA in the antisense direction from the paternal chromosome in neurons (UBE3s). In all other cells, the antisense transcription is incomplete but can transcribe the snoRNA. In neurons, the full lncRNA can provide feedback regulation of UBE3a because of complementary RNA binding (179).

SnoRNAs drive rRNA modification, maturation and editing in the nucleolus (180). SnoRNAs are spliced from introns and are characterised by their highly conserved nucleotide sequences, which are complementary to themselves and their targets, forming RNA duplexes (181). Their complementary sequences allow the formation of hairpin loops, which can direct RNA editing and modification with high specificity (201). SnoRNAs have demonstrated genomic transposition through integration with retrotransposing machinery (200).

SnoRNAs carrying the C/D box domain target RNA for 2'O ribose methylation and H/ACA domains containing snoRNAs interact with phosphouridine transferase dyskerin to establish pseudouridination (181).

When snoRNAs are transcribed antisense to their pre-ribosomal RNA target, concomitant expression allows for immediate hybridisation and regulation through a methylating modification (182). SnoRNAs can also associate directly with a protein, forming sno-ribonucleic proteins (snoRNP), such as the essential methyltransferase fibrillarin (183).

RNA Editing and Alternative Splicing

Alternative splicing (AS) has emerged as a key regulator of gene expression. AS uses deamination to alter exons, influencing the structure, binding properties and modification potential of mRNA and its encoded proteins. An analysis of individual chromosomes shows every protein-coding gene is capable of undergoing AS (183). Adenosine deaminase (ADAR) targets an adenosine editing site of the X chromosome transcribed serotonin (5HT2 C) mRNA and hydrolyses adenosine to inosine, forming a wobble base. Deamination contributes to 32 possible serotonin mRNA isoforms and up to 24 unique proteins (184). Serotonin contributes to epigenetic mechanisms through serotonylation of histones (185). Interestingly, ADAR can edit its own pre-mRNA, creating a new splice site, with a reduced function frameshift to regulate its activity (186).

For pre-mRNA editing, ADAR requires accessing base pairs between intronic and exonic sequences of double-stranded pre-mRNA (187). The 364-kb intron 2 of 5HT2 C hosts four miRNA and complements with itself, forming a loop at the editing site (188). Intron 5 of the gene is a H/ACA snoRNA (187). Deamination of at least five sites is required for the inclusion of the alternatively spliced exon VB and the translation of a full-length receptor (189). The receptor formed by the AS exon VB RNA forms an intracellular loop which is essential for G protein binding (190).

An 18-nt editing site of exon VB on the sense strand pairs complementarily to the C/D box containing snoRNA (HBII-52/SNORD115) transcribed in antisense by the paternal ICR on chromosome 15 (190). The ends of the snoRNA are self-complementary, interacting with non-canonical base pairs (181) and forming a box formation over a splice silencing sequence (190), inhibiting protein interactions on the sense strand, which allows further splicing of intron 2 and recruitment of spliceosome components such as small nuclear RNA (snRNA) (153) (Figure 10.2a).

X Chromosome Inactivation and SnoRNA

The precise complementary pairing of the X chromosome sense-transcribed 5HT2 C pre-RNA with the paternally imprinted antisense SNORD115 suggests that the paternal X chromosome is inactivated in animals capable of carrying the spliced exon VB. In support of this discovery, the loss of paternally transcribed SNORD115 results in severe X chromosome inactivation skewing (191) (Figure 10.2a).

RNA Editing and Disease

Editing 5HT2 C determines the efficiency of the receptor's G protein coupling and the efficacy of an agonist (192). Dysregulated 5HT2 C receptor activity has been implicated in many neurological and psychiatric conditions (188). Differences in the gastrointestinal microbiome have also been shown to influence AS and ultimately the levels of 5HT2 C receptor isoforms (193).

Exosomes

RNA degradation, maturation and surveillance through embryogenesis are tightly regulated by the nuclear exosome complex (194). Exosomes are extracellular vesicles (30–120 nm) which transfer genetic information over long distances. They are excreted by all cells and send chemical messages of protein, mRNA, non-coding RNA (ncRNA) lipid and DNA to their target to regulate cell metabolism, proliferation and differentiation (57). Extracellular vessels also mediate the horizontal transfer of active L1 (195). Exosomes derived from embryonic stem cells transport mRNA capable of reprogramming haematopoietic stem cells, demonstrating the exosomes' role in balancing evolutionary adaptation genome-wide through systemic mechanisms (196).

A growing body of evidence describes the exosomes' involvement in regulating the circadian rhythm (197). Exosomes function as a bridge between the central pacemaker and genetic expression in peripheral cells. Chronic nocturnal shift workers display altered microbiome and changes in exosome composition including *CLOCK* genes (198). MiRNAs in exosomes of shift workers signal circadian misalignment to peripheral tissues (57). MiRNAs can alter epigenetic mechanisms through repressing epigenetic modulators such as sirtuin (199).

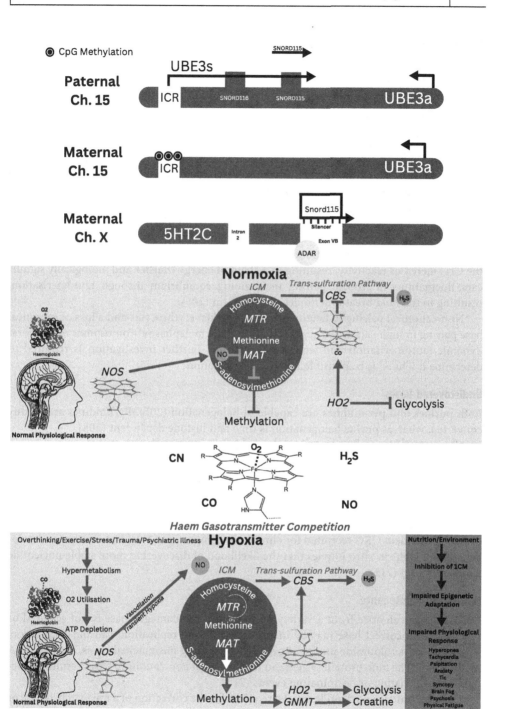

Figure 10.2 Chromosome 15 imprinted control region and gasotransmitters and epigenetic metabolic switching in hypoxia.
(a) Maternally methylated imprinted control region (ICR) of E3 ubiquitin protein ligase 3 (UBE3a) on chromosome 15. Paternal antisense and sense transcription. Antisense SNORD115 complementary pairing with X chromosome 5'hydroxytryptophan 2 C (5'HT2 C), forming a box formation over the splice silencer region, allowing further splicing. Adapted from (307). (b) Epigenetic adaptation and regulation by gasotransmitters in transient hypoxia. Adapted from (26).

Cell Cycle: In Vitro Metaphase Chromosomes

Changes to salt concentrations in the chromosomal media determine the level of compaction for analysis (65). The transfer of condensed chromatin to reduced Na^+ or $Mg2^+$ cation concentrations results in the re-relaxation of the chromosome structure (200). In contrast, increasing salt concentrations leads to a loss of histones, a reduction in UV absorption and a loss of template activity, which is essential for retaining canonical base pairing (201).

In vitro bromination of thymine (5'BrU) replaces the 5'C methyl group and enables thymine to transform from the keto (=O) isoform to the enol (-OH⁻) isoform (202). The reactive hydroxyl enables wobble pairing with guanosine instead of the canonical adenosine (203). Because of increased reactivity, 5'hmU also wobble pairs with guanosine (204).

Thymine is halogenated for fluorescent detection of AT-rich segments of the metaphase chromosome. The increased electro-negativity allows for substantially increased photon quenching and greater differentiation between cytogenetic bands (205). Thymine's loss of the CH_3 increases reactivity, resulting in a chain of energy transfer and biologically significant fluctuations in wobble pairing maintaining equilibrium through tautomerisation, resulting in the fluid breathing model of chromatin (206).

Non-canonical pairing in heterochromatic chicken erythrocytes and a loss of canonical base pairing in high-salt media suggest that compact metaphase chromosomes may rely on dynamic tautomerisation and wobble-base pairing. Further investigation is required to determine if 5'hmU is responsible for this conformation.

Undiscovered Bases

Both purines and pyrimidines are capable of halogenation (207). Pyrimidines are readily converted, whereas purine halogenation is time and histone dependent (208).

Chorine (Cl) is an abundant physiological halogen; its use is essential for chromosome extraction and modulation of structure in vitro (98). Nuclear Cl ion channel *NCC27* is expressed at specific times during the cell cycle, is essential for cell cycle progression and may play a role in the modification of nucleotides (209). Cell cycle progression is dependent on intracellular fluctuations of Mg (210); an increase in Mg concentration occurs during mitosis which accompanies a depletion of ATP, which may be due to the increased activity of ATP-dependent CRC recruited for chromatin compaction (211). Cationation and halogenation of DNA in vitro implies that the likelihood of discovering more stable nucleotide isotopes is high (212).

Nucleotide Maintenance

DNA damage can arise from a variety of sources. If the damaged base is not repaired or replaced, an incorrect base may be incorporated during replication, causing a mutation. BER often works alongside processes prone to generating mismatched bases, such as DNA methylation. The four-protein system can repair several non-canonical bases resulting from oxidating, alkylating or deaminating events (213).

Deamination of a nucleotide may be required for the correction of a mismatched base or the rapid evolution of sequences. Somatic hypermutable genes undergo rapid evolution via the induction of deaminase enzymes for immunoglobin antibody diversification and class switching (214). Precise nucleotide levels are regulated by feedback mechanisms between de novo synthesis, degradation and salvage pathways (215).

Nutritional and Environmental Epigenetics

Molecular Mimicry

Pterin

Many vitamins contain nucleotide motifs and have structurally similar bonding arrangements to other biological molecules (216). Pterin (216) is structurally similar to guanine (217) with many identical bonding arrangements.

Pterin is synthesised from the five-membered ring guanine triphosphate (GTP) to a six-membered ring pterin by the rate-limiting enzyme GTP cyclohydrolase (218). Folic acid is a pterin-containing precursor for the synthesis of GMP and AMP in the de novo purine synthesis pathway (219).

The first step of light-induced folate degradation is the cleavage between the pterin chromophore and the PABA-glutamate moiety, leaving a free pterin moiety (220). Guanine-based purines have demonstrated extracellular signalling and neuromodulation. Extracellular concentrations of purines are dependent on reuptake mechanisms and purines can be released to the extracellular space by neurons and glial cells where they can be hydrolysed, producing different forms to modulate the activity of many different receptors (221).

Guanine nucleotides are traditionally known for intracellular signalling by G protein coupled receptors (GPCR). Over 800 GPCRs have been identified in humans. Because of significant ligand diversity (222), GPCRs are targets of more than 40% of manufactured pharmaceuticals (223). Abnormal function of GCPRs is an inherent factor underlying schizophrenia and mood disorders (224).

Three subunits comprise the G protein: Gα, Gβ and Gγ. In its inactive state, Gα binds guanosine 5-diphosphate (GDP). Upon ligand activation of GPCR, Gα releases GDP and the empty Gα forms a complex with the GPCR. GTP is recruited to the empty Gα subunit, causing dissociation of the subunits and GTP phosphate hydrolysis, resulting in the consequent return of GDP and receptor re-inactivation (225).

Because of folate's role in purine synthesis, folate supplementation contributes to the accumulation of the purine intermediate 5-aminoimidazole-4-carboxamide riboside 5'-monophosphate (ZMP) in the feedback regulation of purine synthesis (226). ZMP is also a direct regulator of 1 CM, demonstrating the crossover between the two pathways (227).

Folic acid and guanine have many overlapping mechanisms because of their similar structures. Folates stimulate GTP binding to GPCR and inhibit GTPase-dependent phosphate hydrolysis, essential for cyclic inactivation (228). The reverse has also been demonstrated, where guanine nucleotides can modulate folate receptors (229).

Folate and its derivatives have been used therapeutically to reduce the production of endogenous CH_3 via the inhibition of 1 CM (230) (Figure 10.2b). Because of cell-specific epigenetic mechanisms, it is currently impossible to determine which cells or organs will be implicated by the loss of endogenous methylation and therefore may result in pathological symptoms due to epigenetic inflexibility (26). The neurotoxic effects of folates are often ascribed to its polyglutamate tail and modulation of 1CM (26); however, feedback inhibition of purine synthesis, modulation of the purinergic system and its contribution to epigenetic inflexibility may also play a role (228).

Riboflavin

Riboflavin is a fluorescent pigment and a core component of flavoproteins responsible for several types of redox electron transport reactions (231). Humans carry more than 40 flavoproteins (232).

Mutations in riboflavin transporters are known to cause riboflavin transporter deficiency and severe progressive neurological disease (233). Riboflavin transport dysfunction is associated with various neuromuscular diseases with distinct motor neuron dysfunctional overlap, such as Madras motor neuron disease (MND) (234), Brown-Vialetto Van Laere (235) and juvenile amyotrophic lateral sclerosis (236). However, in all cases, high-dose riboflavin promotes remarkable recoveries (234–238). Madras is a form of MND with juvenile onset with no known mutations. Despite not sharing riboflavin transporter mutations with other early onset MNDs, riboflavin supplementation promotes remarkable recovery in these patients, suggesting epigenetic mechanisms are responsible (234).

Light irreversibly reduces riboflavin (231) to various metabolites such as carboxymethylflavin, lumiflavin and lumichrome (232). Riboflavin end-products are known inhibitors of flavoproteins (239) and transporters (240), including gastrointestinal absorption by human intestinal epithelial cells (241). Therefore, light-exposed riboflavin in dairy (231) and plant foods (239) may negatively affect these conditions.

Metaboloepigenetics

Accumulating connections between energy metabolism and epigenetic mechanisms have given rise to a new field of research referred to as metaboloepigenetics (73). Epigenetically regulated metabolism is unique to each cell type and drives the cell cycle (242, 262).

Metabolic Switch

During exercise or stress, epigenetic mechanisms enable metabolic switches which modify gene expression to optimise fuel utilisation for the changing conditions (243). In the diseased state, a metabolic switch may be pathological or essential. Following traumatic brain injury, a metabolic switch activates a lactate shuttle to optimise lactate utilisation even in the presence of O_2 (244). A similar metabolic adaptation is seen in cancer cells to meet higher metabolic demands, where histone lactylation is the epigenetic mark of the glycolytic switch for fast cell growth and proliferation (245). Impaired epigenetic mechanisms lead to metabolic imbalances (Figure 10.2b).

Hypermetabolism and Brain Energetics

Impaired brain energetics negatively influences psychological and neurological conditions (246). Critical illness is marked by hypermetabolism and increased protein catabolism (247). Ageing (247), illness (248), psychological stress (249) and trauma (250) are also hypermetabolic states where epigenetic adaptation is essential to meet the increased energy demands of the brain (Figure 10.2b). ATP is a primary fuel source for muscular contraction and neural action potentials.

Brain energy consumption is 12 times higher than skeletal muscle and the amount of ATP stored within the brain is minimal (251). ATP is rapidly depleted in normal metabolism; a metabolic switch to rapidly increase the rate of synthesis is required to match increased energy demands (252).

The mere thought of anticipated exercise is sufficient to stimulate adaptive respiratory and cardiovascular systems (253). For example, the anticipation causes an initial increase of oxyhaemoglobin in the prefrontal cortex due to an increase in neurological ATP utilisation and O_2 demand (254). The neurovascular coupling enables haemoglobin transfer of O_2 to the brain (255) and the concomitant release of NO dilates blood vessels, inducing transient cerebral vascular hypoxia (256). Central chemoreceptors detect changes in O_2, stimulating neurological control of ventilation (257).

Gasotransmitters

Gasotransmitters are a class of signalling molecules that are permeable to cell membranes and can interact immediately with proteins, providing ultra-fast communication between cells and molecules (258). Gasotransmitters regulate hypoxic adaptation and are epigenetically regulated (259).

Gasotransmitters nitric oxide (NO) (260), hydrogen sulphide (H_2S) (261) and carbon monoxide (CO)[258] were once considered noxious toxins and have been well documented. Hydrogen cyanide (HCN) has recently been described as a new mammalian gas transmitter (282) and the potential signalling functions following H_2O phase transitions through thermal aquaporins are yet to be defined (263). Gasotransmitters are known to regulate haem, haem-like moieties (cobalamin) and haemoproteins (279). Gasotransmitters regulate epigenetic mechanisms; for example, NO inhibits 1 CM through S-nitrosylation of the cysteine 121 residue of MAT (264).

In normoxia, haemoglobin O_2 saturation is stable; the O_2-dependent haem oxygenate-2 (HO2) is responsible for the degradation of haem and other haem-containing proteins including nitric oxide synthase (NOS). Active HO2 inhibits glycolysis via redirected activation of the pentose pathway (265). HO2 haem degradation produces CO in the process which binds to the haem moiety of cystathionine β-synthase (CBS) where it maintains its inhibition (266).

CBS is an H_2S generating, rate-limiting enzyme of the trans-sulphuration pathway (266). CBS, HO2 and NOS are all haemoproteins and therefore are regulated by preferred binding affinities of gasotransmitters (259). It has been proposed that HO2 is an O_2 sensor. At the onset of hypoxia, O_2 reduction reduces HO2 activity and consequently CO production (259). The reduced CO and O_2 tension activates CBS and H_2S production (265). In addition, the reduced HO2 activity may allow for greater haem protein availability for NOS and upregulation of NO for the regulation of alternative haemoproteins (259) (Figure 10.2b).

Creatine

With increased metabolic demands, the creatine/phosphocreatine system plays an important role in maintaining ATP by acting as an energy buffer (267). Creatine (N-methylguanidino acetic acid) is a nitrogenous amino acid which can be phosphorylated. The phosphate is liberated by creatine kinase for immediate regeneration of ATP in the absence of O_2 (268). Creatine is synthesised by the SAM-dependent methyltransferase guanidinoacetate methyltransferase (GAMT) (243). and up to 40% of methyl groups from 1 CM go towards creatine synthesis. This demonstrates the importance of 1 CM in optimising energy efficiency.

Abnormal phosphocreatine systems are associated with neurological (269) and psychiatric disease (267). Moreover, hypermetabolism and an impaired epigenetic adaptation to transient hypoxia is likely to result in or exacerbate pathological symptomology of psychiatric or neurological origin (Figure 10.2b).

Nitrogen Balance

Protein is a major source of dietary nitrogen (270), which is essential for tissue growth and repair (244). Dietary protein recommendations are based on nitrogen balance studies in healthy subjects (271). However, for growth and repair, nitrogen consumption must exceed catabolism and excretion (272). Hypermetabolism is associated with a negative nitrogen balance; these patients experience impaired cellular repair, DNA synthesis, muscle wasting, decreased immunity and increased mortality (247). Older adults and those with chronic disease require more protein than standard recommendations to promote recovery from illness and maintain a positive nitrogen balance (270). However, not all protein is created equal. Animal and plant proteins contain different amino acid ratios and therefore have different nitrogen levels (271).

Ketogenic Diets

Ketogenic diets are used to manage neurological and psychiatric disease (246). The endogenous ketone beta-hydroxybutyrate possesses HDACi activity and the TCA cycle ketone intermediate αKG is a substrate for demethylase enzymes (273). The metabolic switch associated with modulation of the glycolytic metabolic pathway provides an alternative brain fuel which may not only manage symptoms but also address the underlying disease mechanisms from the epigenetic level (246).

Evolution and Epidemiology

Radioactivity

Evolution begins at the atomic level. Since the discovery of elemental radioactivity, radioactive isotopes have been used as tracers in the study of biological reactions and pathways (274). Isotopes differ in mass and bonding potentials and therefore must be adjusted for in research. Because of safety issues, their use has recently declined (275). Radioactive and non-radioactive heavier isotopes occur naturally in our environment and contribute to the evolution of biological pathways and epigenetics (276). For example, a large banana contains 18.4 Beroquel (Bq), which is equivalent to one nuclear transformation per second (277).

Biological Adaptation

A model of hypertension describes how changes to environment or diet result in subtle epigenetic change, producing hundreds of molecular changes, dozens of signalling adaptations and a few physiological changes, resulting in either stable adaptive gene expression or pathological mutation and/or disease (278).

Following Darwin's description of natural selection in 1859 (279), scientists have made remarkable progress in understanding how evolutionary processes shape species diversity (280). Since the evolution of *Homo sapiens* 100,000 to 200,000 years ago (281), humans have diversified into many subspecies (282), occupying diverse environmental conditions and using a variety of different dietary staples (283). Genes directly involved in environmental or dietary adaptation essential for the survival of a population are subject to subtle shifts in allele frequencies (284). However, human phenotypes are complex, and only a small portion of genetic diversity can be explained by allele frequencies (280). Human variation is also influenced by epigenetic patterns (285) and epigenetic pathways are influenced by environmental selective pressures (286). For example, the natural selection of 1 CM is observed in populations who live at high altitudes, likely due to the combined effects of increased UV radiation and CH_3 formation owing to greater atmospheric methane concentrations (287). However, there is also a significant correlation with increased psychological disease, including suicide rates in populations that live at high altitudes (288), suggesting impaired epigenetic adaptation following recent relocation may be responsible.

Before the shift to horticulture and animal farming approximately 10,000 years ago, hunting and foraging were the primary methods of food selection (289). Selection of genes associated with the metabolism of starch is seen in populations who depend on cereal grains for sustenance (284). Indigenous Australian are a population of hunters and gatherers that were subject to major environmental and dietary shifts less than 250 years ago (290). This population shows minimal allele adaptive selection, likely due to the limited time required for sequence specific evolutionary diversification (284). However, when it comes to health and longevity, populations like Indigenous Australians who have diverged rapidly from tradition tend to do the worst (290), likely because of impaired epigenetic adaptation due to unpredictable food availability (283).

Industrial advances during the twentieth century led to improvements in agricultural plant breeding which could aid malnutrition in developing countries (291). Wild plants were domesticated, breeding out bitterness and toxins (292). Traits were selected for, increasing growth, nutrition and palatability, while increasing sugar content and modifying gene expression and nutrient density. One-third of foraged plants by Indigenous Australians required various kinds of treatment before they could be eaten and were therefore attractive candidates for domestication. By 1926, there were eight major domesticated crops across Asia, Africa and South America (293).

Some pesticides used to increase crop yields are known endocrine disruptors (26) and interact with epigenetic mechanisms through TF modulation of nuclear hormone receptors (294). Some plant food sources still carry their natural defence phytochemicals to protect against predators and may cause allergy, sensitivity or disease in some populations because of impaired epigenetic adaptation (295). For example, Isothiocyanates are goitrogenic toxins found in brassica varieties and may contribute to thyroid pathology in those susceptible (296). Willardine is an amino acid synthesised from uracil which is found in legumes (297). It is a partial agonist of glutamate receptors (298). Thiaminase is found in fish, herbs (299), maize and some brassica varieties (300) and is responsible for thiamine deficiencies in sheep fed maize silage (301). Thiamine deficiency is associated with chronic neuropsychiatric symptoms (302).

Vitamins and minerals are cofactors for many epigenetic pathways; therefore, the chemical composition of our diets directly influences cellular and microbiome epigenetic mechanisms. Fortification or supplementation with folic acid may lead to inhibition of 1 CM and disrupt the infinite flow of epigenetic modifications, resulting in unpredictable metabolic blockages in those susceptible (26). Fortification with riboflavin may lead to the formation of toxic metabolites, resulting in neurological symptoms, and therefore may also be unsuitable in certain populations or those with certain conditions. It is possible that fortification may be essential for survival in some populations but may be toxically detrimental to others (26).

The heavy metal composition of food due to contaminated soil and H_2O may also negatively influence epigenetic mechanisms (303) through replacing essential cofactors

(26). Animal proteins are not only a complete source of amino acids but also an abundant source of hormones, cytokines and neurotransmitters which influence epigenetic mechanisms in the gastrointestinal tract and beyond (26). Bioactive molecules can be transported across the basolateral membrane individually or combined in exosomes (304).

Because of environmental concerns, global consumption of plant-based foods is rising rapidly, leading to the innovation of new plant varieties, insects and plant-based food products (305). Sudden changes to macronutrient ratios lead to a domino effect of compensatory epigenetic adaptations which are uniquely matched to the individual. Bio-individuality suggests that some populations may have difficulty adapting to abrupt changes in environmental conditions or the molecular composition of new foods. Without epigenetic flexibility, biological pathways may over- or under-compensate, leading to disease.

Over the past two decades, researchers have demonstrated the manipulation of epigenetic mechanisms through the modification of environments, microbiomes, diets, vitamins, minerals and herbs (26). Given the unpredictable nature of the genome, gentle nutritional and environmental modification may be a personalised, non-invasive and sustainable alternative to gene-editing treatments or adjunct for the management of psychiatric conditions (26). However, this should not be done without caution, for the more we understand about the genomic diversity of organisms, it is evident that what may be essential to sustain life in one population may be a poison to another.

References

1. Waddington, C. H., 1939. An introduction to modern genetics. *Physiological Entomology*, 14(4-6), p. 82.

2. Bird, A., 2007. Perceptions of epigenetics. *Nature*, 447(7143), pp. 396–8.

3. Luger, K., Mä Der, A. W., Richmond, R. K., Sargent, D. F. and Richmond, T. J., 1997. Crystal structure of the nucleosome core particle at 2.8 A° resolution. *Nature, 389*.

4. Segal, E. and Widom, J., 2009. PolydA:dT tracts: major determinants of nucleosome organization. *Current Opinion in Structural Biology, 19*(1), pp. 65–71.

5. Singh, V., Fedeles, B. I. and Essigmann, J. M., 2015. Role of tautomerism in RNA biochemistry. *RNA, 21*(1), pp. 1–13.

6. Karwowski, B. T., 2020. The electronic property differences between dA::dG and dA::d goxo: a theoretical approach. *Molecules, 25*(17).

7. Lindon, J. C., Tranter, G. E. and Holmes, J. L., 1999. Chemical reactions studied by electronic spectroscopy. In *Encyclopedia of spectroscopy and spectrometry* 2 (pp. 246–52). Elsevier.

8. Fedeles, B. I., Li, D. and Singh, V., 2022. Structural insights to tautomeric dynamics in nucleic acids and in antiviral nucleoside analogs. *Frontiers in Molecular Biosciences, 8*.

9. Grifoni, E., Piccini, G. and Parrinello, M., 2020. Tautomeric equilibrium in condensed phases. *Journal of Chemical Theory and Computation, 16*(10), pp. 6027–31.

10. Tolosa, S., Hidalgo, A. and Sansón, J. A., 2012. Amino acid tautomerization reactions in aqueous solution via concerted and assisted mechanisms using free energy curves from MD simulation. *The Journal of Physical Chemistry A, 116*(43), pp. 13033–44.

11. Haynes, A. and Tekel, S., 2017. Molecular structures guide the engineering go chromatin. *Nucleic Acids Research, 45* 13), pp. 7555–70.

12. Cooper, G. M., 2000. The organization of cellular genomes. In *The cell: a molecular approach*. ASM Press.

13. Happel, N., and Doenecke, D., 2009. Histone H1 and its isoforms: contribution to chromatin structure and function. *Gene, 431*(1-2), pp. 1–12.

14. Churchill, A. and Suzuki, M., 1989. 'SPKK' motifs prefer to bind to DNA at A/T-rich sites. *The EMBO Journal*, 8(13).

15. McGinty, K. and Tan, S., 2015. Nucleosome structure and function. *Chemical Reviews*, 115(6), pp. 2255–73.

16. Vogler, C., Huber, C., Waldmann, T., et al., 2010. Histone H2A C-terminus regulates chromatin dynamics, remodelling, and histone H1 binding. *PLOS Genetics*, 6(12), pp. 1–12.

17. Freitas, A., Sklenar, R. and Parthun, R., 2004. Application of mass spectrometry to the identification and quantification of histone post-translational modifications. *Journal of Cellular Biochemistry*, 924, pp. 691–700.

18. Krebs, J. E., Goldstein, E. S. and Kilpatrick, S. T., 2018. *Lewin's genes XII*. Jones Bartlett Learning.

19. Bednar, J., Garcia-Saez, I., Boopathi, R., et al., 2017. Structure and dynamics of a 197 bp nucleosome in complex with linker histone H1. *Molecular Cell*, 663(8), pp. 384–97.

20. Woodcock, C. L., Skoultchi, A. I. and Fan, Y., 2006. Role of linker histone in chromatin structure and function: H1 stoichiometry and nucleosome repeat length. *Chromosome Research*, 14(1), pp. 17–25.

21. Bates, L. and Thomas, O., 1981. Histones Hl and H5: one or two molecules per nucleosome? *Nucleic Acids Research*, 9 (221981).

22. Widlund, R., Cao, H., Simonsson, S., et al., 1997. Identification and characterization of genomic nucleosome-positioning sequences. *Journal of Molecular Biology*, 2674, pp. 807–17.

23. Lowary, P. T. and Widom, J., 1998. New DNA sequence rules for high affinity binding to histone octamer and sequence-directed nucleosome positioning. *Journal of Molecular Biology*, 2761, pp. 19–42.

24. Menon, V. and Ghaffari, S., 2021. Erythroid enucleation: a gateway into a 'bloody' world. *Experimental Hematology*, 95, pp. 13–22.

25. Strahl, B. D. and Allis, D. C., 2000. The language of covalent histone modifications. *Nature*, 403.

26. Sedley, L., 2020. Advances in nutritional epigenetics: a fresh perspective for an old idea – lessons learned, limitations, and future directions. *Epigenetics Insights*, 13.

27. Clark, D. J. and Kimurai, T., 1990. Electrostatic mechanism of chromatin folding. *Journal of Molecular Biology*, 211.

28. Ramazi, S. and Zahiri, J., 2021. Post-translational modifications in proteins: resources, tools and prediction methods. *Database (Oxford)*, 2021, baab012.

29. Portela, A. and Esteller, M., 2010. Epigenetic modifications and human disease. *Nature Biotechnology*, 2810, pp. 1057–68.

30. Sadakierska-Chudy, A., Kostrzewa, R. M. and Filip, M. A., 2015. Comprehensive view of the epigenetic landscape part I: DNA methylation, passive and active DNA demethylation, pathways and histone variants. *Neurotoxicity Research*, 27(1), pp. 84–97.

31. Biswas, S. and Rao, C. M., 2018. Epigenetic tools: the writers, the readers and the erasers and their implications in cancer therapy. *European Journal of Pharmacology*, 837, pp. 8–24.

32. Mentch, S. J. and Locasale, J. W., 2016. One-carbon metabolism and epigenetics: understanding the specificity. *Annals of the New York Academy of Sciences*, 13631, pp. 91–8.

33. Farra, A. H., 2010. Methionine synthase polymorphisms MTR 2756 Agt;G and MTR 2758 Cgt;G frequencies and distribution in the Jordanian population and their correlation with neural tube defects in the population of the northern part of Jordan. *Indian Journal of Human Genetics*, 16(3), pp. 138–43.

34. Murray, B., Antonyuk, S. V., Marina, A., et al., 2014. Structure and function study of the complex that synthesizes S-adenosylmethionine. *IUCr Journal*, 1(4), pp. 240–9.

35. Bing, Y., Zhu, S., Yu, G., et al., 2014. Glucocorticoid-induced S-adenosylmethionine enhances the interferon signaling pathway by restoring STAT1 protein methylation in hepatitis B virus-infected cells. *Journal of Biological Chemistry*, *28947*, pp. 32639–55.

36. Pé Rez-Mato, I., Castro, C., Ruiz, A., Corrales, F. J. and Mato, J. M., 1999. Methionine adenosyltransferase S-nitrosylation is regulated by the basic and acidic amino acids surrounding the target thiol.*Journal of Biological Chemistry*, *274*(24).

37. Soderberg, T., 2022. Steric effects on nucleophilicity. In *Organic chemistry with a biological emphasis*. LibreTexts.

38. Dhareshwar, S. S. and Stella, V. J., 2008. Your prodrug releases formaldehyde: should you be concerned? No!*Journal of Pharmaceutical Sciences*, *9710*, pp. 4184–93.

39. Dahl, A. R. and Hadley, W. M., 1983. Formaldehyde production promoted by rat nasal cytochrome P-450-dependent monooxygenases with nasal decongestants, essences, solvents, air pollutants, nicotine, and cocaine as substrates. *Toxicology and Applied Pharmacology*, *672*, pp. 200–5.

40. Burgos-Barragan, G., Wit, N., Meiser, J., et al., 2017. Mammals divert endogenous genotoxic formaldehyde into one-carbon metabolism. *Nature*, *5487*(669), pp. 549–54.

41. Leighton, P. A., 1961. *Photochemistry of air pollution*. Academic Press.

42. Rossi, M., Amaretti, A. and Raimondi, S., 2011. Folate production by probiotic bacteria. *Nutrients*, *31*, pp. 118–34.

43. Chaudhary, P. P., Conway, P. L. and Schlundt, J., 2018. Methanogens in humans: potentially beneficial or harmful for health. *Applied Microbiology and Biotechnology*, *10*(27), pp. 3095–104.

44. Sofia, H. J., Chen, G., Hetzler, B. G., Reyes-Spindola, J. F. and Miller, N. E., 2001. Radical SAM. a novel protein superfamily linking unresolved steps in familiar biosynthetic pathways with radical mechanisms: functional characterization using new analysis and information visualization methods.*Nucleic Acids Research*, *29*(5).

45. Landgraf, B. J., McCarthy, E. L. and Booker, S. J., 2016. Radical adenosylmethionine enzymes in human health and disease. *Annual Review of Biochemistry*, *85*(1), pp. 485–514.

46. Lanz, N. D. and Booker, S. J., 2015. Auxiliary iron-sulfur cofactors in radical SAM enzymes. *Biochimica et Biophysica Acta*, *1853*(6), pp. 1316–34.

47. Fujimori, D. G., 2013. Radical SAM-mediated methylation reactions. *Current Opinion in Chemical Biology*, *17*(4), pp. 597–604.

48. Wang, S. C. and Frey, P. A., 2007. S-adenosylmethionine as an oxidant: the radical SAM superfamily. *Trends in Biochemical Sciences*, *32*(3), pp. 101–10.

49. Brown, A. C. and Suess, D. L. M., 2020. Reversible formation of alkyl radicals at [Fe4S4] clusters and its implications for selectivity in radical SAM enzymes. *Journal of the American Chemical Society*, *142*(33), pp. 14240–8.

50. Shi, R., Hou, W., Wang, Z. Q. and Xu, X., 2021. Biogenesis of iron–sulfur clusters and their role in DNA metabolism. *Frontiers in Cell and Developmental Biology*, *9*.

51. Shimberg, G. D., Pritts, J. D. and Michel, S. L. J., 2018. Iron–sulfur clusters in zinc finger proteins. *Methods in Enzymology*, *599*, 101–37.

52. Sadakierska-Chudy, A. and Filip, M. A., 2015. Comprehensive view of the epigenetic landscape. Part II: histone post-translational modification. Nucleosome level and chromatin regulation by ncRNAs. *Neurotoxicity Research*, *27*(2), pp. 172–97.

53. Rolfe, D. F. and Brown, G. C., 1997. Cellular energy utilization and molecular origin of standard metabolic rate in mammals. *Physiological Reviews*, *77*(3), pp. 731–58.

54. Black, J. C. and Whetstine, J. R., 2012. LOX out. Histones: a new enzyme is nipping at your tails. *Molecular Cell*, *46*(3), pp. 243–4.

55. Adams-Cioaba, M. A., Krupa, J. C., Xu, C., Mort, J. S. and Min, J., 2011. Structural basis for the recognition and cleavage of histone H3 by cathepsin L. *Nature Communications*, 2(1).

56. Sancar, A., 2000. Cryptochrome: the second photoactive pigment in the eye and its role in circadian photoreception. *Annual Review of Biochemistry*, 69, pp. 31–67.

57. Khalyfa, A., Gaddameedhi, S., Crooks, E., et al., 2020. Circulating exosomal miRNAs signal circadian misalignment to peripheral metabolic tissues. *International Journal of Molecular Sciences*, 21(17), pp. 1–25.

58. Okamoto-Uchida, Y., Izawa, J. and Hirayama, J. A., 2018. Molecular link between the circadian clock: DNA damage responses and oncogene activation. *IntechOpen*. https://doi.org/10.5772/intechopen.81063.

59. Lavebratt, C., Sjöholm, L. K., Soronen, P., et al., 2010. Cry2 is associated with depression. *PLoS ONEx*, 5(2).

60. Hirano, A., Shi, G., Jones, C. R., et al., 2016. Cryptochrome 2 mutation yields advanced sleep phase in humans. *eLife*, 5, p. 16695.

61. Terai, Y., Sato, R., Matsumura, R., Iwai, S. and Yamamoto, J., 2020. Enhanced DNA repair by DNA photolyase bearing an artificial light-harvesting chromophore. *Nucleic Acids Research*, 48(18), pp. 10076–86.

62. Su, Y., Cailotto, C., Foppen, E., et al., 2016. The role of feeding rhythm, adrenal hormones and neuronal inputs in synchronizing daily clock gene rhythms in the liver. *Molecular and Cellular Endocrinology*, 422, pp. 125–31.

63. Johnson, C. H., 2013. Circadian clocks and cell division: what's the pacemaker? *Cell Cycle*, 9(19), pp. 3864–73.

64. Potten, C. S., 1998. Stem cells in gastrointestinal epithelium: numbers, characteristics and death. *Philosophical Transactions of the Royal Society B*, 353 (1370), pp. 821–30.

65. Ozer, G., Luque, A. and Schlick, T., 2015. The chromatin fiber: multiscale problems and approaches. *Current Opinion in Structural Biology*, 31, pp. 124–39.

66. Routh, A., Sandin, S. and Rhodes, D., 2008. Nucleosome repeat length and linker histone stoichiometry determine chromatin fiber structure. *Proceedings of the National Academy of Sciences of the United States of America*, 105(26), pp. 8872–7.

67. Adams, M. D., Celniker, S. E., Holt, R. A., et al., 2000. The genome sequence of drosophila melanogaster. *Science*, 287 (5461), pp. 2185–95.

68. Rajewska, M., Wegrzyn, K. and Konieczny, I., 2012. AT-rich region and repeated sequences: the essential elements of replication origins of bacterial replicons. *FEMS Microbiology Reviews*, 36(2), pp. 408–34.

69. Shi, W. and Zhou, W., 2006. Frequency distribution of TATA Box and extension sequences on human promoters. *BMC Bioinformatics*, 7S4, s2.

70. Phillips, D., 1963. The presence of acetyl groups in histones. *Biochemical Journal*, 87(2), pp. 258–63.

71. Shukla, S., Levine, C., Sripathi, R. P., et al., 2018. The kat in the HAT: the histone acetyl transferase *KAT6b* (*MYST4*) is downregulated in murine macrophages in response to LPS. *Mediators of Inflammation*, 2018, pp. 1–11.

72. Shogren-Knaak, M., Ishii, H., Sun, J. M., et al., 2006. Histone H4-K16 acetylation controls chromatin structure and protein interactions. *Science*, 311(5762), pp. 844–7.

73. Nitsch, S., Zorro Shahidian, L. and Schneider R., 2021. Histone acylations and chromatin dynamics: concepts, challenges, and links to metabolism. *EMBO Reports*, 22(7).

74. Linster, C. L., Van Schaftingen, E. and Hanson, A. D., 2013. Metabolite damage and its repair or pre-emption. *Nature Chemical Biology*, 9(2), pp. 72–80.

75. Fan, F., Williams, H. J., Boyer, J. G., et al., 2012. On the catalytic mechanism of human ATP citrate lyase. *Biochemistry*, 51 (25), pp. 5198–211.

76. Xu, Y., Shi, Z. and Bao, L., 2022. An expanding repertoire of protein acylations. *Molecular and Cellular Proteomics*, 21(3).

77. Seto, E. and Yoshida, M., 2014. Erasers of histone acetylation: the histone deacetylase enzymes. *Cold Spring Harbor Perspectives in Biology*, 64.

78. Biava, H., 2022. The chemistry of NAD+ and FAD. In *Biochemistry*, ed. H. Jakubowski. LibreTexts.

79. Kim, J., Lee, S. H., Tieves, F., et al., 2019. Nicotinamide adenine dinucleotide as a photocatalyst. *Science Advances*, 5(7).

80. Feldman, J. L., Dittenhafer-Reed, K. E., Thelen, J. N., et al., 2015. Kinetic and structural basis for acyl-group selectivity and NAD+ dependence in sirtuin-catalyzed deacylation. *Biochemistry*, 54(19), pp. 3037–50.

81. Fellows, R., Denizot, J., Stellato, C., et al., 2018. Microbiota derived short chain fatty acids promote histone crotonylation in the colon through histone deacetylases. *Nature Communications*, 9(1), p. 105.

82. Yang, Z., He, M., Austin, J., Pfleger, J. and Abdellatif, M., 2021. Histone H3K9 butyrylation is regulated by dietary fat and stress via an Acyl-CoA dehydrogenase short chain-dependent mechanism. *Molecular Metabolism*, 53, p. 101249.

83. Brown, T., 2002. *Genomes*. Wiley-Liss.

84. Kearse, M. G. and Wilusz, J. E., 2017. Non-AUG translation: a new start for protein synthesis in eukaryotes. *Genes & Development*, 31, pp. 1717–31

85. Peabody, D. S., 1989. Translation initiation at non-AUG triplets in mammalian cells. *Journal of Biological Chemistry*, 26(49), pp. 5031–5.

86. Echingoya, K., Koyama, M., Negishi, L., et al., 2020. Nucleosome binding by the pioneer transcription factor OCT4. *Scientific Reports*, 10(1), p. 11832.

87. Kujirai, T. and Kurumizaka, H., 2020. Transcription through the nucleosome. *Current Opinion in Structural Biology*, 61, pp. 42–9.

88. Kulaeva, O. I., Hsieh, F. K., Chang, H. W., Luse, D. S. and Studitsky, V. M., 2013. Mechanism of transcription through a nucleosome by RNA polymerase II. *Biochimica et Biophysica Acta*, 1829(1), pp. 76–83.

89. Martin, B. J. E., Brind'Amour, J., Kuzmin, A., et al., 2021. Transcription shapes genome-wide histone acetylation patterns. *Nature Communications*, 12(1).

90. Banine, F., Bartlett, C., Gunawardena, R., et al., 2005. SWI/SNF Chromatin-remodeling factors induce changes in DNA methylation to promote transcriptional activation. *Cancer Research*, 65(9).

91. Mathur, R. and Roberts, C. W. M., 2018. Swi/snf baf complexes: guardians of the epigenome. *Annual Review of Cancer Biology*, 2, pp. 413–27.

92. Josling, G. A., Selvarajah, S. A., Petter, M. and Duffy, M. F., 2012. The role of bromodomain proteins in regulating gene expression. *Genes*, 3(2), pp. 320–43.

93. Farnung, L. and Vos, S. M., 2022. Assembly of RNA polymerase II transcription initiation complexes. *Current Opinion in Structural Biology*, 73, p. 102335.

94. Lambert, S. A., Jolma, A., Campitelli, L. F., et al., 2018. The human transcription factors. *Cell*, 8(4), pp. 650–65.

95. Dancy, B. M. and Cole, P. A., 2015. Protein lysine acetylation by p300/CBP. *Chemical Reviews*, 115(6), pp. 2419–52.

96. Hansen, J. C., Maeshima, K. and Hendzel, M. J., 2021. The solid and liquid states of chromatin. *Epigenetics & Chromatin*, 14(1).

97. Gibson, B. A., Doolittle, L. K., Schneider, M. W. G., et al., 2019. Organization of chromatin by intrinsic and regulated phase separation. *Cell*, 179(2), pp. 470–84.

98. Thoma, F., Koller, T. H. and Klug, A., 1979. Involvement of histone H1 in the organisation of the nucleosome and of the salt-dependent superstructures of chromatin. *Journal of Cell Biology*, 83, pp. 403–27.

99. Worcel, A., Strogatz, S. and Riley, D., 1981. Structure of chromatin and the linking number of DNA. *Proceedings of the National Academy of Sciences of the United States of America*, 78(3), pp. 1461–5.

100. Woodcock, C. L., Frado, L. L. and Rattner, J. B., 1984. The higher-order structure of chromatin: evidence for a helical ribbon arrangement. *Journal of Cell Biology, 99*(1), pp. 42–52.

101. Williams, S. P., Athey, B. D., Muglia, L. J., et al., 1986. Chromatin fibers are left-handed double helices with diameter and mass per unit length that depend on linker length. *Biophysical Journal, 49*(1), pp. 233–48.

102. Song, F., Chen, P., Sun, D., et al., 2014. Cryo-EM study of the chromatin fiber reveals a double helix twisted by tetranucleosomal units. *Science, 344* (6182), pp. 376–80.

103. Farr, S. E., Woods, E. J., Joseph, J. A., Garaizar, A. and Collepardo-Guevara, R., 2021. Nucleosome plasticity is a critical element of chromatin liquid–liquid phase separation and multivalent nucleosome interactions. *Nature Communications, 12*(1).

104. Von Hippel, P. H., Johnson, N. P. and Marcus, A. H., 2013. 50 years of DNA 'breathing': reflections on old and new approaches [For special issue of biopolymers on 50 years of nucleic acids research]. *Biopolymers, 99*(12), pp. 923–54.

105. Hospital, A., Goñi, J. R., Orozco, M. and Gelpí, J. L., 2015. Molecular dynamics simulations: advances and applications. *Advances and Applications in Bioinformatics and Chemistry, 8*(1), pp. 37–47.

106. Szyc, Ł., Yang, M., Nibbering, E. T. J. and Elsaesser, T., 2010. Ultrafast vibrational dynamics and local interactions of hydrated DNA. *Angewandte Chemie, 49* (21), pp. 3598–610.

107. Pal, S. K., Zhao, L. and Zewail, A. H., 2003. Water at DNA surfaces: ultrafast dynamics in minor groove recognition. *Proceedings of the National Academy of Sciences of the United States of America, 8*(14).

108. Lieberman-Aiden, E., Van Berkum, N., Williams, L., et al., 2009. Comprehensive mapping of long-range interactions reveals folding principles of the human genome. *Science, 326*(5950), pp. 289–93.

109. Spector, D. L. and Lamond, A. I., 2011. Nuclear speckles. *Cold Spring Harbor Perspectives in Biology, 32*.

110. Rao, S. S. P., Huntley, M. H., Durand, N. C., et al., 2014. 3D map of the human genome at kilobase resolution reveals principles of chromatin looping. *Cell, 159*(7), pp. 1665–80.

111. McArthur, E. and Capra, J. A., 2021. Topologically associating domain boundaries that are stable across diverse cell types are evolutionarily constrained and enriched for heritability. *American Journal of Medical Genetics, 108*(2), pp. 269–83.

112. Martin, R. P. and Krawetz, S. A., 2000. Characterizing a human lysyl oxidase chromosomal domain. *Molecular Biotechnology, 15*(3), pp. 225–36.

113. Dixon, J. R., Selvaraj, S., Yue, F., et al., 2012. Topological domains in mammalian genomes identified by analysis of chromatin interactions. *Nature, 485*(7398), pp. 376380.

114. Ejlassi-Lassallette, A. and Thiriet, C., 2012. Replication-coupled chromatin assembly of newly synthesized histones: distinct functions for the histone tail domains. *Biochemistry and Cell Biology, 90*(1), pp. 14–21.

115. Harris, E., Bohni, R., Schneiderman, H., et al., 1991. Regulation of histone mRNA in the unperturbed cell cycle: evidence suggesting control at two posttranscriptional step. *Molecular and Cellular Biology, 11*(5).

116. Christophorou, M. A., Castelo-Branco, G., Halley-Stott, R. P., et al., 2014. Citrullination regulates pluripotency and histone H1 binding to chromatin. *Nature, 507*(7490), pp. 104–8.

117. Lio, C. W. J., Yue, X., López-Moyado, I. F., et al., 2020. TET methylcytosine oxidases: new insights from a decade of research. *Journal of Biosciences, 45*(1), p. 21.

118. Woodcock, D. M., Crowther, P. J. and Diver, W. P., 1987. The majority of

methylated deoxycytidines in human DNA are not in the CpG dinucleotide. *Biochemical and Biophysical Research Communications*, *145*(2), pp. 888–94.

119. Hayatsu, H., Wataya, Y. and Kai, K., 1970. Addition of sodium bisulfite to uracil and cytosine. *Journal of the American Chemical Society*, *92*(3), pp. 724–6.

120. Laurent, L., Wong, E., Li, G., et al., 2010. Dynamic changes in the human methylome during differentiation. *Genome Research*, *20*(3), pp. 320–31.

121. Lister, R., Pelizzola, M., Dowen, R. H., et al., 2009. Human DNA methylomes at base resolution show widespread epigenomic differences. *Nature*, *462* (7271), pp. 315–22.

122. Patil, V., Ward, R. L. and Hesson, L. B., 2014. The evidence for functional non-CpG methylation in mammalian cells. *Epigenetics*, *9*(6), pp. 823–8.

123. Straussman, R., Nejman, D., Roberts, D., et al., 2009. Developmental programming of CpG island methylation profiles in the human genome. *Nature Structural & Molecular Biology*, *16*(5), pp. 564–71.

124. Miller, J. L. and Grant, P. A., 2013. The role of DNA methylation and histone modifications in transcriptional regulation in humans. *Subcellular Biochemistry*, *61*, pp. 289–317.

125. Doi, A., Park, I. H., Wen, B., et al., 2009. Differential methylation of tissue- and cancer-specific CpG island shores distinguishes human induced pluripotent stem cells. embryonic stem cells and fibroblasts. *Nature Genetics*, *4112*, pp. 1350–3.

126. Hellman, A. and Chess, A., 2007. Gene body-specific methylation on the active X chromosome. *Science*, *315*(5815), pp. 1141–3.

127. Hervouet, E., Peixoto, P., Delage-Mourroux, R., Boyer-Guittaut, M. and Cartron, P. F., 2018. Specific or not specific recruitment of DNMTs for DNA methylation, an epigenetic dilemma. *Clinical Epigenetics*, *10*(1).

128. Adam, S., Anteneh, H., Hornisch, M., et al., 2020. DNA sequence-dependent activity and base flipping mechanisms of DNMT1 regulate genome-wide DNA methylation. *Nature Communications*, *11* (1), p. 3723.

129. Okano, M., Bell, D. W., Haber, D. A. and Li, E., 1999. DNA methyltransferases Dnmt3a and Dnmt3b are essential for de novo methylation and mammalian development. *Cell*, *99*(3), pp. 247–57.

130. Dong, C., Zhang, H., Xu, C., Arrowsmith, C. H. and Min, J., 2014. Structure, and function of dioxygenases in histone demethylation and DNA/RNA demethylation. *IUCrJ*, *1*, pp. 540–9.

131. Xu, C., Liu, K., Lei, M., et al., 2018. DNA sequence recognition of human CXXC domains and their structural determinants. *Structure*, *26*(1), pp. 85–95.

132. Hashimoto, H., Zhang, X., Vertino, P. M. and Cheng, X., 2015. The mechanisms of generation, recognition, and erasure of DNA 5-methylcytosine and thymine oxidation. *Journal of Biological Chemistry*, *290*(34), pp. 20723–33.

133. Song, J., Rechkoblit, O., Bestor, T. H. and Patel, D. J., 2011. Structure of DNMT1-DNA complex reveals a role for autoinhibition in maintenance DNA methylation. *Science*, *331*(6020), pp. 1036–40.

134. Pradhan, M., Estève, P. O., Hang, G. C., et al., 2008. CXXC domain of human DNMT1 is essential for enzymatic activity. *Biochemistry*, *47*(38), pp. 10000–9.

135. Li, D., Guo, B., Wu, H., Tan, L. and Lu, Q., 2015. TET family of dioxygenases: crucial roles and underlying mechanisms. *Cytogenet and Genome Research*, *146*(3), pp. 171–80.

136. Long, H. K., Blackledge, N. P. and Klose, R. J., 2013.ZF-CxxC domain-containing proteins: CpG islands and the chromatin connection. *Biochemical Society Transactions*, *41*(3), pp. 727–40.

137. Olinski, R., Starczak, M. and Gackowski, D., 2016. Enigmatic 5-hydroxymethyluracil: oxidatively modified base, epigenetic mark or both? *Reviews in Mutation Research*, 767, pp. 59–66.

138. Xu, Y., Wu, F., Tan, L., et al., 2011. Genome-wide regulation of 5hmC, 5mC, and gene expression by Tet1 hydroxylase in mouse embryonic stem cells. *Molecular Cell*, 42(4), pp. 451–64.

139. Lurlaro, M., Ficz, G., Oxley, D., et al., 2013. A screen for hydroxymethylcytosine and formylcytosine binding proteins suggests functions in transcription and chromatin regulation. *Genome Biology*, 14(10).

140. Raiber, E. A., Murat, P., Chirgadze, D. Y., Beraldi, D. and Luisi, B. F., 2015. Balasubramanian S: 5-formylcytosine alters the structure of the DNA double helix. *Nature Structural & Molecular Biology*, 22(1), pp. 44–9.

141. Bachman, M., Uribe-Lewis, S., Yang, X., et al., 2015. Balasubramanian S: 5-Formylcytosine can be a stable DNA modification in mammals. *Nature Chemical Biology*, 118, pp. 555–7.

142. Carson, S., Wilson, J., Aksimentiev, A., Weigele, P. R. and Wanunu, M., 2015. Hydroxymethyluracil modifications enhance the flexibility and hydrophilicity of double-stranded DNA. *Nucleic Acids Research*, 44(5), pp. 2085–92.

143. Chrysanthou, S., Senner, C. E., Woods, L., et al., 2018. Critical role of TET1/2 proteins in cell-cycle progression of trophoblast stem cells. *Stem Cell Reports*, 10(4), pp. 1355–68.

144. Sepulveda, H., Villagra, A. and Montecino, M., 2017. Tet-mediated DNA demethylation is required for SWI/SNF-dependent chromatin remodeling and histone-modifying activities that trigger expression of the Sp7 osteoblast master gene during mesenchymal lineage commitment. *Molecular and Cellular Biology*, 37(20).

145. Allshire, R. C. and Madhani, H. D., 2018. Ten principles of heterochromatin formation and function. *Nature Reviews Molecular Cell Biology*, 19(4), pp. 229–44.

146. Dawson, M. A., Bannister, A. J., Göttgens, B., et al., 2009. JAK2 phosphorylates histone H3Y41 and excludes HP1α from chromatin. *Nature*, 461(7265), pp. 819–22.

147. Larson, A. G., Elnatan, D., Keenen, M. M., et al., 2017. Liquid droplet formation by HP1α suggests a role for phase separation in heterochromatin. *Nature*, 547(7662), pp. 236–40.

148. Kumar, S., Kiso, A. and Abenthung Kithan, N., 2009. Chromosome banding and mechanism of chromosome aberrations. In *Cytogenetics: classical and molecular strategies for analysing heredity material*. IntechOpen.

149. Holmquist, G. P., 1989. Evolution of chromosome bands: molecular ecology of noncoding DNA. *Journal of Molecular Evolution*, 286, pp. 469–86.

150. Lu, Z., Carter, A. C. and Chang, H. Y., 2017. Mechanistic insights in X-chromosome inactivation. *Philosophical Transactions of the Royal Society B*, 372(1733), p. 20160356.

151. Lee, H., Zhang, Z. and Krause, H. M., 2019. Long noncoding RNAs and repetitive elements: junk or intimate evolutionary partners? *Trends in Genetics*, 35(12), pp. 892–902.

152. Mager, D. L. and Stoye, J. P., 2015. Mammalian endogenous retroviruses. *Microbiology Spectrum*, 3(1).

153. Lander, E. S., Linton, L. M., Birren, B., et al., 2001. Initial sequencing and analysis of the human genome. *Nature*, 409(6822), pp. 860–921.

154. Zhang, X., Zhang, R. and Yu, J., 2020. New understanding of the relevant role of LINE-1 retrotransposition in human disease and immune modulation. *Frontiers in Cell and Developmental Biology*, 8.

155. Dewannieux, M., Esnault, C. and Heidmann, T., 2003. LINE-mediated retrotransposition of marked Alu sequences. *Nature Genetics*, 35(1), pp. 41–8.

156. Esnault, C., Maestre, J. and Heidmann, T., 2000. Human LINE retrotransposons generate processed pseudogenes. *Nature Genetics, 24*(4), pp. 363–7.

157. Sanchez-Luque, F. J., Kempen, M. J. H. C., Gerdes, P., et al., 2019. LINE-1 evasion of epigenetic repression in humans. *Molecular Cell, 75*(3), pp. 590–604.

158. Garcia-Perez, J. L., Marchetto, M. C. N., Muotri, A. R., et al., 2007. LINE-1 retrotransposition in human embryonic stem cells. *Human Molecular Genetics, 16* (13), pp. 1569–77.

159. Zhang, X., Zhang, R. and Yu, J., 2020. New understanding of the relevant role of LINE-1 retrotransposition in human disease and immune modulation. *Frontiers in Cell and Developmental Biology, 8.*

160. Terry, D. M. and Devine, S. E., 2020. Aberrantly high levels of somatic LINE-1 expression and retrotransposition in human neurological disorders. *Frontiers in Genetics, 10.*

161. Troskie, R., Faulkner, G. J. and Cheetham, S. W., 2021. Processed pseudogenes: a substrate for evolutionary innovation. *BioEssays, 43*(11), p. 2100186.

162. Mattick, J. S. and Makunin, I. V., 2005. Small regulatory RNAs in mammals. *Human Molecular Genetics, 14*(1).

163. Alles, J., Fehlmann, T., Fischer, U., et al., 2019. An estimate of the total number of true human miRNAs. *Nucleic Acids Research, 47*(7), pp. 3353–64.

164. Friedman, R. C., Farh, K. K. H., Burge, C. B. and Bartel, D. P., 2009. Most mammalian mRNAs are conserved targets of microRNAs. *Genome Research, 19*(1), pp. 92–105.

165. Lorio, M. V., Piovan, C. and Croce, C. M., 2010. Interplay between microRNAs and the epigenetic machinery: an intricate network. *Biochimica et Biophysica Acta, 1799*(10–12), pp. 694–701.

166. Kawaji, H. and Hayashizaki, Y., 2008. Exploration of small RNAs. *PLOS Genetics, 4*(1), p. 22.

167. Watanabe, T., Takeda, A., Tsukiyama, T., et al., 2006. Identification and characterization of two novel classes of small RNAs in the mouse germline: retrotransposon-derived siRNAs in oocytes and germline small RNAs in testes. *Genes & Development, 20*(13), pp. 1732–43.

168. Lipardi, C., Wei, Q. and Paterson, B. M., 2001. RNAi as random degradative PCR. *Cell, 107*(3), pp. 297–307.

169. Czech, B. and Hannon, G. J., 2016. One loop to rule them all: the ping-pong cycle and piRNA-guided silencing. *Trends in Biochemical Sciences, 41*(4), pp. 324–37.

170. Lipovich, L., Johnson, R. and Lin, C. Y., 2010. MacroRNA underdogs in a microRNA world: evolutionary, regulatory, and biomedical significance of mammalian long non-protein-coding RNA. *Biochimica et Biophysica Acta, 1799* (9), pp. 597–615.

171. Milligan, M. J. and Lipovich, L., 2015. Pseudogene-derived lncRNAs: emerging regulators of gene expression. *Frontiers in Genetics, 6.*

172. Żylicz, J. J., Bousard, A., Žumer, K., et al., 2019. The implication of early chromatin changes in X chromosome activation. *Cell, 176*(1–2), pp. 182–97.e23.

173. Soldà, G., Boi, S., Duga, S., et al., 2005. In vivo RNA–RNA duplexes from human α3 and α5 nicotinic receptor subunit mRNAs. *Gene, 345*(2), pp. 155–64.

174. Mohammad, F., Mondal, T. and Kanduri, C., 2009. Epigenetics of imprinted long non-coding RNAs. *Epigenetics, 4*(5), pp. 277–86.

175. Yelin, R., Dahary, D., Sorek, R., et al., 2003. Widespread occurrence of antisense transcription in the human genome. *Nature Biotechnology, 21*(4), pp. 379–86.

176. Newall, A. E. T., 2001. Primary non-random X inactivation associated with disruption of Xist promoter regulation. *Human Molecular Genetics, 10* (6), pp. 581–9.

177. Furlan, G. and Galupa, R., 2022. Mechanisms of choice in X-chromosome activation. *Cells, 11*(3).

178. Tu, Y., Chen, C., Pan, J., et al., 2012. The ubiquitin proteasome pathway UPP in the regulation of cell cycle control and DNA damage repair and its implication in tumorigenesis. *International Journal of Clinical and Experimental Pathology, 5*(8).

179. LaSalle, J. M., Reiter, L. T. and Chamberlain, S. J., 2015. Epigenetic regulation of UBE3A and roles in human neurodevelopmental disorders. *Epigenomics, 7*(7), pp. 1213–28.

180. Weber, M. J., 2006. Mammalian small nucleolar RNAs are mobile genetic elements. *PLOS Genetics, 2*(12), p. 205.

181. Bergeron, D., Laforest, C., Carpentier, S., et al., 2021. SnoRNA copy regulation affects family size, genomic location and family abundance levels. *BMC Genomics, 22*(1), p. 414.

182. Kiss-László, Z., Henry, Y., Bachellerie, J. P., Caizergues-Ferrer, M. and Kiss, T., 1996. Site-specific ribose methylation of pre-ribosomal RNA: a novel function for small nucleolar RNAs. *Cell, 85*(7), pp. 1077–88.

183. Kishore, S. and Stamm, S., 2006. Regulation of alternative splicing by snoRNAs. *Cold Spring Harbor Symposia on Quantitative Biology, 71*, pp. 329–34.

184. Lanfranco, M. F., Anastasio, N. C., Seitz, P. K. and Cunningham, K. A., 2010. Quantification of RNA editing of the serotonin 2 C receptor 5HT2CR ex vivo: constitutive activity in receptors and other proteins part B. In *Methods in enzymology*, ed. P. M. Conn (pp. 311–28). Elsevier Academic.

185. Farrelly, L. A., Thompson, R. E., Zhao, S., et al., 2019. Histone serotonylation is a permissive modification that enhances TFIID binding to H3K4me3. *Nature, 567*(7749), pp. 535–9.

186. Rueter, S. M., Dawson, T. R. and Emeson, R. B., 1999. Regulation of alternative splicing by RNA editing. *Nature, 399*(6731), pp. 75–80.

187. Vitali, P., Basyuk, E., Le Meur, E., et al., 2005. ADAR2-mediated editing of RNA substrates in the nucleolus is inhibited by C/D small nucleolar RNAs. *Journal of Cell Biology, 169*(5), pp. 745–53.

188. Stamm, S., Gruber, S. B., Rabchevsky, A. G. and Emeson, R. B., 2017. The activity of the serotonin receptor 2 C is regulated by alternative splicing. *Human Genetics, 136*(9), pp. 1079–91.

189. Flomen, R., Knight, J., Sham, P., Kerwin, R. and Makoff, A., 2004. Evidence that RNA editing modulates splice site selection in the 5-HT2 C receptor gene. *Nucleic Acids Research, 32*(7), pp. 2113–122.

190. Kishore, S. and Stamm, S., 2006. The snoRNA HBII-52 regulates alternative splicing of the serotonin receptor 2 C. *Science, 311*(5758), pp. 230–2.

191. Butler, M. G., Theodoro, M. F., Bittel, D. C., et al., 2007. X-chromosome inactivation patterns in females with Prader–Willi syndrome. *American Journal of Medical Genetics A, 143A*(5), pp. 469–75.

192. Wang, Q., O'Brien, P. J., Chen, C. X., et al., 2000. Altered G protein-coupling functions of RNA editing isoform and splicing variant serotonin 2 C receptors. *Journal of Neurochemistry, 74*.

193. Van De Wouw, M., Stilling, R. M., Peterson, V. L., et al., 2019. Host microbiota regulates central nervous system serotonin receptor 2 C editing in rodents. *ACS Chemical Neuroscience, 10*(9), pp. 3953–60.

194. Belair, C., Sim, S., Kim, K. Y., et al., 2019. The RNA exosome nuclease complex regulates human embryonic stem cell differentiation. *Journal of Cell Biology, 218*(8) pp. 2564–82.

195. Kawamura, Y., Sanchez Calle, A., Yamamoto, Y., Sato, T. A. and Ochiya, T., 2019. Extracellular vesicles mediate the horizontal transfer of an active LINE-1 retrotransposon. *Journal of Extracellular Vesicles, 8*(1).

196. Ratajczak, J., Miekus, K., Kucia, M., et al., 2006. Embryonic stem cell-derived microvesicles reprogram hematopoietic progenitors: evidence for horizontal transfer of mRNA and protein delivery. *Leukemia*, 20(5), pp. 847–56.

197. Guo, J., Cheng, P., Yuan, H. and Liu, Y., 2009. The exosome regulates circadian gene expression in a posttranscriptional negative feedback loop. *Cell*, 138(6), pp. 1236–46.

198. Khalyfa, A., Poroyko, V. A., Qiao, Z., et al., 2017. Exosomes and metabolic function in mice exposed to alternating dark-light cycles mimicking night shift work schedules. *Frontiers in Physiology*, 8.

199. Forterre, A., Jalabert, A., Chikh, K., et al., 2014. Myotube-derived exosomal miRNAs downregulate Sirtuin1 in myoblasts during muscle cell differentiation. *Cell Cycle*, 13(1), pp. 78–89.

200. Adolph, K. W., Kreisman, L. R. and Kuehn, R. L., 1986. Assembly of chromatin fibers into metaphase chromosomes analyzed by transmission electron microscopy and scanning electron microscopy. *Biophysical Journal*, 49(1), pp. 221–31.

201. Bonner, J., 1965. The template activity of chromatin. *Journal of Cellular and Comparative Physiology*, 66(s1), pp. 77–90.

202. Sinden, R. R., 1994. Introduction to the structure, properties, and reactions of DNA. In *DNA structure and function* (pp. 1–57). Elsevier.

203. Tashiro, R. and Sugiyama, H., 2022. Photoreaction of DNA containing 5-halouracil and its products. *Photochemistry and Photobiology*, 98(3), pp. 532–45.

204. Hori, M., Yonei, S., Sugiyama, H., et al., 2003. Identification of high excision capacity for 5-hydroxymethyluracil mispaired with guanine in DNA of Escherichia coli MutM, Nei and Nth DNA glycosylases. *Nucleic Acids Research*, 31(4), pp. 1191–6.

205. Cremer, C. and Gray, J. W., 1982. Application of the BrdU/thymidine method to flow cytogenetics: differential quenching/enhancement of hoechst 33258 fluorescence of late-replicating chromosomes 1.*Somatic Cell Genetics*, 8(3).

206. Brovarets', O. O. and Hovorun, D. M., 2015. Tautomeric transition between wobble A·C DNA base mispair and Watson-Crick-like A·C* mismatch: Microstructural mechanism and biological significance. *Physical Chemistry Chemical Physics*, 17(23), pp. 15103–10.

207. Kochetkov, N. K. and Budowsky, E. I., 1969. The chemical modification of nucleic acids. In *Progress in nucleic acid research and molecular biology* (pp. 403–38). Elsevier.

208. Tung, F., Tsai, K. H. and Marfey, P., 1972. Bromination of calf thymus chromatin. *Biochimica et Biophysica Acta*, 277(1), pp. 117–28.

209. Valenzuela, S. M., Mazzanti, M., Tonini, R., et al., 2000. The nuclear chloride ion channel NCC27 is involved in regulation of the cell cycle. *The Journal of Physiology*, 529(3), pp. 541–52.

210. Maier, J. A., 2013. Magnesium and cell cycle. In *Encyclopedia of metalloproteins*, ed. R. H. Kretsinger, V. N. Uversky and E. A. Permyakov (pp. 1227–32). Springer.

211. Maeshima, K., Matsuda, T., Shindo, Y., et al., 2018. Transient rise in free Mg2+ ions released from ATP-mg hydrolysis contributes to mitotic chromosome condensation. *Current Biology*, 28(3), pp. 444–51.

212. Joule, J. A. and Mills, K., 2009. *Heterocyclic chemistry*. Wiley.

213. Robertson, A. B., Klungland, A., Rognes, T. and Leiros, I., 2009. Base excision repair: the long and short of it. *Cellular and Molecular Life Sciences*, 66(6), pp. 981–93.

214. Li, H., Li, Q., Ma, Z., et al., 2019. AID modulates carcinogenesis network via DNA demethylation in bladder urothelial cell carcinoma. *Cell Death & Disease*, 10(4), p. 251.

215. Lane, A. N. and Fan, T. W. M., 2015. Regulation of mammalian nucleotide

metabolism and biosynthesis. *Nucleic Acids Research*, 43(4), pp. 2466–85.

216. Luscombe, N. M., Laskowski, R. A. and Thornton, J. M., 2001. Amino acid-base interactions: a three-dimensional analysis of protein-DNA interactions at an atomic level. *Nucleic Acids Research*, 29(13).

217. Pospisil, P., Ballmer, P., Scapozza, L. and Folkers, G., 2003. Tautomerism in computer-aided drug design. *Journal of Receptors and Signal Transduction*, 23(4), pp. 361–71.

218. Suckling, C., Gibson, C. and Huggan, J., 2008. Bicyclic 6-6 systems: pteridines. In *Comprehensive heterocyclic chemistry III*, ed. A. R. Katrizky, C. A. Ramsten, E. F. V. Scriven and R. J. K. Taylor (pp. 915–75). Elsevier.

219. Sato, K., Kanno, J., Tominaga, T., Matsubara, Y. and Kure, S., 2006. De novo and salvage pathways of DNA synthesis in primary cultured neural stem cells. *Brain Research*, 1071(1), pp. 24–33.

220. Gazzali, A. M., Lobry, M., Colombeau, L., et al., 2016. Stability of folic acid under several parameters. *European Journal of Pharmaceutical Sciences*, 93, pp. 419–30.

221. Di Liberto, V., Mudò, G., Garozzo, R., et al., 2016. The guanine-based purinergic system: the tale of an orphan neuromodulation. *Frontiers in Pharmacology*, 7.

222. Prabhu, Y. and Eichinger, L., 2006. The Dictyostelium repertoire of seven transmembrane domain receptors. *European Journal of Cell Biology*, 85 (9-10), pp. 937–46.

223. Duc, N. M., Kim, H. R. and Chung, K. Y., 2015. Structural mechanism of G protein activation by G protein-coupled receptor. *European Journal of Pharmacology*, 76(3), pp. 214–22.

224. Catapano, L. A. and Manji, H. K., 2006. G protein-coupled receptors in major psychiatric disorders. *Biochimica et Biophysica Acta*, 1768(4), pp. 976–93.

225. Brandts, D. R. and Ross, E. M., 1985. GTPase activity of the stimulatory GTP-binding regulatory protein of adenylate cyclase: accumulation and turnover of enzyme nucleotide intermediates. *Journal of Biological Chemistry*, 260(1), p. 266472.

226. López, J. M., Outtrim, E. L., Fu, R., et al., 2020. Physiological levels of folic acid reveal purine alterations in Lesch-Nyhan disease. *Proceedings of the National Academy of Sciences of the United States of America*, 117(22), pp. 12071–9.

227. Ducker, G. S. and Rabinowitz, J. D., 2015. ZMP: a master regulator of one-carbon metabolism. *Molecular Cell*, 57(2), pp. 203–4.

228. Hartley, D. M. and Snodgrass, S. R., 1990. Folate interactions with cerebral G proteins. *Neurochemical Research*, 15(7), pp. 681–6.

229. De Wit, R. J. W. and Bulgakov, R., 2021. Guanine nucleotides modulate the ligand binding properties of cell surface folate receptors in Dictyostelium discoideum. *FEBS Letters*, 179(2).

230. Rosenblatt, D. S. and Erbe, R. W., 1977. Methylenetetrahy drofolate reductase in cultured human cells. I. Growth and metabolic studies. *Pediatric Research*, 11 (11), pp. 1137–41.

231. Sheraz, M. A., Kazi, S. H., Ahmed, S., Anwar, Z. and Ahmad, I., 2014. Photo, thermal and chemical degradation of riboflavin. *Beilstein Journal of Organic Chemistry*, 10, pp. 1999–2012.

232. Mack, M. and Grill, S., 2006. Riboflavin analogs and inhibitors of riboflavin biosynthesis. *Applied Microbiology and Biotechnology*, 71(3), pp. 265–75.

233. Fanet, H., Capuron, L., Castanon, N., Calon, F. and Vancassel, S., 2020. Tetrahydrobiopterin BH4 pathway: from metabolism to neuropsychiatry. *Current Neuropharmacology*, 19(5), pp. 591–609.

234. Nalini, A., Pandraud, A., Mok, K. and Houlden, H., 2013. Madras motor neuron disease MMND is distinct from the riboflavin transporter genetic defects that cause Brown–Vialetto–Van Laere syndrome. *Journal of the Neurological Sciences*, 334(1-2), pp. 119–22.

235. Bashford, J. A., Chowdhury, F. A. and Shaw, C. E., 2017. Remarkable motor recovery after riboflavin therapy in adult-onset Brown–Vialetto–Van Laere syndrome. *Practical Neurology*, 17(1), pp. 53–6.

236. Carreau, C., Lenglet, T., Mosnier, I., et al., 2020. Juvenile ALS-like phenotype dramatically improved after high-dose riboflavin treatment. *Annals of Clinical and Translational Neurology*, 7(2), pp. 250–3.

237. Timmerman, V. and De Jonghe, P., 2014. Promising riboflavin treatment for motor neuron disorder. *Brain*, 137(1), pp. 2–3.

238. Johnson, J. O., Gibbs, J. R., Megarbane, A., et al., 2012. Exome sequencing reveals riboflavin transporter mutations as a cause of motor neuron disease. *Brain*, 135(9), pp. 2875–82.

239. Treadwell, G. E., Metzler, D. J. E., Treadwell, E. and Present, J., 1972. Photoconversion of Riboflavin to Lumichrome in Plant Tissues.*Plant Physiology*, 49.

240. Darguzyte, M., Drude, N., Lammers, T. and Kiessling, F., 2020. Riboflavin-targeted drug delivery. *Cancers (Basel)*, 12(2).

241. Said, H. M. and Ma, T. Y. 1994. Mechanism of riboflavine uptake by Caco-2 human intestinal epithelial cells. *American Journal of Physiology*, 266(1), pp. 15–21.

242. Kalucka, J., Missiaen, R., Georgiadou, M., et al., 2015. Metabolic control of the cell cycle. *Cell Cycle*, 14(21), pp. 3379–88.

243. Brosnan, J. T., Wijekoon, E. P., Warford-Woolgar, L., et al., 2009. Creatine synthesis is a major metabolic process in neonatal piglets and has important implications for amino acid metabolism and methyl balance. *Journal of Nutrition*, 139(7), pp. 1292–7.

244. Kurtz, P. and Rocha, E. E. M., 2020. Nutrition therapy, glucose control, and brain metabolism in traumatic brain jury: a multimodal monitoring approach. *Frontiers in Neuroscience*, 14.

245. Liu, Y., Chen, C., Wang, X., et al., 2022. An epigenetic role of mitochondria in cancer. *Cells*, 11(16), p. 2518.

246. Norwitz, N. G., Dalai, S. S. and Palmer, C. M., 2020. Ketogenic diet as a metabolic treatment for mental illness. *Current Opinion in Endocrinology, Diabetes and Obesity*, 27(5), pp. 269–74.

247. Dickerson, R. N., 2016. Nitrogen balance and protein requirements for critically Ill older patients. *Nutrients*, 8(4).

248. Steyn, F. J., Ioannides, Z. A., Van Eijk, R. P. A., et al., 2018. Hypermetabolism in ALS is associated with greater functional decline and shorter survival. *Journal of Neurology, Neurosurgery, and Psychiatry*, 89(10), pp. 1016–23.

249. Soyka, M., Koch, W., Möller, H. J., Rüther, T. and Tatsch, K., 2005. Hypermetabolic pattern in frontal cortex and other brain regions in unmedicated schizophrenia patients: results from a FDG-PET study. *European Archives of Psychiatry and Clinical Neuroscience*, 255(5), pp. 308–12.

250. Xie, X., Yang, H., An, J. J., et al., 2019. Activation of anxiogenic circuits instigates resistance to diet-induced obesity via increased energy expenditure. *Cell Metabolism*, 29(4), pp. 917–31.

251. Rolfe, D. F. and Brown, G. C., 1997. Cellular energy utilization and molecular origin of standard metabolic rate in mammals. *Physiological Reviews*, 773, pp. 731–58.

252. Baker, J. S., McCormick, M. C. and Robergs, R. A., 2010. Interaction among skeletal muscle metabolic energy systems during intense exercise. *Journal of Nutrition and Metabolism*, 2010, pp. 1–13.

253. Green, A. L., Wang, S., Purvis, S., et al., 2007. Identifying cardiorespiratory neurocircuitry involved in central command during exercise in humans. *The Journal of Physiology*, 578(2), pp. 605–12.

254. Asahara, R., Matsukawa, K., Ishii, K., Liang, N. and Endo, K., 2016. The prefrontal oxygenation and ventilatory responses at start of one-legged cycling exercise have relation to central

command. *Journal of Applied Physiology*, *121*(5), pp. 1115–26.

255. Marina, N., Kasymov, V., Ackland, G. L., Kasparov, S. and Gourine, A. V., 2016. Astrocytes and brain hypoxia. *Advances in Experimental Medicine and Biology*, *903*, pp. 201–7.

256. Crawford, J. H., 2006. Hypoxia, red blood cells, and nitrite regulate NO-dependent hypoxic vasodilation. *Blood*, *107*(2), pp. 566–74.

257. Nobrega, A. C. L., O'Leary, D., Silva, B. M., et al., 2014. Neural regulation of cardiovascular response to exercise: role of central command and peripheral afferents. *BioMed Research International*, *2014*, pp. 1–20.

258. Mustafa, A. K., Gadalla, M. M. and Snyder, S. H., 2009. Signaling by gasotransmitters. *Science Signaling*, *2*(68).

259. Ishikawa, M., Kajimura, M., Adachi, T., et al., 2005. Carbon monoxide from heme oxygenase-2 is a tonic regulator against NO-dependent vasodilatation in the adult rat cerebral microcirculation. *Circulation Research*, *97*(12).

260. Kolluru, G. K., Shen, X., Yuan, S. and Kevil, C. G., 2017. Gasotransmitter heterocellular signalling. *Antioxidants & Redox Signaling*, *26*(16), pp. 936–60.

261. Wang, R. 2002. Two's company, three's a crowd: can H2S be the third endogenous gaseous transmitter? *The FASEB Journal*, *13*, pp. 1792–8.

262. Randi, E. B., Zuhra, K., Pecze, L., Panagaki, T. and Szabo, C., 2021. Physiological concentrations of cyanide stimulate mitochondrial Complex IV and enhance cellular bioenergetics. *Proceedings of the National Academy of Sciences of the United States of America*, *118*(20).

263. Aryal, P., Sansom, M. S. P. and Tucker, S. J., 2015. Hydrophobic gating in ion channels. *Journal of Molecular Biology*, *427*(1), pp. 121–30.

264. Pé Rez-Mato, I., Castro, C., Ruiz, A., Corrales, F. J. and Mato, J. M., 1999. Methionine adenosyltransferase S-nitrosylation is regulated by the basic and acidic amino acids surrounding the target thiol. *Journal of Biological Chemistry*, *274*(24).

265. Kabe, Y., Yamamoto, T., Kajimura, M., et al., 2016. Cystathionine β-synthase and PGRMC1 as CO sensors. *Free Radical Biology and Medicine*, *99*, pp. 333–44.

266. Kabil, O., Yadav, V. and Banerjee, R., 2016. Heme-dependent metabolite switching regulates H2S synthesis in response to endoplasmic reticulum ER stress. *Journal of Biological Chemistry*, *291*(32), pp. 16418–23.

267. Allen, P. J., 2012. Creatine metabolism and psychiatric disorders: does creatine supplementation have therapeutic value? *Neuroscience & Biobehavioral Reviews*, *36*(5), pp. 1442–62.

268. Kreider, R. B. and Stout, J. R., 2021. Creatine in health and disease. *Nutrients*, *13*(2), pp. 1–28.

269. Halbrich, M., Barnes, J., Bunge, M. and Joshi, C., 2008. A V139 M mutation also causes the reversible CNS phenotype in CMTX. *Canadian Journal of the Neurological Sciences*, *35*(3), pp. 372–4.

270. Bauer, J., Biolo, G., Cederholm, T., et al., 2013. Evidence-based recommendations for optimal dietary protein intake in older people: a position paper from the pro-tage study group. *Journal of the American Medical Directors Association*, *14*(8), pp. 542–59.

271. Sriperm, N., Pesti, G. M. and Tillman, P. B., 2011. Evaluation of the fixed nitrogen-to-protein N:P conversion factor 6.25 versus ingredient specific N:P conversion factors in feedstuffs. *Journal of the Science of Food and Agriculture*, *91*(7), pp. 1182–6.

272. Maxwell, J., Gwardschaladse, C., Lombardo, G., et al., 2017. The impact of measurement of respiratory quotient by indirect calorimetry on the achievement of nitrogen balance in patients with severe traumatic brain injury. *European Journal of Trauma and Emergency Surgery*, *43*(6), pp. 775–82.

273. Tsukada, Y., Fang, J., Erdjument-Bromage, H., et al., 2006. Histone demethylation by a family of JmjC domain-containing proteins. *Nature, 439* (7078), pp. 811–16.

274. Kamen, M. D., 1963. Early history of carbon-14 discovery of this supremely important tracer was expected in the physical sense but not in the chemical sense. *Science, 140*(3567), pp. 584–90.

275. Wilkinson, D. J., 2018. Historical and contemporary stable isotope tracer approaches to studying mammalian protein metabolism. *Mass Spectrometry Reviews, 37*(1), pp. 57–80.

276. Dingwall, S., Mills, C. E., Phan, N., Taylor, K. and Boreham, D. R., 2011. Human health and the biological effects of tritium in drinking water: prudent policy through science – addressing the ODWAC new recommendation. *Dose-Response, 9*(1), pp. 6–31.

277. Ball, D. W., 2004. How radioactive is your banana? *Journal of Chemical Education, 81*(10), p. 1440

278. Liang, M., 2018. Epigenetic mechanisms and hypertension. *AHA Hypertension, 72* (6), pp. 1244–54.

279. Darwin, C., 2009. *The origin of species.* Cambridge University Press.

280. Hancock, A. M., Alkorta-Aranburu, G., Witonsky, D. B. and Di Rienzo, A., 2010. Adaptations to new environments in humans: the role of subtle allele frequency shifts. *Philosophical Transactions of the Royal Society B, 365*(1552), pp. 2459–68.

281. White, T. D., Asfaw, B., DeGusta, D., et al., 2003. Pleistocene Homo sapiens from Middle Awash. Ethiopia. *Nature, 423*(6941), pp. 742–7.

282. Stringer, C., 2003. Out of Ethiopia. *Nature, 423*(6941), pp. 693–5.

283. Luca, F., Perry, G. H. and Di Rienzo, A., 2010. Evolutionary adaptations to dietary changes. *Annual Review of Nutrition, 30*, pp. 291–314.

284. Hancock, A. M., Witonsky, D. B., Ehler, E., et al., 2010. Human adaptations to diet, subsistence, and ecoregion are due to subtle shifts in allele frequency. *Proceedings of the National Academy of Sciences of the United States of America, 107*(suppl. 2), pp. 8924–30.

285. Heyn, H., Moran, S., Hernando-Herraez, I., et al., 2013. DNA methylation contributes to natural human variation. *Genome Research, 23* (9), pp. 1363–72.

286. Yafei, W., Lijun, P., Jinfeng, W. and Xiaoying, Z., 2012. Is the prevalence of MTHFR C677 T polymorphism associated with ultraviolet radiation in Eurasia? *Journal of Human Genetics, 57*(12), pp. 780–6.

287. Cordain, L. and Hickey, M. S., 2006. Ultraviolet radiation represents an evolutionary selective pressure for the south-to-north gradient of the MTHFR 677TT genotype. *The American Journal of Clinical Nutrition, 84*(5), p. 1243.

288. Kious, B. M., Bakian, A., Zhao, J., et al., 2019. Altitude and risk of depression and anxiety: findings from the intern health study. *International Review of Psychiatry, 31*(7–8), pp. 637–45.

289. Smith, B., 1995. The emergence of agriculture. *Bulletin of Science, Technology & Society, 15*(1).

290. Valeggia, C. R. and Snodgrass, J. J., 2015. Health of Indigenous peoples. *Annual Review of Anthropology, 44*(1), pp. 117–35.

291. Evans, L., 1996. Domestication of crop plants. In *Crop evolution, adaptation and yield* (pp. 106–7). Cambridge University Press.

292. Moreira, X., Abdala-Roberts, L., Gols, R. and Francisco, M., 2018. Plant domestication decreases both constitutive and induced chemical defences by direct selection against defensive traits. *Scientific Reports, 8*(1).

293. Zohary, D., Hopf, M. and Weiss, E., 2012. *Domestication of plants in the old world,* 4th ed. Oxford University Press.

294. Fahrbach, S. E., Smagghe, G. and Velarde, R. A., 2012. Nuclear receptors. *Annual Review of Entomology, 57*(1), pp. 83–106.

295. Dolan, L. C., Matulka, R. A. and Burdock, G. A., 2010. Naturally occurring food toxins. *Toxins*, 29, pp. 2289–332.

296. Altamura, M. R., Long, L. and Hasselstrom, T., 1959. Giotrin from fresh cabbage. *Journal of Biological Chemistry*, 234(7), pp. 1847–9.

297. Negi, V. S., Pal, A. and Borthakur, D., 2021. Biochemistry of plants N-heterocyclic non-protein amino acids. *Amino Acids*, 53(6), pp. 801–12.

298. Martinez, M., Ahmed, A. H., Loh, A. P. and Oswald, R. E., 2014. Thermodynamics and mechanism of the interaction of willardiine partial agonists with a glutamate receptor: Implications for drug development. *Biochemistry*, 53 (23), pp. 3790–5.

299. Kenten, R. H., 1957. The partial purification and properties of a thiaminase from bracken [Pteridium aquilinum L. Kuhn]. *Biochemical Journal*, 67.

300. Zallot, R., Yazdani, M., Goyer, A., et al., 2014. Salvage of the thiamine pyrimidine moiety by plant TenA proteins lacking an active-site cysteine. *Biochemical Journal*, 463(1), pp. 145–55.

301. Candau, M. and Massengo, J., 1982. Evidence of a thiamine deficiency in sheep fed maize silage. *Annales de recherches veterinaires*, 13(4), pp. 329–40.

302. Chandrakumar, A., Bhardwaj, A. and T'Jong, G. W., 2019. Review of thiamine deficiency disorders: Wernicke encephalopathy and Korsakoff psychosis. *Journal of Basic and Clinical Physiology and Pharmacology*, 30(2), pp. 153–62.

303. Martinez-Zamudio, R. and Ha, H. C., 2011. Environmental epigenetics in metal exposure. *Epigenetics*, 6(7), pp. 820–7.

304. Wolf, T., Baier, S. R. and Zempleni, J., 2015. The intestinal transport of bovine milk exosomes Is mediated by endocytosis in human colon carcinoma CACO-2 cells and rat small intestinal IEC-6 cells1-3. *Journal of Nutrition*, 145 (10), pp. 2201–6.

305. Onwezen, M. C., Bouwman, E. P., Reinders, M. J. and Dagevos, H., 2021. A systematic review on consumer acceptance of alternative proteins: pulses, algae, Insects, plant-based meat alternatives. and cultured meat. *Appetite*, 159.

306. Fowler, S., Roush, R. and Wise, J., 2013. The cell cycle. In *Concepts of biology*. OpenStax.

307. Segal, D. J. and LaSalle, J. M., 2018. UBE3A: an e3 ubiquitin ligase with genome-wide impact in neurodevelopment disease. *Frontiers in Molecular Neuroscience*, 11, p. 476.

Index

Printed in the United States
by Baker & Taylor Publisher Services